Igniting Your Genius

The Startling Fusion of Creativity, Curiosity, Intellect, Passion, and Awe

Curtiss DeMars-Johnson

scarecrow education

The Scarecrow Press, Inc.
A Scarecrow Education Book
Lanham, Maryland, and London
2002

SCAREcrow PRESS, INC.
A SCARECROW EDUCATION BOOK

Published in the United States of America
by Scarecrow Press, Inc.
4720 Boston Way
Lanham, Maryland 20706
www.scarecroweducation.com

4 Pleydell Gardens, Folkestone
Kent CT20 2DN, England

British Library Cataloguing in Publication Information Available

ISBN: 978-0-8108-4181-9

Library of Congress Cataloging-in-Publication Data

DeMars-Johnson, Curtiss, 1951–
Igniting your genius : the startling fusion of creativity, curiosity, intellect, passion, and awe / Curtiss DeMars-Johnson.
p. cm.

1. Health—Miscellanea. 2. Mental health—Miscellanea. I. Title.
RA 776.5 .D37 2002
613—dc21 2001049497

∞™ The paper used in this publication meets the minimum requirements of American National Standard for Information Sciences—Permanence of Paper for Printed Library Materials, ANSI/NISO Z39.48-1992.
Manufactured in the United States of America.

With Gratitude

To my father, Curt, for leading me on long forays deep into the woods and bogs, sometimes at odd hours, sharing the heartfelt rapture of Life! and for sharing his passion and joy for poetry, reading, and stirring music; to my mother, Ruth, for her constant unquestioned love that provided a secure foundation for all the ventures of my life, and for her grace and èlan that everybody feels while in her presence; to both of my parents for instilling a love for excellence and lifelong learning; to my sister Kris for teaching me about responsibility; to my sister Margot, who illustrated the meaning of friendship and the love of teaching; to my brother Rolf who reminds us all that creativity, humor, and art are essential.

To my wife, Reneé, who has been a steady source of support and love through this challenging time of changes and writing. I was encouraged to write in part because of her soulful wisdom, ardent passion, sharp intellect, and profound vision—my helpmate, soulmate, and companion. To my son, Kyle, who has inspired me in more ways than can ever be expressed. More than anybody on this planet, he provided the energy and vision for writing such a book because of his curiosity, awe, sensitivities, intellect, and creativity.

This book is dedicated to all those who awaken:

- the capacity to freshly observe without the presumption that we already know,
- an appreciation for the gifts of those who are different from ourselves,
- the courage and wisdom that allow us to open our hearts to life's possibilities,
- the courage that allows us to trust our own unique combinations of gifts,
- a fundamental gratitude for life,
- the fullness of life's opportunity in the current moment instead of allowing our lives to be entirely governed by past presumptions and future anticipations,
- the capacity to sense emerging novelty, and
- the gift of gently touching the lives of others in healing ways.

This book is also dedicated to those who demonstrate creative ways to:

- face intractable problems, uncomfortable enigmas, dispiriting setbacks, and apparent dead ends without becoming deeply discouraged or cynical,
- view problems, enigmas, setbacks, and apparent dead ends as fresh beginning points for something unknown and new,
- see more encompassing landscapes for life's drama,
- quest for excellence,
- cultivate originality,
- recognize the moment to leap beyond all known bounds and previous safe havens,
- realize when not to leap,
- encourage people to risk going beyond our biases and all prior tendencies,
- gracefully accept guidance along the path,
- find energy and vitality through fresh ideas from unexpected resources,
- find life ever-renewing because of the constant stream of suggestive metaphors, intimations, and cues persistently being born around us,

- become aware of the importance of anomalies,
- see the relevance of what has been forgotten or pushed to the periphery and margins,
- be attuned to the deep structure of surface expressions,
- contend with fear of the dark and the unknown (in whatever forms it takes in one's own life),
- find playful elements in our work,
- manifest the uncanny capacity to make connections and discover emerging patterns,
- sustain one's creative endeavors,
- cooperatively work with others for ends greater than any individual's ego,
- wisely coexist with the ecological needs of the earth and her future offspring,
- discover and embrace the vision, means, courage, strength, and wisdom necessary to pick up one's endeavors again after a severe loss, and
- express fidelity to the greatness of life until our last breath.

Contents

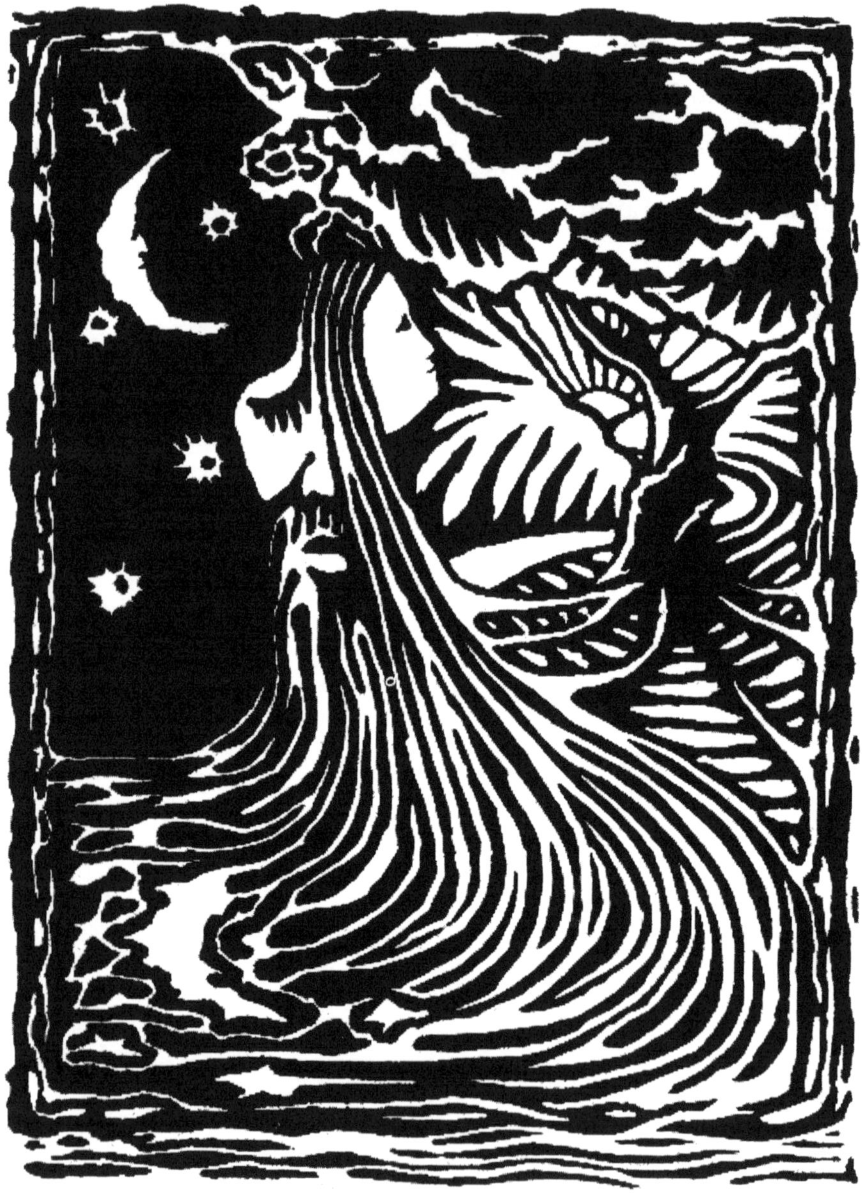

Illustration by Nicholas Quiring

INTRODUCTION

The Unrecognized Treasure

IMPORTANT NOTICE!

Anything written in the introduction of this book may not be necessary to read. The introduction is composed of separate and deeply interrelated sections. Follow the fancy of your eye and the spark of your heart. You do not need to start at the beginning! Creativity, curiosity, intellect, passion, and awe start in the heart. Who can say where the fusion of such gifts begins? Glance through the section titles and sense where your heart is leading you. Start reading any place you desire.

The source for this book lies deep in my experience of inexplicable connections and startling expansion of previously held views, limits, and presumptions. In part, the inspiration for writing this book came from students. Those who had been identified as being problems to the system became the catalysts for the greatest shift in my perceptions of the possibilities for learning and growth. Together we created the means for alternative expressions of passion and intellect. Those who were defined as not being among the brightest youth in the school turned out to possess vast pools of wit, humor, insight, intellect, care, concern, and energy that can all be liberated through a love for learning. When I used the same approach of asking unique, surprising, and stimulating questions to those who had been defined as being the brightest of the students, the same startling explosion of interest, curiosity, fascination, and thirst to learn emerged. Obviously, something extraordinary was at play. At first, this was surprising to me. I realized that there is literally a hidden treasure within all of us.

As we learn to experience our life context, others, and ourselves in creative ways, we discover that we all have within us startling treasures. These treasures are our creativity, curiosity, intellect, passion, and awe. By being attentive to these treasures, we become more able to care for the gift of life. They are like an inner diamond that reflects light in fascinating ways through its various facets (faces) as we learn to change our point of view. The treasures are like gold with an appearance that causes us to feel a sense of inspiring beauty. They are like pearls with a deep luster (sheen or brilliance) that delights, encourages, and entices us. These inner treasures are like a mysterious and profound light that causes us to see everything freshly. Our world is starving for the affirming expression of these gifts of creativity, curiosity, intellect, passion, and awe. As we learn to value these treasures, learning and growth naturally become a way of living for us.

There is also a great poverty gripping the entire human family. Our culture tends to define human characteristics in broad compartments that result in a tendency to hold these treasures in separate mental and culturally defined boxes. An effect of this fragmentation is that we fail to grasp our potential for transforming the way we encourage learning. This fragmented view causes us to misconstrue and underestimate the importance of whole-brain learning, multiple forms of intelligence, an integral holistic manner of learning and growth, and the importance of the varied gifts of diverse people.

What we fundamentally don't see in ourselves, we fail to expect in others. This results in diminished expectations for all kinds of group processes taking place in our homes, classrooms, work sites, voluntary associations, sites for play, and public gathering places. We all unnecessarily suffer from impoverished expectations and vision related to learning and growth while paradoxically we are unaware of what is being lost. If the world proves repeatedly while deeply impressing the message that an individual's or group's vital expressions are worthless, undesirable, or if significant persons actively, consistently, and directly discourage the spirit of venturing the risks of creativity, most people eventually adapt to these enervating cultural, organizational, group, or community expectations. Being dispirited means that we, for many reasons, fail to manifest our combination of gifts. The dispirited person or group may conform to some set of cultural standards and focus on getting through life rather than making a creative difference. Instead of conforming, dispirited individuals and groups may also react to this inner frustration with actions that hurt and limit others. Most commonly the tragedy is that the voice, creativity, and particular collection of gifts (genius) of the dispirited person or group are not expressed and paradoxically, this absence is not missed by others who are unaware of their own diminished condition. Being inspirited is to experience the wonder, intelligence, and passion focused in creative ways that stimulates growth and learning. Everybody profoundly benefits from the presence of inspirited persons and groups. We all suffer tremendous and incalculable loss as people and groups become dispirited.

The following dynamics contribute to the diminishment of our regard for our inner resources and the active suppression of our most precious inner treasures. These dynamics are low expectations, cultural and systemic biases, lack of imagination, fear of facing our core challenges, the anxiety related to change, power struggles, the absence of an awareness of alternatives, contradictory community expectations, conflicting organizational goals, expediency, and discouraging presumptions related to learning.

Learning to see life, others, and ourselves in fresh and sometimes startling ways is the birthplace of wisdom, care, and wonder. Seeing life's opportunities and ourselves in this fresh light generates the necessary passion for venturing the risks associated with genius, originality, insight, invention, and innovation. Genius has been defined as extraordinary intellect irregularly occurring in rare persons. Genius can be experienced in a very different light. Genius arises when a comprehension emerges that alters our way of experiencing a challenge, intellectual problem set, our sense of self, our place in the community, the role of others in society, or our relationship to those who are different from us or from our view of life. Genius is also the manifestation of our unique combination of creativity, curiosity, intelligence, passion, and awe that can be shared with the wider community. Genius is the crystallizing influence that inspires individuals and sometimes entire groups to leap beyond what is assumed to be natural and necessary. So often these kinds of expressions are squelched and stymied by those who find it difficult to face the necessary ambiguity, uncertainty, and risk that accompany the emergence of the immeasurable and indefinable ignition of creativity and intelligence.

This book illustrates a way of playing with our gifts. Humor is included in the text because humor often accompanies expressions of joy for life itself. As we learn to suspend our dependence upon certain beliefs, change our point of view, or see a challenge or situation with a totally fresh outlook (the heart of creativity itself), we become amazed. We behold life in awe rather than presume that our knowledge is sufficient already. Awe bursts all confines that limit the greatness of life and its opportunities. Awe is a matter of the heart. All life-altering learning reflects passion stemming from the deepest place of our heart.

When learning is viewed as a mechanical process involving some segmented compartment of established human knowledge, we arrest and stifle the amazing experience of directly sensing the depths of insight, wisdom, and knowledge. Every community activist, employee, student, employer, administrator, university president, department head, professor, school principal, teacher, writer of curricula, parent, and concerned person would benefit from a truly fresh look at the effect of our tendencies to construe (image, present, or cast) knowledge as a segmented and discrete object unto itself. This mysterious fusion of creativity, curiosity, intellect, passion, and awe is the dawning moment of opportunity for learning and growth. We come face-to-face with a vast, interconnected, and interwoven greatness of comprehension that had eluded us until this dawning moment of insight.

Our companies, nonprofit organizations, schools, professional associations, community groups, and faith communities would all conduct their shared life in vastly different ways if organizational dynamics were to reflect, embrace, and honor this fusion of creativity, curiosity, intellect, passion and awe. With this embrace, along with its ambiguity and uncertainty, there is a richness and depth that is no longer squelched and stymied in a regular systemic fashion. Entire organizations, entrenched bureaucracies, and tired or troubled groups that have gone through strings of development consultants can all find the means to incorporate the effects of this fusion stemming from creativity, originality, fresh insight, novel solutions, alternative ways of seeing the same challenge, enlarged awareness, alternating contexts, and seeing old and abiding problems in a vastly different kind of light.

This unpredictable and extraordinarily rich fusion emerges only as we permit ourselves to examine a process that shapes our lives in every moment. This process is the manner in which we all learn. We've all been deeply conditioned at the root levels of our consciousness to split, divide, segment, and fragment what we presume is our base of knowledge of life. The manner in which we process what we presume to know hinders and hobbles us in innumerable ways that largely escape our conscious attention. We may walk our pets on leashes, but we are the ones tethered to a strong strap that never was necessary.

Just as we think of our organizations and ourselves as being very resourceful, intelligent, and efficient, we are actually spinning in spirals around the axis of our limiting presumptions. Every rotation or cycle, the spiral closes on itself imperceptibly and progressively. Eventually, the creative energies dissipate or become consumed by our internal unwillingness or incapacity to leap beyond the core presumptions that have been unconsciously stifling us. This creative energy is necessary for adapting and evolving in light of ever-changing contexts. It is entirely possible to open ourselves to this fusion of creativity, curiosity, intellect, passion, and awe. The only way this can occur is if we are willing to examine unconsciously held, highly conditioned, and personally cultivated root presumptions related to what we think we know and how we learn. If we are willing to enter this process, then the structures we create will be altered and, in many senses, liberated.

All the little seemingly fragmented pieces of learning suddenly burst into full splendor, and we become grasped by something greater than what we had suspected. It is amazing what is possible for any group at any time in its life cycle if people awaken to the potential for this kind of fusion of human energy. It is all already there inside of each of us. We are so conditioned to respond to challenges in set patterns that we stifle the expression of originality in others while we nip its expression prior to us consciously recognizing its beauty and wonder within ourselves.

One of the greatest gifts and contributions any person or group can make is to foster, create, nurture, and sustain environments within which people gain a passion for opening themselves to greater and vaster horizons of human comprehension. It is in the self-interest of every organization to realize this potential. Anyone impassioned to learn and grow will be enamored by life. Anyone who is taken up by the wonder of sheer existence will honor life. If we want to change the world and do something about the ugly, disastrous, and momentous currents affecting all of us, we can support those people who have the gift of giving birth to learning environments for all different kinds of people.

All of us can become partners in the venture of learning. We need to create safe sanctuaries in which this kind of learning can transpire. Diverse forces suppress such learning within every organization and individual. Those who are willing to take the risks of significant leadership need to be supported and honored and not viewed as bothersome aberrations that need to be put up with temporarily so that a group or organization can project the image of being sensitive or responsive.

We are startled by our individual and shared breakthroughs, insights, odd juxtapositions with surprising interrelationships, leaps of revealing genius, inspiring bursts of intelligence, unleashed constructive passion, invigorating creativity, and unspeakable moments of awe. We are startled because of what becomes possible for us to realize, know, sense, learn, behold, share, create, understand, imagine, see, relate to, value, and experience. It's as though we suddenly leaped from a two-dimensional black-and-white world into a full-color, multidimensional world of surprises and delight. Instantaneously, it's as though there are hundreds of kinds of ice cream instead of just plain vanilla. Why should we convince others and ourselves that sugar, salt, and pepper are the only options in life when saffron, ginger, cinnamon, coriander, nutmeg, and other marvelous spices are awaiting our attention?

One of the most startling features of directly experiencing this fusion of gifts is that we start to see things we never noticed. We begin to notice many things that had always been present but which escaped our conscious attention. The Fusion Effect is so powerful and transforming that we realize that what we had presumed we were seeing in beliefs, intuitions, situations, emotions, intellectual constructs, other people, and all our other ways of experiencing life were actually great illusions upon which we had built our lives. Stemming from this Fusion Effect is the Fusion Paradox.

This paradox has many forms. One form of the Fusion Paradox is that our illusions aren't really illusory, but they are possible versions or renditions of life that are encapsulated in our conditioned fragments of a larger whole. When these fragments are allowed to evolve and fuse with other facets of our experience, these pieces play their role in a much greater scheme of things. This is the emergence of discovery, invention, and originality. Everything in life, without exception, can be fresh if we open ourselves to this possibility. Life is always renewing itself. We've grabbed a piece of its whole and clutched onto it as though it were the whole. The challenging aspect of this insight is that everything without exception changes. It is only an illusion we create that we can hang onto something as though it were set in a form accurately portraying the entire picture.

Through the Fusion Paradox, we find our place in the ever-evolving miraculous process of life. We learn to participate in this greater drama. We can learn to cease presuming that we are separate entities needing to struggle, control, dominate, and exert our influence for the end of establishing our own secure, set, and dependable place on our own terms. Our place is no longer a set idea, object, or goal. Rather, our place becomes the unfolding process itself. This is not idealistic dreaming. It is the basic way life works. Without the pretense of exerting all our vital energy in preserving what we believe we must hold onto, we can open our hearts to the startling presence of limitless creativity, curiosity, intellect, passion, and awe. These are inherent capacities within us all. This deepest and most significant learning is always a matter of the heart and mind. It is only the heart that can cause us to be open to what is greater than anything the mind alone can grasp, hold, or define.

Another form of the Fusion Paradox is that whatever it is we are giving attention, loyalty, or credence to reflects the presence of a larger whole, but we don't have the wisdom and means to interpret its incredible depth. This isn't because something is wrong with us. It is the consequence and reflection of the greatness of the array of our gifts that is potentially available to us all. The insight strongly suggests that as we learn to work creatively with groups we each control but gifts that through the Fusion Effect can positively ignite unexpected creative resources. Life is so rich with potential that it is impossible to have all the richness in view all at once. We can only continue to open ourselves to its depths and continue to learn and grow.

Another form of the Fusion Paradox is that this persistent learning and growth occurs even in our deepest recesses and sanctums that hold our most basic presumptions. In any instance, as we open ourselves to having our basic presumptions transformed in the light of a more encompassing context, everything in our lives changes. As everything changes, we have to be open to embracing our new self, orientation, and presumptions. The paradox has to do with the seeming impossibility of living in this manner. For anyone or any group that takes seriously the implications of the Fusion Effect and the Fusion Paradox, it's as though we've been touched and transformed by something that is greater than our comprehension. On one level, it can be valiant, noble, romantic, or courageous to embrace the notion that we all can learn and grow throughout our lives. It is a very different experience to realize the import of the persistent, deep, structural transformation of our most basic presumptions, biases, orientations, ways of processing issues, feelings, manners of relating to others, and definitions of our place in life. The paradox is that this seems impossible, but it is only impossible if we resist the Fusion Effect and opt to hang onto set and staid prior tendencies. This resistance vexes us all. Entrusting ourselves to the effects of the Fusion Effect blesses us. To be vexed and hexed by the illusion of security enforced on our own terms or to be blessed and empowered by an unending learning and growth process is our choice. This inclination takes place in the deepest part of the heart. This inclination determines our fundamental orientation to all the issues of our lives.

Another form of the Fusion Paradox is that as we approach our deeper presumptions, assumptions, values, orientations, core sense of identity, and crux (base) of our worldview, it requires increasing energy to change. Surface changes require of us about as much energy as changing clothes. Change at the deepest core of our being requires of us tremendous energy, risk, faith, and courage. As this change occurs repeatedly, it is almost as though we require an infinite amount of energy. What occurs through the Fusion Effect is a liberation of energy, vision, direct experience of a greater way to lead our lives, and the creative means to sustain ourselves. These resources allow us to participate in groups with sustained discipline creatively, intelligence, and compassion.

Another form of the Fusion Paradox is that we can dabble around the edges of growth and learning while convincing ourselves that we are brave souls at the rarely reached limits of human knowledge. We can then portray ourselves as being adventurers into the great beyond. In actuality, we are grasping an idea that we barely are familiar with and use it to establish our place in the wider community as a renowned and prescient seer and wise person. The paradox is that many people may succeed in this ploy. They become deeply mired in the admiration of their own cleverness, vision, and intellect. The image is marketed. People react to this projected image. This fosters dependent relationships that only limit what is possible in the wider community. One truly living in the light of the Fusion Effect and Fusion Paradox is persistently opening one's basic core of identity and security. This disallows any self-serving "use" of this effect and paradox. One can serve the community through one's experience of the Fusion Effect and the Fusion Paradox, but in this kind of service, there is no pretense or false facade or public persona that needs to be projected, reinforced, and defined. This selfless service encourages a surprising integration of the insights and wisdom in cooperative workgroups and learning environments. The Fusion Effect allows for the persistent emergence of fresh resources and alternatives.

Another form of the Fusion Paradox has to do with the manner in which the mind and heart function at the most rudimentary roots of our awareness. Enigmas, riddles, ironies, challenges, apparent dead ends, setbacks, what seem to be sidetracks and diversions, and paradoxes are all portal opportunities. Life is profoundly greater than any instance of an idea, insight, feeling, formulation, pattern of interaction, way of processing our work, imagining our future, projecting our assumptions, analyzing our goals, interpreting our experience, regarding others, or valuing the Earth and her ecosystem. By necessity of this profundity beyond measure, any grasp we have of our greater context in which life emerges is riddled. It has holes. It is incomplete. It is never the whole, because the greater context is always presenting itself to us in changing and evolving ways and because of its sheer magnitude of dimensions that elude our ego's mistaken notion that our intellects can capture and define what we are focused upon. These riddles are a reminder of life's greatness, not our poverty of gifts and resources.

Another aspect of the Fusion Paradox is that we are part of this larger whole. We contribute to what everything else shares in. What we enact and how we learn matter greatly. This aspect of the Fusion Paradox comes with its own warning. We must be aware of the persistent potential challenge related to the fact that technological innovations can and often do far outstrip our ethical capacities to realize the consequences of such technological innovations. This is a consequence of the Fusion Effect. Since we can't know in advance the effects of our learning and growth, neither can we ever know in advance the consequences of our technological innovations. This requires of us extraordinary care and sensitivity. It does not require of us resistance to all significant technological change.

The Fusion Effect and the Fusion Paradox present us all with tremendous possibilities. Nothing is set. We are able to change. We are able to recognize and benefit from an inexhaustible resource of creativity, curiosity, intellect, passion, and awe. There is no end to this resource.

Life benefits when we learn to honor all expressions of this greater whole in which we live. Common and ordinary encounters carry with them hidden treasures that can astound us. No matter what our age, life can continue to fascinate us with an endless depth of intrigue, insight, and startling connections. All of us are full of kernels and seeds of wonder and awe. All of us have unique ways of manifesting our intelligence. Intelligence has many facets that can surprise us and be an asset to the wider community as we learn to share our gifts. Life itself beckons us to explore, widen our perspectives, be surprised with ourselves, share our gifts with others for the sake of the wider community, and be delighted with the sheer fact of being alive. Even if we don't feel creative, curious, and venturesome all the time, sample this book and you will experience an invitation to experience yourself and your world in a refreshing manner.

This book is meant to inspire a way of looking at others, the world, the universe, and ourselves in ways that create options for our shared future. Our future is open to us. We need to cultivate and encourage people who can rise to the challenges of a hopeful future. We can't directly eliminate in the wider community cynicism, low expectations for life, narrow thinking, destructive biases, violence in all of its many forms, and fatalistic attitudes. We are able to use our own gifts, and we are able to inspire that similar quality of wisdom and genius in others.

What provides breathing space, a moment of options, and a place for growth is our capacity for the fusion of curiosity, creativity, passion, intelligence, and awe. The effect of this fusion is that something emerges that had not been entirely anticipated or known in advance. The emerging consequence is greater than the sum of its parts. Another form of the Fusion Paradox is that we realize what had been taken to be separate discrete things (creativity, intellect, awe, curiosity, passion, intuitions, feelings, mind, and heart) never were separate aspects of our lives. How can there be a fusion of what is already whole? The paradox is that what we experience as a fusion of separate discrete facets of life is actually the release of incredible energy and creativity. This release and creativity only occurs when the mind's strictures and filters are released so that we realize the greatness of the context in which this fullness and wholeness are already fully intact and available to all of us. Communities, groups, organizations, and individuals all can encourage this surprising and marvelous process. The instant we begin to identify, resonate, and associate with this depth of fullness, we become transformed. How can we live in ignorance of our most basic resource for living? What occurs in this coalescing and crystallizing of genius and wisdom is the emergence into conscious attention of gifts that we have been oblivious to.

We can learn to value this capacity as a means of honoring the greatness of life. Learning and teaching devoid of these facets of our human nature will serve the limited end of getting people through some system. This learning and growth can never inspire the kind of outlook and passion needed for the great challenges of our times. The aspiring heart and awakening mind will never have the hunger for the fullness of life fed with the junk-food diet of narrowly conceived learning borne along in a limited vision of growth. What is possible when people share their passion, creativity, curiosity, intelligence, and awe is immeasurable, unpredictable, fascinating, encouraging, and startling.

Our world is becoming increasingly complex. We need people who are flexible and adaptable. Beyond flexibility and adaptability is the tremendous need for innovation, creativity, and inventive critical thinking. Whether we call it genius or wisdom, we all have it in some special form. By allowing this quality of life to flourish, we will become awakened to possibilities, creativity, intelligence, joy, compassion, and the goodness of life in surprising and life-affirming ways that create fresh options for our future.

Our future is open to us. We need to cultivate and encourage people who can rise to the challenges of a hopeful future for everybody. We can inspire learning in which wisdom and genius in others and the similar gifts within ourselves open our hearts and minds to value the gift of life in such a way that persistent encouragement for shared growth becomes a metaphor for treasuring the life reflected in all people and all other creatures interdependently existing on this planet.

As the environment creates and fosters a passion for learning, individuals and groups will flourish in unexpected and surprising ways. How we relate to others is profoundly important. The Fusion Effect causes a startling awakening and encouragement as it integrates individual and group gifts. One surprising consequence is that people become more willing and able to communicate across well defended lines of division related to power, gender, social rank, race, ethnicity, economic status, educational attainment, age, and religious and political affinities. Our biases don't magically disappear, but their relative importance and power to prevent life engendering creativity is at least tempered as we experience ourselves and others in a new light. The Fusion Effect and Fusion Paradox can inspire fresh intelligence, intention, creativity, and compassion. This can result in ingenious and courageous leaps of human spirit while this freshness can also provide a crystallizing spark of opportunity for dealing with fear-based antagonisms and reactions. The creative edge of change is not a neat, well-ordered, pre-arranged, and perfectly secure niche. There is always a degree of vulnerability as we venture the risk of engaging what is fresh and transforming. We live in times of huge and unprecedented change affecting every aspect of our lives. We can react with fear and loss of nerve or we can engage our challenges inspired by resources and alternatives that only become apparent through the Fusion Effect. People will be encouraged to take risks, become leaders, and give voice to issues that need addressing. People can be inspired to share their genius and thus provide for others insights as to a greater comprehension, depth, and sense of unity that reveals to others that we actually do have options. People can be empowered to venture the risk of failure. The entire community and world benefit when brave souls value what others presume is unimportant, unnecessary, impossible, or merely foolish. Instead of losing face, these brave-of-heart individuals find the internal courage and wisdom to express what they feel, sense, intuit, see, experience, realize, know, and think—even while others remain silent in the face of circumstances that demand attention, care, and courageous expression of concern. This kind of courage needs to be cultivated and supported by the larger community. Learning and growth are ultimately communal affairs.

Our corporations, government, non-profit organizations, school systems, voluntary associations, religious organizations, and families can all tap into this limitless creative resource. Every group can benefit: debate teams, artists cooperating on a project, people working together for peace and justice, boards of directors for nonprofit organizations, planners for a parade, sports teams, and children trying to figure out how to get more candy on Halloween. We are all able to persistently learn and grow. Productivity and effectiveness in business, education, government, religious communities, and service organizations are always directly linked to the kind of learning and growth encouraged within the culture of a group. The viability of a society is dependent upon the quality of learning that occurs in the diverse kinds of families and peer groups that are the place of fundamental growth and character formation. Because of these concerns, the following story is of great importance.

Certain people have a tendency to peer beneath the surface of what appears to be set, natural, and necessary in life. They burrow beneath the surface of things. They often find alternatives to what others hold as unquestioned conclusions and unexamined biases. Some of these courageous and curious people venture the great risk of taking small boats on big oceans. Far beyond safe harbors on the wind tossed seas some of these intrepid explorers find a place in the open stretches of pathless waters to dive deeply into the depths of the ocean. Inexplicably, each explorer sense the genius loci (location that has a particular allure and spirit) that indicates that this place and time is the opportunity to dive deeper than ever imagined possible. They go for it. They make discoveries that surprise even the most imaginative of the lot. They discover a great variety of treasures down in the unfathomable and unexplored depths. These treasures include diamonds, gold, pearls, and a startling spark of light. These dauntless (daring) pioneers are generous souls who share everything they discover.

Imagine diamonds being brought to the surface. Everybody receives a special diamond. Those who discipline themselves to behold the depths of wonder in these diamonds learn how to experience their talents and life through an astounding emergence of a crystallizing influence. This crystallizing influence is a continuing comprehension of unimagined creativity and intelligence. These disciplined few behold the burst of creativity inflected (given character) through them as they see life reflected in this surprising crystallizing influence. Few people choose to discipline themselves. Those who do learn about the crystallizing influence gain great insight about their gifts they have to offer others. Although they've been distributed to everybody, these diamonds lie around mostly unused collecting dust.

A massive number of chunks of gold are raised up from the bottom of the ocean. There are so many of them each person on the earth is able to have a portion of this treasure. Each piece's shape, sheen (reflected appearance) and texture is unique for each person. Curiously the shape, sheen, and texture of each unique gold piece inspires a sense of beauty in every person who is willing to follow their inner passion to affirm what they truly feel to be inspiring in life. If you open your heart to this treasure, the only condition is that your life will be changed in unpredictable ways. Most people do not follow this inner inspiration because of their unwillingness to risk the venture of profound change and transformation. Although everybody has the gold, people forget about the real gift of being inspired by this precious treasure. Most of these gold pieces wind up in the back of closets beneath old shoes that nobody wants to throw away quite yet.

In the deepest trench of the ocean, there is a cavern that goes back into the Earth's crust several miles. At the far end of the cavern, there is a deep shaft with a huge room at the bottom. In this room are pearls. When they are brought to the surface, the pearls look normal except that they are the size of a baseball. At first, they merely look like pale white plastic mass-produced balls. These pearls are given to everybody. They become so common most people forget they're in the house.

A few persons discover that under certain conditions the pearls become translucent. Their luster (brilliance) changes when we focus our attention with unbroken depth, clarity of intention, heightened expectation of new understanding, and an openness of heart to the unknown. As we look at a pearl, we start to see deeper layers and levels of connections and insights that we never thought possible. In order to continue seeing these deeper layers of wisdom one has to commit to following a rigorous journey that challenges us to find the meaning of these insights.

Only those who respond to the appearance of fresh depths of comprehension directly experience this effect. If we don't embark on the journey and enter these depths, this direct experience of unexpected depths of wisdom ceases almost as though its potential is only a fiction or trick of memory. All we are left with is a dull large sized pearl and diminished possibilities. Most people think these stories of the pearls inspiring transforming insights and wisdom are ridiculously untrue—after all the pearls are so common!

The most unexpected treasure from the depths of the ocean might turn out to be a special form of fire. Deep in the dark ocean waters, there is a cavern lit up by light within which we are able to see with great and stunning clarity. The magnificent surprise is that in this light we see a surprising treasure-trove (collection) of unsuspected inner gifts. People are greatly surprised to see themselves in new ways that they would never have believed before arriving in this place.

A discernable and surprising genius becomes manifest that is like a fire illuminating what we had not seen before. The treasure is our genius. The genius manifests because of a fusion of inner resources that can be shared with others for the benefit of life. These people see themselves like they have never seen themselves and life before. We see that we are being continuously and marvelously transformed in this light. The sparks of genius can be shared with others. The co-mingling of these sparks ignites unexpected and tremendous energy that encourages everybody to venture the risks of creativity. There is awe and spontaneity springing up in surprising ways and in unexpected moments.

As we become aware that these sparks are within us, we feel stronger, more courageous, more focused, and able to see our emerging options. So much energy is liberated that we begin to interpret life through the lenses of abundance of opportunity rather than the scarcity of viable options. In this special light, we grow a deeper appreciation for our gifts and for the gifts of others. We discover what we have to share with others. Entire groups of people learn to share these sparks. As they share these sparks, they all become infused with something greater than their individual contributions and the sum of their previous expectations.

The ones who take the pilgrimage into the depths return with sparks that are freely distributed to everybody on the face of the earth. To experience the spark's effect of inner discovery, we must each open ourselves to an unbroken stream of subtle (fine) cues (clues) that suggest to us that there is a vastly greater context for our individual and shared lives. No one can convince another person that they also have these sparks inside and that these sparks can be shared to the benefit of everybody. Groups and entire cultures can learn how to inspire venturing the risk of this journey.

Whether we call it genius or wisdom, we all have the inner treasure of the:

- diamonds revealing a crystallizing influence of unimagined creativity and intelligence only if we discipline ourselves to behold the depths of our individual and shared gifts,
- gold disclosing unexpected inspiration and beauty only if we open our heart to transforming experiences whose effects are unpredictable,
- pearls divulging unexpected depth of wisdom, connections, and patterns only if we embrace the rigorous journey of accepting the challenge of responding to the meaning of these insights,
- sparks illuminating and clarifying the presence of unrealized gifts only if we open ourselves to an unbroken stream of subtle intimations of a vastly greater context for our individual and shared lives.

By allowing these inspiriting and inspiring qualities of life to flourish, we will become awakened to unimagined possibilities for the expression of desperately needed wisdom, courage, inspiration, clarity, creativity and intelligence. Since we are now globally so deeply interconnected in terms of culture, economics, environment, and politics, more than ever we need to discover the existence of these gifts and to honor their diverse expressions. We can experience diversity as a tremendous gift rather than a problem of divergence and conflict. Compassion is the direct result of living in this manner. Compassion can be taught and encouraged. It is as basic to any curriculum of life as is reading, writing, and arithmetic. It is as essential as breathing.

Our lives are intertwined in ways that enable us to conspire (from the Latin roots—to breath together) together to inspire (from the Latin roots—to breath into) and illumine (from the Latin roots—to see what is lit up) the persistent possibilities for cooperation in creative ventures.

As we conspire together, we share our deepest gifts. As we inspire each other, we are drawing forth from the depths of our individual and shared human capacities that benefit all of us. As we experience the illumined way of living cooperatively, we discover opportunities that were dormant and unexpected.

Since we are globally interconnected and inextricably intertwined, there is the stark and poignant (touching) reality that we also have a capacity to injure each other and violate each other. Everybody is touched by what we all choose to manifest in our lives. Our response to the presence of these life-affirming treasures is of vital importance. Responding to what is best within us is the only way to honor and revere the gift of life. We need to support those people who take the risks of encouraging others to find their inner voice, creative spirit, special genius, and means of living in a responsible and responsive manner. We can encourage a sense of safe sanctuary in which all persons can experience sufficient security that we all become able to experience the ignition of this irrepressible genius and wisdom. Some of these inner treasures are:

- the ardent commitment to create and nurture safe sanctuaries and secure environments for all people from which they are able to explore and express their humanity,
- an open mind,
- an irrepressible playfulness,
- personal responsibility for our actions,
- belief in the inherent potential within every person,
- an expectancy that we can all rise to what is best within us,
- life honoring attitudes,
- the charm of giving credence to our dreams and movements of our hearts,
- love for persistent learning and growth,
- a taste for adventure,
- the joy of questioning reality presumed by others to be set and necessary,
- the glorious gift of saying Yes! to life's unutterable magnificence and unfettered potential,
- an idealism that empowers us to continue creating,

- a realism that enables us to remain relevant and effective partners in transformation and growth,
- a faith that life lived for the sake of the whole is worth taking significant risks,
- a wit abut us (perceptive ease of being) that allows calmness, discernment, clarity, and keen perception even in the midst of crisis, pressed circumstances, short time frames, and important decisions,
- the mysterious internal diamond, gold, pearl, and spark that continuously seek expression through us,
- the capacity to experience the Fusion Effect with others for the good of the entire community,
- a compassionate heart,
- a steady integrity while we are at juncture points in which what has been isn't any longer and what will be has yet to be born,
- an intuitive sense that there are always yet undiscovered. more inclusive, and more revealing contexts within which to comprehend this hallowed (revered and honored) gift of life,
- an eye for beauty, a heart open to inspiration, and a spirit that never ceases to aspire.

Honor the unfolding story of your life and be courageous and wise in encouraging others to awaken to their own gifts. With every bit of passion you can muster and in every circumstance possible support the leaders who are willing to risk the venture of cultivating the gifts of creativity, curiosity, intellect, passion, and awe. Find and encourage these teachers, counselors, administrators, artists, scientists, community volunteers, writers, religious leaders, community organizers, workers for justice and peace, politicians, and people of generous spirit and good will. These are the ones inspiring people to see the complexion and emerging nuances of developing gifts as they are being given birth. These are the ones illuminating the immeasurable value and inexpressible tenacity of the inner spirit that is always seeking greater expression, fullness, and wholeness. These are the ones helping affirm the mysterious irrepressible passion for life and the wisdom of living for the sake of the whole. These are the ones illustrating and encouraging others to cultivate a caring understanding for those who don't perfectly match our own cultural conditioning and orientation. These are the ones touching the very wellspring of life wherein we all receive our existence.

Their path is a delicate one that requires of them risks, originality, and vision. They take leaps of faith hoping to spark a response from imaginative people. To these people we can express no greater form of gratitude than to continue manifesting our gifts while encouraging others to find and express their own unique blending of gifts. Sharing these gifts ignites a brilliance of light in which we see opportunities yet unexplored in pathless lands and seas that only the intrepid (brave) will venture into. We need to be encouraging each other to risk the venture of finding, expressing, and sharing our gifts.

Remember to laugh, twit yourself, and be a little ridiculous as you read the book. Don't take yourself or me (the author) too seriously. If we're too heavy in the accumulated mass of past assumptions or in attitudes that stifle us, we'll never fly.

This book is designed for inquisitive people of all ages. Curious and motivated elementary, middle school, high school, and college students will enjoy this book. Adults who know how to savor their curiosity, intellect, and creativity can enjoy this book. Venture a little risk in dabbling with topic areas that perhaps you've never thought about before. Take a full leap into the challenges of other questions. These treasures can be valued only if we experience an inner sense of joy in our own unique learning and growth. Others can't impose it upon us.

If you're a child or adolescent, don't worry that this book is part of a plot by your parents or teachers to make you into something they want you to be. Creative leaps are so vast that nobody can predict outcomes. If you've comprehended anything related to the Fusion Paradox, you are already coloring outside the lines of the coloring book of life. Imagine things that have never been before which might be if you believe in your own brightness. Find anyone in your life who can encourage you to be bold, courageous, wise, and adventuresome. Don't forget to look in places others never thought of:

- In senior citizen communities, there are people whose intellect is fully intact. Some of these persons carry tremendous wisdom.
- People in the neighborhood may be excellent resources. Some persons have had strokes or suffer from debilitating illness. If a person

looks different, this doesn't mean that he or she couldn't be a marvelous guide and encouraging presence of genius.

- Many quiet people are extreme introverts. Some of these people may be amazing resources for growth and learning. Paradoxically, don't assume extroverted individuals aren't capable of deep insight and profound wisdom.
- People who speak a different language might be the ones who can inspire you to grow beyond your present assumptions and biases. Teach the person what you can about your native language. Have them teach you their language.
- As you've been affected by gender bias, don't forget that people of the opposite sex have many gifts to offer you. Learn how to cross the lines that divide us. Often these lines are based on race, neighborhood, religion, educational or income level, ideology (strongly held unexamined beliefs), and age (something that happens to us when we're not looking). There are people around you who are living libraries of insight, information, and wisdom. You'll be amazed at what you experience when you begin to seek out these hidden resources in your community.
- Younger people are often thought of as being inexperienced, callow (immature), and naïve (simple). Remember that when we see life through the eyes of somebody else, our worldview is expanded. Don't forget that younger persons can also be excellent resources. This includes newborn babies.
- Imagine if a brother or sister were a resource! If you can't bring yourself to do this, then observe them carefully. Something in their unique mix of gifts can contribute to the richness of your life.
- If you're a teenager, find some loving and benign (good) adult who can help mentor (guide) you. It is such an odd thing that our own parents have so much to teach us, but for most teenagers or post-teens, parents just aren't the first candidates in line for an open discussion of life's greatest issues. If you're like most young adults, try a little trick. Just for a few moments, blank out from your mind anything that you don't like about your parents and fill in the blanks with as many wonderful qualities as you can think of. You may discover that they've had a tremendously positive impact on

your life. Parents can try this same experiment (for your own parents and for your children). It's an interesting little trick for leaders getting a little tired at the end of the day, year, or career.

- People who work jobs that you consider beneath your level of pride may be people of wit, humor, intellect, and wisdom. Just because a person is working a low-paying or unglamorous job doesn't mean that they don't have rich inner resources.
- If you live in a very isolated area, think of ways that you can get other people to pay for your participation in special events, camps, courses, adventures, seminars, or retreats. Find a mentor who will help you in these efforts.
- Go live in a completely different culture for a while. If you can't afford to fly overseas, then right in your own country there are diverse cultures.

Create your own path. Explore it. Enjoy your life and your learning!

If you're a parent, read this book yourself. Reflect on its content. Share your reflections with your offspring. Do not buy this book in order to make your child successful, brighter, more competitive, able to pass examinations, look smarter in front of the teacher, or be more likely to get into the right school. This book will not teach your child everything she or he needs to know at a certain grade level. At any major bookstore, there are at least ten miles of bookshelf space taken up by these kinds of improvement books. Find the treasures of diamonds, gold, pearls, and sparks within yourself and within your child. This is the beginning and root of inspiring learning and growth. This is the commencement point of finding your own curiosity and creativity. If you enjoy your own beauty and brightness of life's spark, others around you will feel this curiosity and passion. This will assist others in discovering their unique combination of gifts (genius). Encourage expression and experimentation. Do not get caught up in trying to have your children be something you consciously or unconsciously want them to be. Maybe you'll choose not to show this to your kids (especially if you really desire that they continue to draw neatly inside the lines in the coloring book of life). As you want them to discover their own inner treasures and means of expression. Share your own curiosity, musings, dreams, ideas, and insights with your children.

If you're an adult without children, you're never too old to be ridiculous, preposterous, unpredictable, original, creative, and ingenious. Some persons in their eighties, nineties, and older are some of the brightest persons who are the most creative cutting-edge people. Savor your wisdom and thirst for refreshing ways to express life's wonder. Be fully alive! Don't let age or cultural conditioning dispirit you. Experiment with the way you have taught yourself to think about life's truths and necessities. Sense the presence of your gifts in a fresh manner. Surprise and delight yourself!

Don't be shocked if there are some moments of inner turmoil related to the great question of whether or not you really want to learn and grow over the course of your entire life. You may be an adult who has unconsciously, through repeated behaviors, fallen into patterns of not growing throughout life. Be that refreshing presence. Until you draw your last breath, you can be learning and growing, if you are willing to take certain risks of the journey into your evolving self. This journey requires both work and play. It affords (grants) the opportunity to avoid the kind of sadness in life related to having regularly said no to life's invitation to venture and sally forth (set out) into terra incognito (uncharted lands). Keep seeking to enlarge your sensitivities, mind, and the stage upon which you lead your life. Share your wisdom with others. Be a community resource for those seeking or needing a benign and inspiring guide.

If you're a teacher, first recognize the treasures within yourself. Is your spark burning brightly? If your spark is burning brightly, then you'll be able to see the same qualities in others. You'll be able to see these diamonds, gold, pearls, and sparks as means to create an atmosphere that inspires curiosity and creativity in ways that are not entirely tame, neat, controllable, or expected. Unleash the energy contained in these treasures and see what happens to your school (and your own life)! Such unleashed creativity might cause some unexpected career shifts for you as the school experiences waves of original and innovative thinking and cooperative exploration. If you keep these energies of curiosity and creativity pent up, channeled, and controlled, you'll be complimented with comments about how orderly and well behaved the students are. Release the energies of the diamonds, gold, pearls, and sparks. You'll see lives changed. This will remind you of why you went into teaching in the first place. Don't retire with a host of accolades (positive recognition) for how your students conformed so well to the needs of the system.

If you're a principal, department chair, or an administrator of any organization, how aware are you of the routines that others are forced into that suppress the manifestation of creativity, compassion, and intelligence? Continually invent ways to liberate others to take risks that may foster environments that inspire people to want to learn and grow. Go out of your way to encourage others to express and nurture optimism and experimentation with current presumptions. Find some enlightened persons who can help teach that all of us in our own manners are capable of finding productive places in society and the workplace. Use all available resources to encourage everybody to discover and express their own combination of gifts (genius). Respond to opportunities to demonstrate in your own actions the necessary discipline, creativity, intelligence, intention, and compassion that encourages the emergence of these vitally needed gifts.

If you're a young child who's learned to read early, find others who can help you with some of the conceptual material contained in this book. Almost all the big words are immediately explained in parentheses. Be tickled with wild delight as you continue to explore this great world.

For everybody alive enough to want to read a book like this, enjoy the reading, exploring, supposing, imagining, fact finding, mind exploration, stepping back and looking at things (including yourself) askance (at an unusual angle of view), suspension of judgment, seeing first then defining odd and unexpected connections, emergence of surprising patterns, middle-of-the-night insights, vivid and lucid (clear) dreams, illuminating intuitions, original thoughts, revealing feelings, ingenious leaps of comprehension, Eureka! moments (aha!), and the cultivation of the necessary willingness to combine work with play.

STRUCTURE OF THE BOOK

The book uses original questions to startle the reader's mind to leap to broader, more inclusive, and significantly different ways of viewing an issue or the humanity of another or our own humanity. The book is not based on answering questions, because its main purpose is to stimulate creative responses to questions, passion to seek out related questions that lead to further depths of curiosity, and critical thinking skills.

Most sections of the book are very brief. A few of the sections, which deal with the most puzzling and paradoxical material, are extended. These sections deal with the very limits of human comprehension in such a manner that we commence questioning our definitions related to limits and what is presumed to be natural and necessary. Some sections are extremely practical, while some are highly speculative. The book covers ordinary issues of everyday life and topics related to the most mysterious and baffling aspects of life. The book's format encourages the reader to explore different forms of intelligence, varieties of creative responses, and diverse ways of caring for the gift of life.

The book is about empowerment. It is also written to encourage character formation. The five basic focal points of the book are empowerment, character formation, and the encouragement of creativity, intellect, and compassion. All five focal points of the book are critically important features for integral holistic learning. There are no separate sections on each of these five focal points. All of these facets of our lives reflect the presence of genius within individuals, small groups, organizations, and in the wider community (that encourages such dynamic exploration of the heart and mind).

The passion for learning and growth must include our whole human range of gifts. The heart and mind are not separate functions. Any institutions that, by their behaviors and systemic bias, exclude the heart or mind or value one over the other are missing the opportunity to inspire the passion for lifelong learning and a fundamental curiosity that is rooted in a sense of awe and wonder for life itself.

If you would like to respond to any of the sections, please write the author in care of the publisher. I would love to write subsequent books along this same line. You can make original contributions also. Everybody has original thoughts. Send them in, and they will be considered for inclusion in a subsequent book. Your genius is needed in this world. Write me or find some means of connecting with others who are willing to take the risks of the journey into uncharted regions.

A–Z

ACCELERATION

Is it possible to accelerate without gaining any velocity? Hint: find out what occurs when an uncooked egg is dropped on a hard surface. Find other examples.

Extensions

Is it possible for something to accelerate almost to the speed of light without an increase in mass? Hint: some things in nature have mass and others don't have mass. Learn something about Higgs bosons. Find out what f = ma means.

AGING AND HEALTH FOOD

Why is it that, as young kids grow older, so many of them find that the numbers and kinds of foods they enjoy are reduced? Is it physiological? Is it because of peer group pressure? Are there foods that adolescents like to eat but refuse to consume because others make fun of the targeted food? Maybe our taste buds change as we grow up. Is it an evolutionary thing? Maybe children's genes are instructing them not to eat broccoli, carrots, oranges, and nonhamburger types of foods. Maybe we are about to discover the gene that makes us cringe at the thought of certain foods at certain ages. Next time anybody quizzes you on your food habits, try this line: "It's a necessary evolutionary thing." Look as though you really know what you're talking about.

Extensions

There are many assumptions that people make about each other. Is it true that most adolescents become very narrow in their choice of foods as they get older? Do adults really know what they are talking about when it comes to food nutrition? Do adults always eat the way they want their children to eat? Sometime take a sneak look at what adults are eating when it is presumed that the kids aren't around. It might be surprising in ways you don't expect. Maybe they really do eat all their vegetables!

Challenge yourself and others around you to list as many patterns in life that people assume to be true, but that with closer examination turn out to be false assumptions. Look for examples of where false and true assumptions are mixed together.

Example: Because someone has lost three soccer games in a row, are they going to lose the next one also? What are some true and some false assumptions that are mixed together? There may be specific reasons for these losses, and it is therefore reasonable to expect that the next game will probably result in a loss. Three of your best starters may in fact be too sick to play. Even when most players on the team believe they will lose the next game, is this necessarily a true assumption? More frequently, a mind-set gets us thinking that past patterns will repeat, and then we get down on ourselves. We lose our spirit and belief in ourselves. We set ourselves up to lose.

Test for assumptions. Watch for the mixture of true and false assumptions. Always be aware of the emerging assumptions of your own or of any group. What are some assumptions from your past that affect what you are willing to believe about yourself and your prospects in life? The deeper you delve for these assumptions, the closer you'll get to actual core images of yourself that affect you every moment of every day. Once we've learned to examine these core assumptions about ourselves, it is far easier to see what assumptions we are making about other people all the time. In any five-minute period of any interaction with others, be mindful of the assumptions you are making about yourself and others. At the end of the day, try listing all of these assumptions. The journey into self-knowledge will surprise you and make you wiser.

Yet even deeper in our minds are our presumptions. We accept these unconscious patterns as being true. These patterns shape us in innumerable ways. These presumptions are so fundamental to the way we exist that we literally don't see them. They are out of sight. Example: if someone attacks me, I must get him or her back. Another example is that we are all separate individuals who need to compete for scarce resources against others who are outside our immediate circle of people with whom we identify. The only way to discover our unconscious presumptions is to continue to learn and grow in a fuller sense of what life is and what our basic identity is. Only with this greater wisdom may we look back and see what our presumptions were in the previous and more limited context.

AGING AND TRAVELING

If you were traveling in outer space at a speed that was 95 percent of the speed of light, would this affect your aging process? Would you live for a longer period of time? Always ask, "Relative to what?" In this case, length of life is relative to time as we experience it on Earth. As you are traveling at this speed, would one calendar year, one day, one hour, or a minute seem to be normal?

If you were to be gone for fifty Earth years, would you return having aged fifty Earth years? Is it possible to leave the Earth older than somebody else and return from space younger than the other person who stayed on Earth?

Extensions

What happens to something's mass if it accelerates to the speed of light? If you were to travel near the speed of light and if your mass increased, would this mean that you'd gained weight? What other things might happen to a human being if one were to travel near the speed of light? Remember that mass and weight are not the same thing. Weight is relative to the effect of gravity. Only those particles without mass travel at the speed of light. If the entire universe were traveling at the speed of light, what would this speed be relative to? Wouldn't every object have infinite mass? Would the infinite mass of a planet precisely equal the infinite mass of a marble or a pen? Might the infinite mass of a planet be different from the infinite mass of another object, such as a feather? Can one infinity be greater or less than another infinity? Draw a picture of what you think you'd look like traveling near the speed of light. Find some resources that will help you understand mass. Be very patient with this question because it is one of the fundamental mysteries of the universe. You may not get a simple answer, but you will become more informed about the vital role of mass in the universe.

AIR—HOW MUCH?

Does air weigh anything? Wave your hand through the air. Does it feel as though there is anything there that is substantial and that amounts to much weight?

Air pressure at sea level is 14.2 pounds per square foot. Does one cubic foot of air weigh anything when it is not pressing against anything? Now try to figure out the surface area of your body. (*See* "Hairs on Your Head.") Once you have approximated the surface area of your body, multiply this figure times the average air pressure at sea level. Can you believe how much pressure is exerted on you every moment of your life because of air?

Extensions

Try to figure out the surface area of any other irregular object (like a basketball with a huge bump on it, or your foot, hands, feet, fingernails, and toenails). Look up the surface area of the Earth. What is the total air pressure exerted upon the surface of the Earth? What might be the effect on the Earth if suddenly all air pressure were to be released? Would the oceans and the land suddenly move? What would the waves look like the instant all air pressure was released? Would you want to be around if such a thing were to occur? The sight might astound you. What keeps all the gases in the atmosphere in place? Why don't they float away into space? Why don't they all accumulate about a foot off the ground with a vacuum above one foot? If this were the situation, how would that affect us? How might we have evolved? What would it have felt like to be an apatosaurus with such a long neck? Draw a picture of a giraffe and an apatosaurus living in an atmosphere that is one foot high. If the atmosphere were one foot high, how dense would the air be? Would our lungs have to be different? If so, how? How would we play basketball? How might life have evolved if the life-yielding air were entirely located one hundred feet above the ground?

Learn to look at given sets of circumstances and change some piece or factor. For instance, what would the game of baseball be like if there were only three innings each game with nine outs per team? What would the life in our country be like if there were no racism? Imagine if women and men lived on an equal basis. Examine any set of circumstances and learn to imagine some critical part of the situation being completely different.

AIR AND DEEP BELIEFS

Have you ever seen air? Is it a fair comparison to say: Have you ever seen God, hope, love, or truth? We see the effects of certain things. Has anybody ever seen mass or energy? Has anyone ever seen a stationary photon or a quark? If we try to understand matter and energy without mass, we run into some major problems. What are some things in your life that are of great importance but that can't be directly experienced with our five senses?

Extensions

We human beings have greatly diverse ideas and values related to the way we believe we should be living together. One may take a belief for granted without considering other possibilities, while someone else who is equally observant and bright may have totally different beliefs. For example, many people believe in God. Many people who believe in God have greatly differing ideas of what God is. These beliefs become so central to their lives that they can easily assume all others should believe exactly what they believe. Try talking to others about their belief in something that is central to their lives, like their belief in God. Try to keep track of the common points shared by others, as well as the differences. There are many things in life that we take for granted, hope in, and dream about. What happens to you and others whom you observe when absolutely core values and beliefs are directly challenged? There are many patterns of responses. What are the most common ones you observe? What is the relation between a belief, an assumption, and a presumption?

Just because we believe in something that can't be directly experienced with the five senses doesn't mean that it actually exists. Just because many people tend to believe in the existence of something doesn't make it a fact. For instance, there have been many people throughout history who have believed that people of other races or the other gender are inferior. They believed that this quality called *inferiority* was genetic and that it existed out there in others as a fact of nature. Because so many people believed it, does it exist? In what sense does it or does it not exist? Many people have recently questioned from a scientific view if race is even a useful category.

What are other examples of strongly held beliefs that differ greatly between various people? What are some of the challenges related to communicating our beliefs to each other? Is it offensive for some people to talk about their deepest beliefs? Is it challenging for some people to talk about or describe what they believe so deeply? There is an old saying that you do not talk about sex, politics, or religion in polite conversation. Look up the word *polarize*. When people talk about controversial or core issues, sometimes the positions and conversation become polarized. When an encounter is becoming polarized, people become defensive. They try to prove the weakness and vulnerability of the other's positions, values, and beliefs. Regard for the other person is frequently lost. The atmosphere begins to feel like some kind of war is going on. What happens to the emotions in such circumstances? Why does this happen so frequently? What is the effect on individuals and groups if some or all of the people in the group tacitly (in an unspoken manner) never attempt to discuss any issues of prime importance?

Observe the different contexts in which opinions expressed between persons become polarized. What are the patterns that you notice? What happens to people when they are beginning to become polarized? Once the conversation has become polarized, is there any way to bring people back to some common ground so they can begin communicating more clearly and kindly? What kinds of feelings are in evidence when people become polarized? Do we need to be defensive around people if they have different experiences from our own? What occurs when people are able to grow closer together while talking about highly valued topics that reflect great diversity of beliefs and feelings? List as many of the qualities of this kind of conversation as you can. Keep mental or paper notes on what encourages encounters that build a sense of community, trust, and understanding.

If God were the source of compassion, why would the topic of God's reality be so touchy for so many persons? How could it be that what many people consider being the source of all life could also be the source of so much controversy?

ALCHEMIST'S DREAM

Alchemists are people who tried to convert various common substances into valued or useful substances. For instance, they tried to turn lead into gold. German alchemist Hennig Brand discovered phosphorus. Alchemists are thought to have identified at least four other elements: bismuth, arsenic, zinc, and antimony. Were they early scientists looking for order and patterns in the universe, or were they merely looking for magic? Some people look upon alchemists as being persons who studied magic but, in fact, they were looking for useful patterns in nature. They were operating on the base of knowledge available in their day.

Extensions

Who are the modern-day alchemists? Example: An old man living behind my house when I was a child collected junk. He collected anything he thought could be used in the future—like old washing machines, old radios, and curious looking automobile parts such as fender ornaments and hood ornaments. He had a barn full of old pieces of horse and wagon trailers. His collectibles were from many different decades. Looking into his garage was like peering into the past. The kids of the neighborhood never did get into his barn, but occasionally a few of us would get brave and sneak up to the big double doors and pull them open until the locks stopped the doors. We could only see through a little crack, but what we saw made the risks worthwhile. He sold the stuff to others who needed particular items. He never opened the double set of doors facing the alley while kids were around. We were all perfect angels. Therefore, I didn't understand his hesitancy. He turned the raw material of junk into valued objects for others.

What are some other examples of modern alchemy? What do some people creatively do with new tree stumps? For years, people have woven old rags together to make beautiful rugs. Look around at what is common, ordinary, and discarded. Could some of this stuff be turned into valued things? Instead of throwing old asphalt or cement chunks from old roads into big holes to sit there for a few hundred years, observe the process of these materials being used to make new roads right at the same spot. Refuse has been turned into a vital, locally available commodity. What are we throwing away right now that could possibly be used for a productive end? What about used toothpaste tubes, film canisters, and old tires? What about people? With a change of attitude and perspective, might certain highly undervalued people become sources of wisdom, insight, love, and ideas? There are many people in nursing homes who are mentally alert with vast experience. Who talks and listens to them? Who are others who are undervalued? How could we all become resources for each other? Look around your community. There are people with unrecognized talents. Look up the word *nanotechnology*. We are in a dawning age of unprecedented technological breakthroughs related to the manipulation of molecules and atoms. Are we getting closer to being able to turn base elements such as lead into gold? What would the effect of this be?

ALIENS—PROVED OR DISPROVED?

Many people believe that there are extraterrestrial aliens visiting our planet. Many others believe that this is a myth or hoax. What do you believe? Some people believe that their brothers and sisters are aliens from another planet. Is there a way to prove or disprove the theory that extraterrestrial aliens have visited our planet?

Extensions

People believe many things that can't be proved or disproved (like the existence of aliens on our planet). What are some other examples of beliefs that cannot be proved or disproved?

ALLOWANCE TIME

Do you believe that children and adolescents should get an allowance? Why or why not?

Extensions

Should children and adolescents get a set allowance whether they have done any work or not? Should allowances be directly related only to work performed?

ALPHA ORDER

Alpha order means that things are organized in alphabetical order. Get out any phone book. Look up the private residential listings. These listings are in perfect alpha order. Now go to the business section. Are entries organized in alpha order? Figure out the system of what goes first. To begin with, go to the beginning of each letter of the alphabet. It appears as though spaces and hyphens are treated equally. List out the rules that you can detect or discover for putting entries in order. The rules are not a simple alpha order. There is logic to the system. These include subrules related to the primary rule of alpha order. What are these subrules? Go to the government pages and figure out the ordering system for entries. The telephone book is one example of a printed form (hard copy) of a database (source of information).

List many kinds of databases (different ways to collect information). What are the internal rules for ordering, accessing, and manipulating information? If a database is a collection of information, you need to know how to understand its own order or organization. We most often link the idea of a database with collections of data in the form of names and numbers that are useful in some fashion. There are other databases. Our bodies carry information as to how we have eaten, exercised, slept, and reacted to certain diseases. The body itself is a database. A tree is a database. It possesses information. One cubic foot of earth carries information. All of these databases contain their own manner of storing information. They each encode data differently. Look around and see how many different kinds of databases surround you in this very moment.

Extensions

Imagine different collections of living beings or things. List different ways to order or categorize a group of randomly selected animals. Take any other collection and list as many ways to categorize them as possible. Taxonomy is how structure is organized. Nomenclature refers to the names chosen to represent anything under consideration. Raw data needs to be organized in order for it to be useful to anybody. Raw data might be the names, addresses, ages, gender, preferred hobbies, and preferred kinds of movies and reading materials of five hundred people. Will they be listed by alphabetical order only? Might it be useful to break down the data by preferences, age, and gender? Learn to be very careful about the taxonomy and nomenclature you choose, because this will greatly influence the kinds of questions you are able to ask and the kind of answers you will derive (get).

ALWAYS DOING SOMETHING?

Have you ever relaxed and enjoyed a moment of not doing anything? What does it feel like? Do you think this is good for your body and mind? Is this the same as being lazy?

Extensions

Is it possible to be doing nothing?

AN AND *A*—WHEN TO USE?

Grammatically, the words *an* and *a* are called indefinite articles. When do we use the articles *an* and *a*? For instance, a boy and a girl ran past me; a cow trotted past a boy and a girl, a turtle blew by the cow while an aardvark tried to catch up to all the others just when an owl looked up and tried to figure it all out. The Standard English usage would dictate that we use *an* when the next word begins with a vowel sound and *a* when the next word begins with a consonant sound. What do we do with the word that follows *a* or *an* that begins with the letter *h* (a history book, an honor)? If the *h* sound is silent, use the article *an*. If the *h* sound is pronounced, use the article *a*. Try these combinations: "A horse ran past me while a hysterical bus driver and a hypocritical doctor spoke loudly about not eating a hamburger in front of a hive of bees." "An honorary degree was given to the new person at a university—an utterly bad mistake because it was an unprecedented action." "It was a eureka moment and an uplifting experience when an uplink was successfully completed between two computers." "We have discovered that this was not a unanimous decision." Because the sound of the opening syllables are different, some of the words that begin with the letter *u* are preceded by the word *a* and others are preceded by the word *an*. What is the difference for the words beginning with an *h* and the letters *u* or *eu* (a *h* and an *u*, a *eu* and a *u*)?

Extensions

Keep your eyes out for exceptions to rules. Go check out how to spell words with *ei* or *ie* letter combinations. Under what conditions is the letter *y* used as a vowel? What are the rules and what are the exceptions? For many things, there are apparent accepted norms. Look for the anomalies, exceptions, and odd instances in which the example of a norm is applied differently than expected. Sometimes there is no logic or rationale for these exceptions, and sometimes there is a larger framework that illustrates an enlarged set of operating principles. An example would be that Newton's laws for the movement of large-scale objects are defined by one set of explanations while the characteristics of subatomic particles are defined by a different set of explanations. Look for the larger, more-inclusive contexts. This requires you to step back and continually seek a larger picture of reality. Don't forget to look to the periphery and edges of what is known and accepted. We often find unexpected relationships, associations, and connections there at the edges.

ANALOGIES

One of the most useful means to understand difficult or complex processes or events is to use analogies. Analogies extend what you know by comparing something familiar with what is unfamiliar. Something in one context helps you comprehend something in another context. Analogies enable us to make leaps of intellect and imagination. Assume that you know how to play soccer very well, but you've never skated in your life. Another person who is both a good skater and soccer player might draw an analogy by saying, "When you get on your skates, it is like moments when you're playing soccer. When you're going after the ball, you're moving quickly in a chosen direction by alternating from one foot to the other. You're not thinking of exactly how you're going to push off with one foot and hope to land on the other. You do it. Now that you have your skates on, try pushing off on the inside of one foot and then do it again with the other foot. Concentrate on that soccer ball over there on the ice." Whether the analogy is perfect or not, it is always an attempt to extend what is known. Be careful of soccer balls on ice rinks. When you see soccer balls on an ice rink, you know somebody has been reading this book—or when you see ice skates being worn on a soccer field, you'll know somebody drew an invalid inference from this book that the author didn't imply.

When you are faced with something very complex, draw analogies between the new challenge and something you know well. The phrase "drawing an analogy" means that you need to exercise your intelligence and imagination while painting a picture in your mind that includes two different things or processes that are similar in some way. Often these similarities are not apparent to others. Extraordinary originality may emerge as you begin to notice similarities and differences in many things. What are some analogies you can draw between things you know well and things you don't know much about? It is extremely useful to image complex processes. Look at a basketball player standing near the hoop going through the motion of shooting a shot without a ball in his or her hands. They are seeing and feeling something that others aren't seeing or feeling. Painters see (image) the subject in a certain way and then proceed to create some work of art reflecting their picture of the object. If you are being asked to do something that is new, you can create pictures in your mind of what you know from personal experience and then find something in common with the new challenge.

Extensions

Art is a great means of picturing complex phenomena. A single tree in a forest among other living plants is an extremely complex ecosystem. Imagine as many ways as possible to draw a tree in situ (in its context). Try to use as many points of view as possible. Don't forget to draw from the perspective of being inside the vascular system of the tree, or from the inside of the leaf as it is being bathed in fresh sunlight. Have you ever seen a leaf with sunlight streaming through it and toward you? From this angle, the leaf looks translucent. From the opposite side of the leaf (the side from which the light is radiating) the leaf looks to be opaque. See the picture of the tree from as many views and perspectives as possible—as a single thing, member of an ecological niche (place), at one point in time, or over the course of time. What about drawing a tree from the air the way a bird would see it, straight down, or try picturing the tree from the Earth looking up through the root system. What we choose to emphasize as foreground or background and as the framework are very important. With all these different perspectives, the complexity of the organism is appreciated. Also, with all of these multiple perspectives, we start to see connections and analogies to different things or processes in other contexts. Always do everything possible to be resource rich.

Learn to see complex phenomena as a picture. If you're memorizing a poem, scientific facts, code structure, lists of names, or a group of clients' or friends' interests, learn to see the entire complex as a picture. Pictures can be accessed from different places in different ways. The picture is like the tree, and the particular facts are like the leaves—they all have a place to go. They all interrelate in manners that are not directly apparent.

ANALYSIS AND SYNTHESIS

How do you personally come to understand something well? Do you break it into little pieces and then analyze each piece? Alternatively, do you look at it as a whole to see how it works? Do you prefer to pick things apart or look at processes as a whole in their natural settings?

There are two distinct ways of looking at something you want to learn about. One of them has to do with breaking the subject down into basic pieces (analysis). Another has to do with putting together data, information, intuition, and feelings into a useful or understandable format or picture (synthesis).

If you visit the Lego Imagination Center at the Mall of America that is south of Minneapolis, Minnesota, you can see the many huge figures made out of Legos. Somebody might say that in order to understand the figure (say it is a fifteen-foot-high dinosaur), you need to break it down into pieces, perhaps in a laboratory. Another person would say that in order really to understand how it works, you need to observe the giant Lego figure in its setting (its environment) and see it in action.

Give different examples of when one approach is appropriate, or when the other approach is better. Might we need both methods in many circumstances?

Extensions

Is there any such thing as being totally objective (removed, neutral, observing without bias, being independent from the subject being observed)? What is an example of where an observer alters the environment being studied? Does relating to certain environments alter us? Is subjective knowledge inferior to objective knowledge? Are there forms of subjective knowledge (such as intuition, feelings, insight, and leaps of imagination or intellect) that far exceed the value of objective knowledge? Pretend you are a scientist studying dancing. One approach would be to go to many dances and get into the dancing yourself. At other times, you might sit there and take notes or videotape the dances. Another approach might be to procure (get) many videotapes of people dancing. You could sit in your laboratory and logically, statistically, cross-culturally, historically, mathematically, and sociologically analyze the raw data on the tapes. One would utilize (use) a more subjective approach, while another would involve objective methods only. Are both approaches appropriate in different kinds of settings? Which would you prefer?

ANGER'S SUBSOIL

If we carefully pay attention to the moments in which we are just becoming angry, we can discover that there are some underlying experiences and feelings at play. Try to examine the relation of loss, fear, and threats to anger. What are the various forms of anger you've experienced? Learn to study your emotions very carefully. It is entirely possible to learn to see the initial movement within us that results in strong emotional reactions. In this instant of the first emergence of a reaction, we can learn to see what we are associating with this movement. We can also learn to see in that initial moment that some things we are symbolically representing to ourselves result in strong emotions. We discover that emotions are not there all by themselves. Slow down. Learn to observe your inner workings. Wisdom will emerge that you never imagined possible.

Extensions

We can go through our entire lives without ever putting our anger into a larger context that helps us understand our deeper impulses and reactions. Wisdom is revealed to us as we learn about our deeper material. Is anger ever nice? Can it be civil and respectful of life? Can it honor basic commitments related to love? Is anger something that is so primitive that it vents and rages against all things? Is it good to contain anger? Does it help us to grow as human beings if we allow our anger to take whatever course we feel like in the moment? Do we ever deceive ourselves by telling ourselves that we shouldn't feel angry because we are above such things? What forms of anger can sustain and nurture life?

ANIMALS' SENSES

We have five senses, which are sight, touch, taste, smell, and hearing. Look up some articles on the senses that other animals have. Can humans know how other animals experience their senses? Might other animals have other senses? What about insects and microscopic life-forms—might they have senses similar to ours?

We generally think of senses as some quality that resides in individuals. Alter your fundamental framework: might groups be able to possess and benefit from shared communal senses? Observe colonies of insects and think about this question. How could an Africanized queen bee (which matures more quickly than a North American queen bee) know that she must kill the other queen bees before they are mature enough to kill her? Might there be kinds of senses that deal with time, inaudible sounds, feelings, intuition, health, survival, or changes in the cultural environment that are not detected by most people? Which animals can see the furthest? Which can see with the greatest clarity? Which can see with the greatest range of color? Find out about differences and commonalties of the other senses of animals. Learn about the incredible sense of smell in animals of the sea.

Extensions

Are *Homo sapiens* the only intelligent animals on the face of the Earth? If not, what are other intelligent animals? How do they display this quality we call *intelligence*? Learn about birds on the Galapagos Islands, off the coast of South America. There are no woodpeckers on these islands. Therefore, if birds want to eat grubs burrowed into the wood of trees they have to use tools to help them. Study how different animals use their senses and intellect to accomplish almost impossible goals. Don't just look at individual animals or insects. Look at how the senses are used and the intellect is applied by small and large groupings of living things. What are the smallest living creatures that display the presence of intelligence? Sit and observe an ant colony sometime. It is amazing! Just be careful where you are sitting.

ANOTHER WAY

Have you ever faced a challenge that, no matter how hard you work at it, you can't resolve? Observe some people who want to have friends so badly that they drive others away. Frequently they smother others with their own internal needs. The closer these persons try to get to other people (physically and emotionally), the further others back away. Some people have such intense internal needs that these needs prevent any real relationships from developing. For these persons, the immediate (or presenting) challenge is friendship. On that level, the issue can't be resolved. These people first need to gain inner peace, self-confidence, and a healthful sense of self-love. Then friendships can start to happen, because they will have changed the level at which they are dealing with the challenge. They will have redefined the challenge, and refocused themselves. What are some other examples of challenges that seem to be impossible to solve on one level, but are relatively straightforward in resolution on another level?

Extensions

When you feel stuck or challenged in any kind of relationship, step back from the intensity of trying to solve the problem. Take a wider look at what is happening within yourself and in the social field of your life. Too frequently, we try to change the world around us without examining what is happening in the world of our own inner emotions and ideas. Something needs to be changed, but this something may be ourselves and the way we look at the world. We may need to change how we define our own self-identity. Be kind to yourself. Use your imagination. Love who you are.

Try to apply this method of changing the way you look at a challenge to math problems, term papers, relationship issues, or sports. You have the capacity to alter your understanding of the framework or context, the structures, dynamics, and names commonly used to define the particular challenge.

For instance, you're with a group of persons and you've been given the challenge of doing a science project related to how the heart works. Instead of immediately jumping to the resources with diagrams of the heart and full descriptions of the heart processes, sit back and redefine the terms of the challenge. What are the various definitions of heart? Why is the heart a symbol of love? Why did the ancient Egyptians throw away the brain and save the heart when they were preparing a person's body to make a mummy? Look at the process in terms of mechanics. What are other examples of pumps? What are other examples of one-way valves? What are other examples of multichambered devices that are input-output devices? How does the human heart compare to the hearts of other animals? Look at the heart in terms of electrical processes. There are some rather unusual cells in the heart. How have other cultures looked upon the heart? What are some mythical stories from different cultures related to the heart? What are some fallacies and inaccurate assumptions many people hold about the heart? How do we care for the heart? How do we abuse our hearts? How is the heart similar and dissimilar to other muscles in the body? What kind of special quality allows the heart to beat with such regularity? If you take two certain heart tissues, they will beat with different rhythms. Place them close enough together and they will begin to beat in rhythm with each other. There is a field at play. How do the emotions we carry around inside of us affect our heart?

ANTARCTICA—ICE AND RAIN FORESTS?

How could there be oil under the ice in Antarctica or under the desert sands of the Mideast? Hint: oil occurs in regions that were once rain forests.

Things weren't always as they appear now, yet people have a tendency or unconscious presumption to assume that the way things are now is how they always were. In addition, we can easily assume that the way things are now is the way that they will be in the future.

For instance, one morning I parked my car in my reserved spot next to my office. When I parked the car, there were two other cars parked at angles on either side of my spot instead of straight between the lines as they were supposed to be parked. I parked my car between them. After the two other cars left, my car was still parked at an angle in a straight parking spot. Some people kidded me about not knowing how to park my car, because they didn't know about the cars that were there before I parked mine. Be careful in your analysis and in the assumptions you make about how things appear when you first look into a circumstance or challenge.

How could there be glaciating marks under the sands of the Sahara Desert? We like to look at our world and presume that what we see is accurate and stable over time. Glaciers and the Sahara Desert don't fit well in our images of the world. One part of us always knows that things always change. Another part of us needs stability, and we depend upon things being the same. How does this interplay affect us?

Extensions

Is it a safe assumption that, since certain patterns occurred in the past, they will continue in the future? Example: The sun has risen every morning for as long as the planet has spun. Does this absolutely mean that it will rise tomorrow? What are some examples of patterns that last just long enough that we get adjusted to them? When these patterns no longer occur, what do we experience? What are other examples of patterns we know are not permanent but upon which we've become dependent?

ANTIGALAXIES

NASA sent up a sixty-story-high, helium-filled balloon (39 million cubic feet of the lofty stuff) twenty miles up into the atmosphere carrying an instrument that weighs five thousand pounds. It is called the BESS project (Balloon-borne Experiment with a Superconducting Solenoidal Magnet). What would really blow the socks off these researchers is if they detect the presence of more complex atoms, such as antihelium. The reason would be that other simpler particles such as antiprotons could have their presence explained as the result of the collision of ordinary particles (regular everyday matter). An instance of antihelium could not be produced by a collision of regular matter. This discovery would suggest the existence of antigalaxies composed entirely of antimatter. You thought the Fourth of July fireworks were cool, imagine if an antigalaxy were to collide with a galaxy composed of matter? The fireworks would really fly. Unfortunately, so would we (not in all directions as pieces of matter but as 100 percent radiant energy). What do you think of the possibility of the existence of antigalaxies? Try to imagine what would happen to this oversized balloon filled with helium if it really were to encounter even a single particle of antihelium! What would be the result of this collision? What would the result look like?

Extensions

What will scientists be looking for next? How about extraterrestrial intelligence? Look up the SETI (Search for Extraterrestrial Intelligence) project. You can download a screensaver for your computer from this group. What are the various possibilities for intelligence becoming manifest to us? What could constitute (make up) intelligence that we could detect?

ANTIPARTICLES

Matter in our universe is composed of particles with many different properties. One of these properties is charge. At one point in the development of the universe (in the first fraction of a second after the big bang), there might have been an even balance of subatomic particles with opposite kinds of charges. For some unknown reason, our universe evolved in such a manner that we primarily only have one kind of matter. Particles with the opposite charge are called antiparticles. Find the latest information on antiparticles. Is it likely that these particles will ever be a significant source of energy for any purposes?

Extensions

Research the different sources of energy. Certain kinds of energy are related to certain chemical reactions. An example of an energy source is gasoline. Gasoline and other derivatives of hydrocarbons (hydrogen and carbon molecules) provide energy through chemical reactions. The sources of these petrochemicals are the ancient forests from the time of the dinosaurs. The decomposing (rotting) materials of the forest (biomass) became compressed and transformed into oil. See if you can find the various forms of energy we derive from petrochemicals. Also, research what has been the effect on the Earth of using these chemicals. What is the effect on our bodies of the vapors of these chemicals (like inhaling gasoline vapors while filling your car)?

Another form of energy is nuclear. Why don't these explosions (chain reactions) continue? What limits them? What causes them to spread out to a certain area (consume so many atoms) and then dissipate (stop)? Why wouldn't this reaction simply continue until it had used up all the atoms in the air and the Earth? How can the waste materials from nuclear energy be safely stored? Do we possess the technology to store this material safely *and* in a 100 percent ecologically sound manner? If we can't store it safely until it becomes nontoxic, then ought we be using it? The issues related to nuclear energy are becoming more complex. Learn as much as you can because all of our futures will be affected in some way or another by the use of nuclear energy. How do you pronounce the word *nuclear*? Listen to how most people pronounce the word *nuclear* and then look it up in the dictionary for the proper pronunciation.

Another potential source of energy is from antiparticles. When chemical reactions are compared to antiparticle reactions, chemical reactions are very inefficient. If we were to explode a single pound, a million tons, or a billion tons of TNT, only a miniscule amount of the matter's mass has been converted to energy. Nuclear reactions convert less than 1 percent of its original matter's mass into energy. That's not very efficient.

When particles and antiparticles come into contact, they instantaneously annihilate each other. Their matter's mass is converted into radiant energy. In this kind of energy source, 100 percent of the mass is converted into energy. Can this process of converting mass to energy be reversed and convert pure energy into mass? Is there ever any mass without matter? If not, can we derive (get) matter from pure energy? Might the entire universe have evolved from pure energy? Compare the efficiency of antimatter and matter reactions to chemical and nuclear reactions.

Is this energy source science fiction or is it a real possible source for energy in our futures? We know how to produce antiparticles in laboratories (CERN in Switzerland, for example). What is energy? What is matter? Compare this answer to what is mass. Don't settle for answers that are too simple.

Are there certain fundamental building blocks of knowledge, such as time, mass, matter, energy, or infinity, that can't be defined fully and completely? If so, why? If our building blocks can't be defined, can we really know anything? What is the role of assumptions? How are assumptions useful to our everyday lives? Maybe we can define these basic building blocks of human knowledge, but only in simple terms that make us think and feel that we really know what we are talking about. Try a test. Go up to any science teacher and ask what these fundamental building blocks of human knowledge and reality mean. Keep probing for deeper answers. Eventually, the teacher may have to refer you to another resource. This does not mean that they do not know what they are talking about. It does mean that the collective wisdom of all humankind has difficulty understanding the meaning of these basic building blocks of human knowledge. There are many other building blocks of human knowledge similar to time, infinity, mass, and energy. Develop a list. Find people who are willing to have the limits of their knowledge tested. Explore with them issues related to the edges of our understanding of the universe and life. These can be precious and useful relationships relative to your growth and learning.

ANTS AND THE RAIN

Why don't ants drown when it rains? Remember the kind of homes in which they live! Usually ants live in the soils of the Earth. When rainwater gushes into their homes, why aren't they all suffocated? Perhaps the holes leading into the tunnels in the ants' homes are too small for raindrops to seep in. When the diameter of a tube is much smaller than a raindrop, the water may not run down the tube even though gravity is encouraging it to do so. Also, there are some very interesting properties of liquids inside vascular systems (any of the tubes inside living organisms). Look up some information on the surface tension of water. Perhaps raindrops have surface tension that remains unbroken even as the drop sits on top of an entrance to an ant home.

Extensions

How can animals survive in the deserts? How can humans survive breathing oxygen when this gas is so corrosive? We tend to think of certain forces as being toxic or detrimental (harmful) to life. Extreme heat would tend to overheat our bodies. Other corrosive gases and liquids kill living things. Then there are always exceptions in nature. Different life-forms adapt to extreme environments in incredible ways. How do animals in the desert adapt to little water, few food resources, and high heat? How have the lungs of mammals evolved to benefit from oxygen instead of being corroded by oxygen? Adaptation is an incredible device of nature. Find our more about it. Find different examples of life-forms surviving, adapting, and thriving in the most extreme of environments (deep in the ocean with high pressure and no light, extreme cold, high altitude, or an extremely toxic environment).

APPLE CORPORATION LOGO COLORS

What is the order of colors in the Apple Corporation logo? How is it similar to the colors of the rainbow and how is it different? Use your knowledge of the order of the colors of the rainbow (red, orange, yellow, green, blue, indigo, and violet) to analyze if there is any order or reason for the arrangement of colors in the Apple logo. A mnemonic device is a tool for memorizing things. In this case, Roy G. Biv is the mnemonic device that my third-grade science teacher taught us.

Extensions

What are other mnemonic devices, such as a name, formula, or rhyme? Try making up a name like Roy G. Biv for the order of the planets in the solar system. Try applying this technique for memorization on different groupings. This can be used in art, math, science, debate, memorizing large groups of names, and for many other things.

Sometimes, when we observe some thing, we may sense that there is pattern at play. We can use many different techniques and different kinds of intuition to determine the existence of patterns. One way is to compare something to another known pattern. In this case, we are comparing the Apple logo to the order of colors in the rainbow. Intuition comes into play when we sense the discovery of some comparison. Some unexplained interconnection of things in nature or in our minds might suggest a relationship is at play. For instance, the vascular system of trees is composed of tubes running up and down the tree trunks. These small-diameter tubes are similar in diameter to the width of the tunnels in ant homes. Something might suggest to us a relationship between liquids running up and down the vascular system of trees and the possibility that water may not flow into ant homes. The relationship is not immediately obvious. The two phenomena are right there in front of us. The tree may be a few inches from the ant home, but it takes a dose of intelligence and a splash of intuition to awaken us to a possible deeper relationship. Always be open to this process of the emergence of deep interconnections that aren't obvious.

Our context for understanding is always enlarged when these relationships become obvious, plausible (reasonable), or imagined and conscious.

List some things that you've observed that may have a pattern at play. Compare these patterns to other known patterns. You can extend your knowledge of your world in this manner. There are many times in which there are patterns right in front of us and we fail to understand or observe them. One reason for missing some pattern is that it develops so slowly we do not see its evolution (for example, the change of some mole on the skin surface over time). Another reason for missing patterns may be that we are not expecting there to be any, so we are not looking for any (a friend being chemically dependent). The more we can be aware of the patterns around us and within us, the wiser we become. Another way that people fail to observe patterns at play is when we abhor (object to) something so much that we deny its existence—like when someone has evidence of some form of severe bad health and we deny it. This is based on the ancient irrational belief that if we close our eyes to something it is no longer present.

Another reason we miss patterns is a mass of accumulated presumptions that are largely unconscious. What we pay attention to is what we presume to be of greatest importance. Over the course of time, we develop a narrow point of view, and we miss a tremendous amount of what is occurring in others, in ourselves, between us, and about us in our environments. These presumptions set up patterns in the deep structure of our psyche (mind). The presumptions act as a filter. Learn to observe your inner workings and you will eventually be able to see this filtering process at play (only after you go deep enough into your core presumptions). There is a very great paradox at play. How can we consciously be aware of our unconscious presumptions? There is only one answer—from outside the system and mechanism that produces the core presumptions in the first place. It is entirely possible to see some of our core presumptions from within their network or system of patterns. It is not possible to see the core, bedrock, or central presumptions operating in our lives in real time (the current moment) unless we step outside the systems of patterns. In one perspective, this is impossible, but it is only impossible if we remain completely associated, identified, and resonating with the presumption. What we are dependent upon and beholden to determine what appears to be possible. By refocusing and revisioning our fundamental orientation, we experience tremendous counterpressures to conform, retreat, and return to what is generally accepted. This is the leap of genius. It is an amazing thing to directly experience how we construct, project, and produce, in every sense, our view of the world within, about, and shared between us. How do we get outside the system of patterns and presumptions that filters everything we call reality? One example is when we are standing inside a room filled with mirrors. If we stand in just the right place, we can almost see an infinite regression (pattern) of reflections proceeding away from us to infinity. We can't see the regression. For one reason, our visual acuity (sharpness) is not sufficient or great enough.

The more important reason we miss seeing what would otherwise be interpreted as infinity (the vanishing point) is that something is in the way. What blocks our view? Try it for yourself. When you discover what is blocking your view, then realize that this is perfect metaphor for what blocks our larger view of greater contexts. Hint: what makes it possible to see the mirrors also prevents us from seeing what is interpreted as an infinite regression. Our presumptions and our identification with these presumptions are extremely powerful. Incidentally, the word *identification* is a major clue as to how we can leap beyond our current presumptions. There are many other reasons we miss emergent patterns that are manifesting themselves. List as many of these patterns as possible, and then list the reasons we tend to miss many of them.

It is rather interesting to note how different logos have evolved over the course of time. Look at the Ford Motor Corporation's logo, and then try to find the ones that have been used in the past. Carefully examine any logo and try to figure out the various symbols used in the fine details. Are there any coded messages in any of the logos? Where do we find the coded message "e pluribus unum"? Try to find the coded message "annuit coeptis" or "novus ordo seclorum." You've all seen these messages. You've held them in your hands. Once you have found them, find out exactly what they mean.

AS TIME PASSES BY

When I was an adolescent, one of my favorite songs had the line, "As time passes by, I realize just what you mean to me. . . ." The truth of this little line has proven itself over and over again as time passes by.

One day I received in a box a most special gift. A sister of mine had taken a large box full of old 8mm home movies and edited them. Subsequently, she had them recorded onto tape for our video player. I decided that I was going to sit down and view all three tapes from beginning to end (that's a lot of popcorn!). At the beginning were shots of grandparents, great-uncles, great-aunts, uncles, aunts, and many family friends who all looked so incredibly young. It's an amazing thing to see people as they were when they were young whom you've known only in their older years. How old do you have to be to be old? Remember—relative to what? The videos went through the period of our parents' lives without children, with young kids, and then suddenly (a few hours later) with teenagers! I viewed the tapes after my father had died.

When I finished, I had this powerful sense of being connected to my family and the fact that I am one player in a huge drama of life and love that started long before me. It also came to me how life is so brief. Here was my dad, a young man, much younger than my current age, coming home from World War II, a wounded veteran who sprang back into life ever so fully. My mother, who always carried with her an indescribable quality of aliveness and love, obviously had these same qualities at a much younger age. He's gone. Death has ended his continuing story. Life is so beautiful and so short. Is this a depressive way of looking at life? No!

Realizing that life is brief emphasizes the points:

- Express your love appropriately, don't wait.
- Never take for granted that you'll see your loved ones again.
- Do the things in life that are most valued.
- Don't wait around thinking that you've got unending time.
- Leap for the big brass ring on the merry-go-round of life (don't just half-heartedly reach for it—leap for it)!
- Give yourself to the fullness of life in the current moment.

How do you open yourself to the fullness of life?

Extensions

What are the many things that change when we consciously live with gratitude? What changes when we take the gift of life for granted? What are the examples of both ways of living that you've seen in your life and in the lives of others?

ATOMS—HOW MANY ARE IN THE LAKE?

Refer to "Waters of Lake Superior," then return to this section. Try to figure out the number of atoms contained in the water of Lake Superior. If you've worked through the section "Waters of Lake Superior," you may have an answer as to how many cubic inches of water are contained in the lake. Once you have this number, figure out how many atoms are in one cubic inch of water. There are many resources available to you to figure out this answer. Once you have the number of atoms figured out, then attempt to imagine and figure out the width of one atom. If you were to take away or eliminate the space between atoms contained in Lake Superior, how much volume would this lake's water take up? Guess in advance. Would it be the size of a baseball, the size of your bedroom, or the size of ten thousand 747 jets? Then try to imagine if we could eliminate the space between atoms and the space within atoms (the space between the nucleus and the electron orbits). How large would this matter be? What kind of matter might this resemble? If you take the diameter of one of the atoms in the water molecule and compare this distance to the distance between the center of the same nucleus and its electrons, this is a ratio of two numbers. Compare this ratio with the ratio of the diameter of the sun and the distance between the center of the sun and its farthest planet. How do the two ratios compare? Which forces of nature would have to be altered in order to accomplish this task? What would you look like if this reduction process happened to your body?

Method: We are dealing with very large numbers representing small entities. Is there such a thing as a large number that represent tiny things? Look up negative exponents. You will need certain tools to understand these very large and very small numbers. Up to this point, you have been looking at numbers with a whole lot of zeroes behind them. Now you must switch over to the use of scientific notation. Scientific notation will help you with the very big and very minuscule (small) numbers. First, look up scientific notation. In scientific notation, there are two sets of numbers. The first number is always between 1 and 10. This first number is multiplied by some power of 10. For instance, 10 to the second power is written 10^2. This means 10 times 10. Ten to the third power is written as 10^3. This means 10 times 10 times 10, which is a thousand. Thus, 4,430 is written in scientific notation as 4.43×10^3. In a few minutes, you can know the basics of scientific notation. You will also need to learn how to multiply numbers written out in scientific notation.

Go to an encyclopedia and look up *atoms*. See if you can find a measurement of the width of various atoms. It will be a very small number. The units of measurement will not be in atoms per inch. You will have to learn how to convert between various units of measurement. Learn how to compute arithmetic averages. It is simple once you know the method. We imagine many things to be greatly complex because we simply don't understand them. The trick is learning how to feel comfortable with learning about complex things. Once we feel comfortable learning, we need to become proficient (effective and efficient) at knowing how to discover various methods or tools that will assist us in the learning process.

Once you have the average width of an atom figured out, how many of these atoms of water would fit in an inch? Once you have this figured out, then learn how to compute a cubic inch. Go to the puzzle on "Waters of Lake Superior" and find out how many cubic inches of water there are in the lake (an approximate number). Multiply the number of atoms in one cubic inch times the total number of cubic inches of water in Lake Superior. Now try to figure out the proportion of space within an atom compared to its matter contained in its nucleus. Then try to find out the distance between atoms in water molecules. Once you have done this, try to figure out how large the matter would be if we eliminated the space between atoms and the space within atoms.

Extensions

To get a sense of how small atoms are, we can generate numbers that reflect the number of atoms given a known thing such as your body, a chocolate chip, or a drop of water. Take the tiniest thing you can think of and then try to figure out how many atoms are in it. When we realize how many atoms there are all working together, it is amazing that the universe functions so well. If all the nuclei of atoms were to become instantaneously twice as big or half as small, would we be able to discern (recognize) the alternation? Would a mile still be a mile? If every atom became a million times smaller or larger instantly, would we notice? What would that transition feel like? Are there actual transitions in nature that are instantaneous? Get used to playing with basic ideas of the universe and life that seem to be set. This can lead to some very interesting and unintended insights and discoveries. This is exactly how some of the greatest discoveries in history were made. Play with your ideas, assumptions, presumptions, biases, and perspectives in a disciplined manner. The results can be amazing!

ATOMS AND SPACE

If atoms and molecules are mostly space, how is there anything in the universe that appears to be solid? Also, why can't things simply pass through each other if all things are mostly space?

Extensions

There are particles that pass right through the Earth without being affected by the Earth whatsoever. What are they? Hint: these particles do not possess mass. The Fermi labs in Chicago will soon be conducting an experiment with these particles. They will produce them in their labs and then transmit them under the state of Wisconsin. The particles will pass under the extreme southwestern tip of Lake Superior, and then they will pass through detectors located deep in a mineshaft in northern Minnesota. These particles will continue on their journey, exiting the Earth approximately at Knife Lake in northern Minnesota. Similar particles are passing through your body every second.

ATOMS AND THE BIG VACUUM

If atoms are mostly space, does it seem reasonable that there must be a vacuum in between the electrons and the nucleus? Is this a correct assumption? Why have we heard of the big bang but not the big vacuum? Is the term *vacuum* being used correctly? If every atom has a vacuum inside of it, does it have negative air pressure? Why isn't all the air on Earth sucked inside all the atoms? If this vacuum creates negative pressure, why isn't all the matter of the universe sucked into this space? Couldn't larger atoms suck in smaller ones?

Extensions

Watch out when people start to use terms that sound right, but have something wrong in the way they are being used. Sometimes we have a feeling that something is wrong with what we are reading or hearing but we are not able to determine exactly what is wrong. If a question isn't asked in a useful and precise manner, can there be a true and accurate answer? One version of this kind of ill-formed question is, "Have you stopped abusing your pet?" It is asked in such a manner that only a yes or no answer is allowed. Either way you answer, you appear to be a terrible person. Lawyers are famous for asking such questions in trials. The range of possible answers doesn't include the domain (area) of your experience. The range of possible answers doesn't include anything that you consider real. This is called a forced option situation. When others control the circumstances in which forced options arise, we need to learn to be very careful. What are other questions that, when asked, only allow for misleading, confusing, or ambiguous answers? Is it possible that atoms do have some kind of negative inner pressure? On one level, some questions make no sense, but when we alter them, suddenly there might be great significance to the question. How do atoms attract other atoms to themselves? What is the process at play that causes them to hang out together?

AUTOMATIC STUFF

What are some automatic behaviors or feelings you revert to (return to) when you feel embarrassed in front of others or feel threatened by others? Do these behaviors and feelings always serve you well? If they are automatic, are you even aware of them? How can you become more aware of your automatic reactions? If someone hurts you or hurts somebody you dearly love, are anger and retribution necessary reactions? There is the phrase, "Don't make me do this!" People have uttered this phrase when they are placing blame on others for the violence they are about to inflict on that person. Responsibility is being projected outward. Do outer circumstances dictate your reactions? Must you be reactive in the first place?

In between every action and reaction, there is a space in which you have time to shape your responses. The existence of this space is what allows you to exercise creativity and the power of choice in a given set of circumstances. Observe yourself in some intense set of circumstances. The more you learn to observe yourself, the more you will become aware of this space that exists between every action and reaction. We derive great freedom because of this space. Look up the terms *nexus* and *nodal point* and compare their definitions relative to the issue of this space between every action and reaction. The next time someone does something that evokes some kind of strong feeling, like love, hate, adoration, disgust, gratitude, or anger, remind yourself to be focused on that incredibly subtle but powerful moment or space in which there are creative options and real choices. Nobody else will be aware that you are doing this, and your self-understanding will increase greatly. Once you learn to observe yourself at this subtle level, you will experience with amazing clarity how others around you are locked into certain ways and behaviors that are not at all necessary.

Extensions

If someone were to observe your reactions to others, what would they see? If somebody is being very kind to you, how does it make you feel? There could be two opposite and equally unnecessary responses: I deserve these compliments, or I don't deserve any of these positive reinforcements. Why not just savor (enjoy) the moment and say thank you?

A VERY BIG BANG

What is probably the biggest natural bang in the Earth's history?

- Would it be the largest volcanic eruption in history?
- Would it be the meteor that struck the Earth 64.9 million years ago and probably wiped out the dinosaurs?

Hint: when we think of big bang, we think of an explosion that is sudden. Might there be a big bang that is very slow and without perceptible sound that is occurring within our atmosphere or in the Earth?

Think about the Indian tectonic plate slowly slamming into the southern shores of the Asian tectonic plate. Tectonic plates are the large landmasses that literally float around the world driven by forces related to upheaval of magma from under the surface of the Earth and the sinking of molten materials back into the Earth. This grand slam has resulted in the huge Himalayan Mountains, and this process is still going on. Since it is possibly the largest bang in history, is there any sound? Might there be sound created by mountains emerging from the Earth, but it is such a slow process that nobody hears it? What about another very slow process ripping apart the landmass from which we got North America and Europe? Big bangs do not need to be loud and quick. Some may be slow and soundless.

Another possibility might be a huge slam to the Earth that possibly created the depths of the Pacific Ocean. What could have hit the Earth that would be that powerful? Hint: some people think that this occurred billions of years ago. The body that hit the Earth may have become the closest celestial body to the Earth. What is your guess? Now if you think you know what some of the greatest bangs (explosions) were in the history of the world, what might be the greatest implosions? Would they make a sound?

Extensions

Photographers can take pictures using a method called time-lapse photography (shown in movies of flowers blossoming, plants poking up from the ground, or clouds racing overhead during the course of a day). Photographers do this by taking a picture once every few seconds, once every few minutes, or once every few hours. The result is that processes that usually take long periods of time appear to be sped up on the film. Usually we do not sit around for twenty-four hours watching the sun and the stars from one position. The camera can do this when a timer electronically controls it.

Imagine trying to set up a moving picture of plate tectonics. If you were able to set up such a recording eye that would take pictures of the Indian tectonic plate slamming into the Asian tectonic plate, how frequently would you have to be taking the pictures—once every few seconds, few hours, once every few weeks, once every fifty years, or once every thousand years? Who would be around to make sure the equipment was operating properly? Who would be around to see the results? What are examples of other processes that would be interesting to observe in this sped-up format?

Hint: try to determine how fast the Indian tectonic plate is moving. One hint comes from a report of a section of California moving approximately as fast as your fingernails grow (extend your knowledge base by using analogies). Look at other phenomena that are recorded using time-lapse photography. Start out with about ten examples of time-lapse photography and then determine how often these pictures were taken. Then, based upon all the information, estimate or guess the rate at which you'd need to have the camera taking pictures of the Indian tectonic plate in order to record its movement. Remember that you are talking about geologic time.

Want another brain builder? Try to figure out where you would position the camera. Do you think the camera would need to be a fixed position relative to the moving plate of India? What happens if the Asia plate were also moving? Then where would the camera be placed?

What might be the opposite of time-lapse photography? Give it a name and figure out what it could be used for. Think of something moving very rapidly. If we were able to record the movement of subatomic particles, could we determine the location and velocity of the particle at the same time? Think of a baseball traveling at just below one hundred miles per hour racing at the strike zone of a batter. Imagine a film showing the intricate path and motion of the ball in great detail. If we could record this process, do you think the shape of the baseball would change at the moment of impact with the bat? What would an armor-piercing shell going through a plate of solid steel that is one foot thick look like? Imagine a slow-motion movie of the effects on the painted surface of two test automobiles slammed together, at high speed, head-on. Imagine other unusual processes to observe.

AWKWARDNESS: A PART OF LIFE

Under what conditions have you ever felt awkward? There is physical and social awkwardness. An example of a socially awkward set of circumstances might be if you were a religious leader and you were asked to do the funeral of a person you did not know. Halfway through the service, you forget the person's name. You are desperately looking around the flowers for a nametag. This could be socially awkward. (This really did happen to a good friend of mine—only once .) Have you ever gone to bed exhausted and wound up tripping on something? Being physically awkward doesn't feel good. List the ways that you have ever felt awkward. What are the patterns?

Extensions

Do you think that people who appear to have it all together and be in control ever feel awkward? Do we make others out to be more perfect than they really are? Do we ever do this as a way of putting ourselves down? Do we ever point out, make fun of, or emphasize the awkwardness of others so that we can feel better about ourselves? Why has slapstick humor proven to be so durable and lasting? What are other feelings associated with awkwardness?

BACK TO THE FUTURE

Are there different ways of interpreting time? Is there a way that you can imagine that would allow you to live life not in a straight line from the past to the future? (*See* "Dimensions—How Many?") What happens in a linear fashion is only one way of looking at the universe and life. Could time just be a useful tool for creating a certain picture of the universe and life? Just because something is useful doesn't mean it actually exists independently of us. If any of this might be valid (true, given a certain set of assumptions), might we be able to imagine experiencing the future as part of the present, and the past as part of the future?

Extensions

How many different kinds of things can you list that might be projections of human intelligence and imagination? These would be things we most often assume are out there in nature or the universe but really are creations of our mental powers. They are not independent of our human perceptions. We convince ourselves that they are out there so that we can feel that we possess an adequate knowledge or control of our environment. What about ghosts? What do they explain to the believers in ghosts? What about aliens that seem to be ever so popular today in our books and movies? Many people certainly believe aliens exist here on Earth. Why is this belief so popular? What is the attraction? Because people believe something, is it really out there? Just because people believe that something is not there, does this prove anything? Just because there are survivalists who ardently believe that every government agent is out to squash liberties by participating in a plot against Americans, does this very projection of fear and antagonism create reactions that reinforce the survivalists' view that they are a besieged and threatened minority? Consider the belief among many young infants that if they cover their faces, either what they don't want to see goes away or others are no longer able to see them. This is my favorite example of people believing things about the universe and life that aren't necessarily true. What are some adult behaviors that are roughly equivalent to the behaviors and beliefs of infants relative to covering their faces and closing their eyes?

BALLS

How are basketballs and Ping-Pong balls made?

Extensions

Think of the most unusual things and try to imagine how they are made; then find out how they are actually created.

BARKS AND MEOWS

Everybody knows that dogs bark or woof and cats meow, right? Not so! Ask persons from a culture other than your own what sounds these two critters make. See if it sounds like bark, woof, or meow to them.

Extensions

What are other sounds in nature whose names are like the sound? What are examples of sounds that we make for other senses such as something that feels, tastes, smells, or looks marvelous?

BEETHOVEN'S TENTH

No, this is not about a tenth inning in baseball. No one named Beethoven has ever played for the Yankees. Beethoven composed nine symphonies. Before the famous composer died, he was working on a tenth symphony. A researcher has discovered this work in progress. Could we take what we know of Beethoven's other compositions and extend the knowledge in such a manner that it would allow us to infer (project) a possible rendition (form) of the entire tenth symphony?

Extensions

Does any pattern from the past give us a guarantee that the pattern will be continued into the future? What are some patterns that seem never to change? What are other patterns that are evolving? Give some examples.

BELOVED DOGS

Pets are not human; therefore, they do things that are foreign to us. One thing that is exasperating for dog owners is the behavior of rolling in dead things (fish along beaches, dead animals in the woods, etc.). Why do dogs love to do this? Do they love it or are they compelled to do it? It has to be a behavior related to genetics and survival in the wild, but yuck! What are other pet behaviors that are interesting and baffling?

Extensions

Just in case we like to think of our own species of humans as being too sophisticated to do such repugnant (weird and disgusting) behaviors, think of the number of times you've seen people picking their noses! How many times have you seen the noses being picked and then people pick up food? How many times have you noticed this behavior, but have not seen it as being remarkable or unusual? If a dog rolling in dead stuff is a genetically related behavior having to do with marking territory, what genetically related drive might nose picking by humans be related to? Did Sigmund Freud have anything to say about this drive? This is not just a crude or uncouth (unacceptable) question. Other human behaviors are very common that nobody in polite conversation would ever bring up. Can you imagine someone asking, "What kind of genetically driven impulse is it that causes anyone to chew his or her fingernails?" Now, a real social deviant is the one who chews their toenails! In the course of one week, note the various forms of odd human behaviors that really might be related to genetically driven instincts.

BENT TOWARD WHAT?

There is a lot in life that happens to us that is not sweet, comforting, caring, sensitive, or thoughtful. People act as they do for many different reasons. Some people are cynical—living with an attitude that the values of others are stupid or worthless, that anyone trying to improve things in life is wasting time, and that any acts of compassion (love) are really gestures (actions) of selfishness. Cynicism is very common in life. Look about you. What are the examples of cynicism that you observe? What are the signs of a person who is cynical?

Some people find it easy to hate others. Observe the examples of hate. There are different causes. Take careful notes on what you have observed. Once you have noticed different kinds of hatred, try to discern what the various categories have in common and how they differ. It is safest for you not to be too closely associated with someone whose life has been consumed with hate. Their toxic energy may well have affected a group of persons around them, and you may not be able to identify who these people are in advance. Hate twists and contorts. It can also destroy and maim (injure). Another thing to be aware of is that once a person's life has been twisted and contorted by hatred, prejudice, or fear, in a sense, they become like a mystery. You can't go inside their heads and figure them out. If the same forces do not consume you, you can't fully understand the one who is consumed. What you can know are some general patterns at play in the lives of people who are ridden with fear, hate, and prejudice.

Observe some persons who are well practiced at the art of lying. Notice what happens to people around them. If the friends want to remain friends with this person, notice how constellations of lies seem to grow and are supported by the group. What happens to persons who start telling the truth? There are so many layers to lies and truth telling. Lies range from outright conscious manipulation of facts for the sake of one's own self-gain to group delusions in which entire groups believe what they say. Entire cultures, societies, and nations can also adapt to and learn to live with huge lies. Sometimes the biggest lies are the most difficult to spot. Find as many examples of different levels of severity of lies and different levels of truth telling. Are there examples of truth telling that are self-serving and damaging to others? Are there examples of truth telling that cause great risks to the one daring to name issues that others pretend do not exist?

One of the greatest mysteries I have ever seen in life is how some people can suffer long-term tragedies or violence and yet eventually grow into contributing, affirming, caring, and loving members of the community. They find a way to heal. These people who have grown back into life don't forget what has happened to them. They learn more about life and live with a deeper wisdom. Oftentimes they become advocates dedicated to teaching others about how we need to change our behaviors and values. Others experience some setback in life and they never recover. The experience remains a primary focus point through which everything else is interpreted and experienced. Sometimes these setbacks are minor compared to the massive tragedies suffered by others who do grow back into life. Observe examples of such healing and brokenness. What could account for this huge difference in response to the challenges of life? We all choose to open ourselves to life in such a manner that either we will move toward healing or we will sink deeper in the muck of our own suffering (that often gets projected onto others). Those who find the ways to be healed become creative and compassionate people; those who become entrapped by their own past imperfect experiences project confusion, complexity, and suffering. What makes the difference? It has to do with the manner in which we incorporate (include) the past in our current lives. It also has to do with our willingness to take further risks required of us if we are to continue in the venture of being alive.

Many people live in circumstances that could be very debilitating (crippling). Some of them live with hope in their hearts. What is it that sustains persons in times of trouble, turmoil, chaos, or loss? Find as many examples as possible of persons or communities that have sustained themselves with hope in greatly challenging circumstances and times.

How is it that some persons live with a basic sense of inner security while others apparently seem to live with an abiding (constant) sense of insecurity? Some people are insecure when all the outer circumstances seem to indicate that they are successful, comfortable, and relatively free from the challenges that others face. Some people exude (give evidence of) an inner sense of security even though the outer circumstances of their lives look as though they are falling apart. Search for examples of such dynamics.

Life's circumstances always affect us and in different ways. Our bent in life is our bias or tendency. We are each unique. Explore these splendid (fascinating) differences and things we hold in common. Who could ever be bored with life? Then again, some people are bored with so many opportunities surrounding them, while others are intrigued by life with few outer exciting opportunities.

Extensions

How does the energy of someone who is cynical, hateful, broken, hopeless, or insecure affect others around him or her? What can we do to cultivate (create) attitudes and values that encourage an affirming outlook on life as well as compassion, healing, hope, and a sense of security?

BETWEEN A BUG AND AN INSECT

What is the difference between a bug and an insect? Are all bugs insects? Are all insects bugs?

Extensions

Which insect is capable of flying to the highest altitude? What is the fastest insect moving on the ground? Which is the fastest flying insect? Are there any underwater insects? If so, which ones go the deepest? What living thing can move through the ground at the fastest rate? Are there any insects that eat dirt? What is the difference (if any) between earth, dirt, and soil?

BIMONTHLY WHAT?

If something occurs bimonthly, how often does it occur? If something is biannual, how often does it occur? If something is biweekly, how often does it occur? How often is something that is semiweekly, semimonthly, or semiannually?

Extensions

The prefixes that precede other words belong to a whole family of prefixes that denote something related to numbers. Figure out other prefixes that refer to numbers.

BIASES—NECESSARY?

What does it mean to have biases? Could we live without biases? Is it bad or good or neither bad nor good to be biased in some manner? How do biases relate to our tendencies to discriminate? (*See* "Discrimination.") Are some biases hurtful to you or others? What are some biases that aren't hurtful to you or others?

Extensions

Is there a way of living in which we could be perfectly neutral on any given topic of concern or life challenge? If we could be neutral, would this be the same as being objective? Are there circumstances in which being neutral or objective would be good, and are there circumstances in which being neutral or objective would cause, extend, or deepen unnecessary suffering?

BIG BANG

Did the big bang take place in space or in time? No! It was an explosion of space-time. When we think of space and time, most of us tend to think of these qualities of the universe as being separate things. Einstein demonstrated conclusively that space and time are one single entity called space-time. When we think about the universe before the big bang, it is very difficult for us to imagine nothing being in the space we call space. In fact, space-time unfolded or emerged as the big bang exploded.

Imagine that if there were a great bang, the matter and energy from which it sprang might have been something like a ball. It must have had some kind of edge. If it were spherical (like a ball), it would have had a diameter (measurement across its width). If it had an edge or surface and a diameter, just beyond the surface would have been a most mysterious kind of space. Can you imagine what it must have been like to be three feet away from the edge of this matter and energy ball? Was there any time before the big bang?

Brain teasers: You've probably heard about black holes in the universe. These black holes are the remnants of old stars that have died and collapsed into themselves. They are also entities at the core of at least some of the galaxies. Physicists tell us that these black holes have such a powerful gravitational pull that they pull in other matter, energy, and even time and space into themselves.

If black holes suck in all the surrounding matter, energy, time, and space, the original matter and energy of the big bang must have been like one giant (or very small and greatly compacted) black hole that affected the entire universe. There would not be any time outside of itself and there would be no space beyond itself. Even though we say these things in order to be consistent, it would still be awesome to view what it looked like. There is no such thing as time before or after the big bang! If there was no space beyond it, into what did it expand when it did explode? Try digesting this idea before breakfast!

Extensions

Might it be possible that the universe is constantly being born from a dimension that is simply not seen from our four-dimensional space-time orientation? Who says that there are only four dimensions (beside almost everybody)? Space as we view it may be infinitely greater than we know right now. In an infinitely small point (called a point of singularity), there might be another infinitely great space. (*See* "Star Count" and "Dimensions—How Many?")

BIG-ANIMAL STORIES

Were there animals in the past that were much smaller or much bigger than their present-day descendants (for example, giant beavers)? Find as many different animals that are still alive today whose ancestors in ancient times were of vastly different size (bigger or smaller).

Extensions

What could account for the difference in sizes of the present-day animals?

BIGGEST SECRET OF ALL TIME

The most obvious thing in life is the least obvious to most people most of the time. Sometimes we encounter:

- a sense of awe
- a different view of normal everyday life
- a sense of rising above the details of life in which we are absorbed almost all of the time
- life in a new manner
- a tremendous sense of beauty that stays with us
- a realm of experience that words cannot describe
- a sense of joy
- a feeling of peace
- a leap of insight and understanding that is revolutionary, revealing, and surprising
- a wisdom that allows us to see things in such a vastly expanded context that we are stunned
- a feeling of being surprised and startled by deep intuition
- an insight in which we can see extraordinary splendor in what is utterly ordinary and common

Who can explain such moments? You may have seen roses hundreds of times in a garden, and then one time you really see a rose and its beauty in depth. It is startling and surprising. You have seen clouds thousands of times. Suddenly, you have an experience out of the ordinary. You see a cloud or set of clouds with astounding clarity. This clarity is not the same as visual acuity (sharpness of image). Clarity has to do with understanding, wisdom, and insight. This clarity has to do with the meaning we ascribe (give to) something. A person with whom you've had many contacts over the course of many years is experienced in a vastly different manner. A recurring (repeating) context is experienced in a vastly different way. A concept, life challenge, or career issue you've struggled to understand suddenly is clearly grasped, just when you were least expecting it. We see ourselves, others, things, and our basic relationships in a new light. The stage of life has been expanded and enriched. Who can explain such things?

It seems that these special experiences related to beauty and wonder open to us because we are receptive and ready. The greatest secret is that we carry this beauty and wonder inside of us all the time. Certain combinations of outer circumstances and inner dynamics occasionally arise that cause us to get in touch with these feelings and insights. We can experience others and ourselves in a radically new light. We can experience our life context in a manner that astonishes us. We can experience the depth of creativity available to each of us. We can experience the beauty of our own genius (our unique combination of gifts, sensitivities, insights, skills, and passions). We possess these treasures. They are our source of creativity, peace, and joy. If you want to be creative, find this place of serenity and beauty within yourself. When you are at peace, your mind and emotions are quiet. You see the world differently. You have the power to be creative. Practice this art. Startling and wonderful experiences will flow from this insight. This source of discovery, new insights, and original questions shakes old assumptions.

How can we stabilize our lives in this place of peaceful creativity? There is no one answer. People experience their own personal gateways into this magic garden in their own manners. Creativity by definition stirs things up. Peace has to do with acceptance of how things truly are. Is the word combination *peaceful creativity* an oxymoron (two words juxtaposed with opposite or contradictory definitions)? If peace has to do with inner calm, integrity, and depth of wisdom, and creativity has to do with fidelity (commitment) to what is true in life, then peace and creativity are necessary twin faces of the same thing—our capacity to be fully alive. "Peaceful creativity" also has to do with the capacity to generate wider life-affirming options for ourselves and others. As we manifest this peace and creativity, we gain greater attentiveness, awareness, and sensitivity through a refined and subtle view of the relation between everything in this more inclusive context. Here are some hints to discover this place and practice the way of "peaceful creativity":

- Take risks.
- Venture beyond what is given by one's group of primary affiliation or culture.
- Process (go) farther on a journey that leads you to your current horizons of understanding.
- Find the courage to look beyond.
- Take the time to actually see what's there over the boundaries you've accepted as being natural and necessary.
- Embrace future possibilities and the wisdom of those who are significantly different from you in some fashion.
- Grasp the significance and intimations of anomalies, the unexpected, the improbable, and the impossible.
- Follow your sense that there are greater associations, relationships, and connections that reveal a more encompassing wisdom.
- Let go of or alter certain prime assumptions.
- Come back to a center point that is home to you.
- Experience creativity within the context of an ever-unfolding and revealing journey.
- Sense the presence of security and well-being in the course of venturing beyond accepted horizons or limits.
- Envision your source of meaning and purpose.
- Express in actions and commitments your deepest meaning and purpose.
- Live in that place of your deepest and truest experiences and wisdom.
- Adapt to those dynamics that are changing and evolving.
- Pursue questions in tenacious (sticking to the task), creative, and original ways.
- Live courageously in finding answers that may not be what you were expecting or desiring.
- Accept the possibility that you might find answers for which others are not ready.
- Question all authority and question all those who find it easy to challenge all authority. (An interesting paradox: certain questioning creatively empowers everyone to grow beyond the confines of current ways and structures while other questioning can be for self-centered and self-serving ends that only implant seeds of confusion while preventing encounters that could clarify issues.)
- Listen carefully to those with whom you disagree.
- Reexamine what most others have accepted as natural, necessary, logical, reasonable, valid, sound, and unassailable (unquestionable).
- Consider that you need to start all over on some project, even when you've invested a massive amount of time, energy, and resources.

- Stay on the same course for different reasons than those that initially impelled you on this course.
- Choose a radically different course if this is what life reveals to you.
- Seek a broader context that yields serenity (inner peace) and wisdom, which results in greater stability and wholeness.
- Let go of or work through your hurt, anger, pain, hate, and righteous indignation related to some past traumas and dramas.
- Resist cynicism (a negative assessment of our human capacity to live toward a greater good).
- Distinguish between the discomfort of being temporarily nowhere (because you are in between some sets of understandings) and the anguish of feeling caught or stuck in a place that does not offer you life.
- Act with courage if you are temporarily in an in-between place as part of your growth and learning.
- Act with courage to ask for help from loved ones if you ever find yourself truly trapped in a place or way of living that is detrimental (harmful).
- Choose to honor the gift that you have a right to not merely survive in life, but that you have a right to thrive in life.
- Resist hate and violence in any of their forms.
- Learn continually how the effects of our behaviors and values may be causing violence to others.
- Resist losing courage.
- Resist security derived from simply following sentiments popular with entire groups, communities, and societies.
- Awaken from illusion (socially reinforced appearances of things as being true that are actually false or things that appear as good that are detrimental [bad]).
- Awaken from delusion (personal internal mental twists and contortions of what we desire to be true, but at some deeper level we know or are capable of realizing that are not true).
- Embrace a larger comprehension of life and the universe that reveals to us the source of compassion, awe, and wonder.
- Seek justice for all living beings (including life-forms that are not human) as an integral (vital) aspect of compassion, awe, and wonder.
- Find a supportive and nurturing community.
- Give yourself generously and consistently to the needs of others without forgetting your own fundamental needs.
- Trust the way "peaceful creativity" will transform your attachments and aversions.
- Cultivate a guiding faith that people and communities are able to rise toward what is best within them.
- Identify with and act out of the faith that gives you life.
- Practice compassion in all things at all times without exceptions.

These are some hints related to the source of "peaceful creativity." Take any one of these points and try living that way for five minutes. Then reflect on what you have learned. Amazing things can occur in and through our lives because of this kind of practice.

Extensions

What provides this wisdom, courage, strength, vision, and awareness is a matter of faith. Your faith matters. There are many kinds of faith in this world. Faith is that quality of life so fundamental that no one can define it for others in its specifics. Generally, it is that quality of our lives that empowers us to go on in life in spite of the turn of outward events and contexts. Our faith is what abides with us. Ultimately, creativity and genius are intimately related to our faith. Our very capacity to affirm the goodness of life and our ability to persevere (go on) in life is deeply related to our faith. You are the only person on Earth who can answer what is faith for you. Matters of faith deal with what is ultimately true. Your faith matters. Others around you have tremendous wisdom related to this topic. Only you can find the answer in the deepest place of your heart using your highest intelligence, creativity, and genius. Your faith ultimately directs how you interpret the past, who you are in the present, who you will become in the future, and what you will contribute to life.

BIG WORDS

One large word is antidisestablishmentarianism. What is the root word? If you don't know the terms *prefix* and *suffix*, look them up right away. How many prefixes and suffixes does antidisestablishmentarianism contain? Try to figure out the meaning of the word. Hint: it is a popular word because it is so long and so odd. It is archaic (not used in regular communication any longer or of historical significance only).

Hint: if you can't find the word in your dictionary, one strategy (means of solving a problem) is to find the root of the long word in a dictionary. The root may have several meanings. Thus, when you are dealing with roots of words, you are dealing with a complex issue from the very beginning. The root for the term *antidisestablishmentarianism* would be *establishment* or *establish*. Look it up and see how far you get. Try an encyclopedia if the dictionary doesn't work. You might define the meaning of the prefixes and suffixes. Put them all together; what are the possible definitions of antidisestablishmentarianism? Why did anybody ever use such a long word? Couldn't some shorter and simpler word convey the same idea? This particular long word has a historical context from which its meaning arises. Another possible way to derive the meaning of some complex words is to locate a dictionary with a section for Indo-European Roots. This will give you much more detailed information on the history of the particular word. One such dictionary is the *American Heritage Dictionary* (third edition). What are other words with a great number of prefixes and suffixes?

Extensions

The process described in the preceding paragraph is a specific form of a more general problem-solving process that can be described as follows: Observe a complex phenomena. Ascertain (determine) the core or multiple interacting cores (centers, bases, initiating forces, primary causes) of the process. Is there an initial primary cause that precedes all other dynamics (factors or variables)? If there is one primary cause, everything else is secondary. Now go on to define the secondary or subsequent dynamics of the situation.

Might there be many initiating causes that subsequently interact with each other? Might there be some situations or processes that have innumerable (too many to count) initiating causes? What would be an example of such a process? One example: Why is one cloud scudding (moving) across the sky in a particular direction and at a specific speed at this time? In this example, what are some of the initiating causes? List as many complex processes as you can think of. (Many researchers have used supercomputers to construct models for such complex phenomena.)

BLIND LIFE

How many years has life existed? When we talk about life, we are describing organisms that reproduce and require energy to survive. Your answer will be an approximation because we aren't exactly sure when the first single-celled creature emerged on Earth. What proportion of the time that living organisms have existed have these organisms had the sense of sight? Were there more primitve forms of what we now call "eyes"? When did eyes come into existence? Did other senses make up for the lack of visual perception? Can we know what we are missing if nobody tells us we are missing it or if we have never experienced such a thing before? Can we sense the possibility of a more inclusive context in which we could face our life challenges even though we can't specifically name or know the nature of what is currently absent?

Extensions

Might there be other senses that we are evolving right now? Might some people already manifest some of the early precursors (initial or not yet fully developed) of these emergent senses? These would be unusual gifts that are statistically aberrant (rare). Might it be possible to have the gift of such a sense, but since we as individuals or we as cultures are not ready to expect the emergence of this gift, therefore we fail to see it? There are many things manifesting themselves in our presence that we fail to appreciate, see, or experience. Once these new senses are developed, will we be able to experience our world in a more complete fashion? What might these senses be? Might they be totally new senses, or might they be enhancements of our existing senses (like being able to smell food ten miles away or seeing a much broader spectrum of light than right now)?

Are there some senses, skills, talents, or abilities that we could be losing (devolving) at this time? Is it possible that cavemen and cavewomen were able to smell cooking meat or the presence of tofu twenty-five miles away?

BLUE MOON

The usual definition of a blue moon is a full moon occurring twice in one month. I once heard someone contend (assert) that a blue moon occurs when there are two months in one season each having two full moons. Find the cultural and scientific reasons why people for hundreds of years have been using the phrase "blue moon."

Extensions

Find some of the songs that include the term *blue moon*. What do you suppose are the themes of most of these songs?

BODY MOTION

When a body of any kind is moving, determine whether it is moving because of forces being exerted on it from outside or moving because of its own internal forces (or a combination of the two). Try taking a small carton and filling it less than half full. Jiggle it around in a circular motion. Let it go on a wet smooth countertop. What do you observe? Does it look as though it is moving around because of its own internal energy?

Extensions

What are some other examples of things moving inexplicably that defy our understanding? Could there be internal chemical reactions? Could there be an interplay (interaction, exchange) between forces from outside of the object acting or interacting with things going on inside of the object? Some people have portrayed themselves as possessing the power to bend spoons with nothing but their thought. Might this be the first sign of our emergent evolutionary power? Imagine an entire race being able to bend spoons. Now try to envision the next step beyond spoon bending. Might this spoon bending be entirely rooted in prestidigitation (deliberate deception using misleading visual cues)?

BONNIE AND CLYDE EFFECT

The first time I ever experienced an entire group wanting somebody to be hurt occurred while I was watching an old movie entitled *Bonnie and Clyde*. These two were bank robbers during the Great Depression in the 1930s. They also killed many innocent persons. They weren't world-class, real nice people. The story was woven in such a manner that by the end of the movie when Bonnie and Clyde are shot in slow motion the audience was cheering. For an instant, I felt great that these horribly bad people were getting their own (receiving what is just and fair). I didn't cheer, but there was a relief. There was resolution to the inner tension created by the story. Then the crowd reaction horrified me. The identical thing happened in an early section of the movie *Patriot*. Set during the Revolutionary War, the British redcoats had just taken the movie star's son hostage. In a subsequent (later) scene, the father and his other sons attacked the group holding his son hostage. When one of the British soldiers was killed with a hatchet (hand ax) to his forehead, cheering and clapping spontaneously broke out all over the movie theater on that dark stormy night. This kind of reaction from the crowd makes me pause and realize that the storytellers manipulate us in many ways. Contexts with an emotional charge do in fact affect our point of view.

How is it that people can shout with joy when a member of "their" team smashes another player from the other team? How is it that people can feel good when others are being hurt? The Bonnie and Clyde effect has something to do with it. Once we have made another person into an object of derision (hate), we can manipulate that object in any manner that we wish. We want the power of the story to make us feel better. We want the story to relieve us of the burden of injustices. We want the story to give us quick, painless, and unambiguous (clearly understood) resolution to all problems. Have you ever been affected by the Bonnie and Clyde effect?

Extensions

The power of stories is tremendous. Think of some stories that have stirred up powerful emotions for you. These stories can be presented in the form of talks, speeches, movies, soundtracks, plays, musicals, physical enactments without words, art pieces, and graffiti. Try to learn as much as you can about the elements of persuasion. Sometimes we are being persuaded without being consciously aware of the process at play. This is called subliminal stimulation. The good news is that we always have the capacity to reflect on what we are experiencing. There is a rich and productive interplay between our feelings and thoughts. We are powerful and creative beyond our wildest dreams. This power and creativity can be used for the welfare of all people or it can be used for selfish and destructive ends. We need to be careful what kinds of stories and influences we project that in fact do affect others. We need to be mindful what kinds of stories, cultural influences, and peer group pressures are being exerted upon us.

BOREDOM?

I can understand how somebody could be angry, sad, upset, happy, lonely, loved, or pleased. How can somebody be bored with living when there is so much in life to be fascinated about? With so much in life to learn, how could anybody be bored? Is the appearance of boredom a socially reinforced thing that certain people find cool?

Extensions

There is a life impulse and a passion for living within each of us. Sometimes, in some people, this passion for living becomes diminished. What might account for this diminishment? What is hope? Define it for yourself in your terms. What is it like to feel totally alive and enthusiastic about living in the present moment? Have you ever awakened to a beautiful day and you feel inside that it is more than just a beautiful day—that something inside is excited and joyful? Describe this feeling.

BOSE-EINSTEIN CONDENSATE

Condensation is a process of joining atoms and molecules together in a more dense, transformed material. For instance, gas can condense into a liquid.

Recently, some scientists from the University of Colorado-Boulder created what had previously been theorized to be a possible state of matter called the Bose-Einstein condensate. Now we have a new state of matter in addition to solids, liquids, gases, and plasmas. Plasmas are high-temperature states of matter created in different ways for different scientific purposes. How will this new state of matter be used? Keep your eyes out for this phenomenon. Look it up and do some research on the topic. You might get some very surprising results. Where would you find resources for such important unfolding knowledge? Do you have access to the Internet? Try it. If someone says that there are only three states of matter, you know better.

Extensions

It is a gift to be able to analyze a new discovery. For instance, did atomic scientists know how the atomic bomb would affect human life? Did people have any idea of the impact on human life when they discovered the human genetic code, fire, or the wheel? Try to randomly list the top ten or fifteen discoveries or inventions that have most deeply affected the lives of the most number of people. Take three or four discoveries or inventions and try to trace as many of the effects as possible. You could also do this with very positive and very negative actions of individuals or groups. One way to do this is to trace lines with interconnected circles (called nodes) connecting one cause with one effect. Start out with some relatively simple process like learning how to brush your teeth. Then proceed on to increasingly more complex processes like the election of a liberal versus a conservative president, the declaration of a war, or the discovery of gasoline. Then try to imagine certain processes like people learning how to live peacefully on Earth, people learning how to share resources, people learning how to live in an ecologically sound manner so as not to destroy the Earth. What would be the effects of these processes?

Starting at one point, trace the effects of any of these processes. Draw a line toward the right, up, down, or left, and then mark its end with an effect of some discovery or change. For instance, we might start with the discovery of toothpaste. From the encircled word *toothpaste* draw a line and encircle the words *fewer cavities*. Anything that is a direct result of toothpaste would have a line drawn directly back to the encircled word *toothpaste*. Then there are effects stemming from *fewer cavities*. This is a form of imaging or graphing. Try to imagine another way of tracing these processes. There are many different ways. One way to graph or illustrate the effects of some significant change is to use more than two dimensions. When you are tracing on a flat sheet, you are using only two dimensions (width and length). Now try to imagine how to use three dimensions.

Create a mobile (with effects stemming from the preceding root cause). Identify five basic effects of the invention of the wheel. Each of these five effects would have a string going down to whatever is the effect. Pick some object to represent the effect. Attach a stick to the end of each of the five strings horizontally. Now, from each of these five effects, identify two or more effects that you can hang on the stick that is attached to the end of the string from one of the first effects. Now all of the original five strings have sticks hanging horizontally on their ends, each of which has two or more strings hanging down. The relative importance of the effect can be represented by the object's size. On each object, place a descriptive label. Good luck trying to balance all the effects in this mobile.

Another way of representing causes and effects would be to tie strings in an entire room connected to little boxes that each represents some cause or effect. Do your entire room. Do your parent's bedroom. Do your children's rooms while they are away. Do it together as a party challenge. Everybody will be glad you got this book.

Another three-dimensional way of graphing or illustrating the effects of some discovery or change is to use a technique I saw used in an underground mine exhibit. There were many layers of tunnels in the mine. Each layer was etched onto a piece of large glass. The layers of glass were placed on top of each other in a large case (about a half-inch separated each layer). As one looks at the case from the side, or straight down from the top, one can see the interconnection of all the layers. Practically and cheaply, how could this be reproduced? Don't use glass (it's too brittle and dangerous). Plastic would work almost as well. Each of the layers could represent a different effect of some change. Each layer could represent a period of time. Each layer could represent a phase (aspect) of some complex process.

One way to graph variables might be to trace various levels of the process you are graphing on pieces of paper. One layer or piece of the process could be assigned to one sheet of paper. After every sheet has been traced (remember to start out very simply), get clear acetate sheets from a business supply store and use a photocopier to copy each of the sheets of paper. Use some transparent spacer blocks to connect and separate each of the acetate sheets. See if there is any way to project these images onto a screen. By focusing on different depths, is there a way to emphasize one layer at a time? Is there a way to show them all at once? You might be able to take a picture of the project and focus on various levels by adjusting the focus on the lens of your camera.

There are some effects of a discovery or effects of a process that can be quantified. When this is the case, then graphing becomes possible. With two variables, you can graph two dimensions of an issue. Call the variables x and y. Learn how to graph two variables. If you were driving a car on a flat surface at a certain rate of speed, what would be the effect of speeding up to twice the speed on fuel consumption? One variable would be speed and another variable would be fuel consumption.

Now learn to graph three variables (x, y, and z). Trace the effect of the speed of the car, the speed at which the engine's pistons are turning over, and fuel consumption. An entire large room can be laid out with three strings, with each string representing one variable (x or y or z). Then you can map the locations of various effects of primary causes with numbers. The distances could represent time, space, magnitude of impact or importance, or any other quantifiable aspect of the process being described.

Experiment with your own ideas of how to graphically display the relation between various factors.

BRUSH THAT TONGUE

People have been told to "hold your tongue." It has to do with being circumspect (careful) with what you say to others. Try to figure out why anyone would want to brush the tongue. Hint: after you've eaten spicy or any kind of food that may give you bad breath, you may want to practice this art of tongue brushing. Don't do it with your dog's hairbrush. Use your toothbrush. Be forewarned—if you get back too far on the backside of the tongue, you may induce (start up) the gag reflex (initiating a regurgitating reaction that can lead to vomiting). Only brush the front part of the tongue. After eating some smelly food like Limburger cheese, try this tongue-cleaning tactic. If you could totally clean your mouth, would this ensure that you would have great fresh breath? Why or why not? What are the sources of bad breath? Is bad breath only caused by food?

Extensions

Find different reflexes of our human bodies. List them. There are some rather interesting reflexes. Try to find the "basal mammalian reflex." It was discovered in a most interesting fashion.

CADILLAC'S VISION

Cadillac has a system for enhancing the view of the driver in dark and dim light circumstances. It uses infrared technology to project the image of the space in front of you in the dark. This system allows you to see more clearly what is beyond the illumined area of your headlights. Find out how this system works.

Extensions

What would happen if you activated this system in broad daylight or if you activated it for an area right beyond the illuminated area of your headlights and suddenly this area was filled with light from floodlights (say from a baseball stadium)? What would appear on the projection area? What would happen to your eyeballs—if anything? What would it be like if you had a large field that many animals visited at night and you had a large bay window overlooking this field? Now imagine hooking up this same system so that the images of what was out there in the dark were projected onto a glass window. Would this be rather nice entertainment in the evening?

CAN I SEE THAT PICTURE?

There are certain things I'd love to see pictured:

- the inside of a functional heart
- the look on somebody's face when they first see their newborn child
- the stuff from which the big bang exploded one second before the explosion
- the bottom of the deepest trench in the ocean
- the inside of the deepest cave in the bottom of the ocean
- the real first human being
- the view from the inside of a leaf viewed outwards

What are the pictures you'd like to see? Which ones would you like to have in your room?

Extensions

What are other media formats that would be enjoyable to have available? What about time-lapse photomicrographs, holographic imagery, regular movies or videos, or infrared formats? Name as many formats for visual and/or audio presentation that you can think of. Now with an extensive list, try to imagine what unusual things you'd like to view. Don't forget shots from the Hubble space telescope.

Try to imagine seeing a photograph of the Earth. It is an average-resolution (sharpness or clarity) photograph, and it is about two feet high and wide. Right in front of your eyes, the resolution begins to improve significantly every five seconds. You are amazed at what is occurring. Eventually, you are able to see individual animals and humans. Then you can clearly read what kind of insignia and emblems are on the clothing of the people. Soon you're able to see ants and spiderwebs. You even get to see a dewdrop on a spider web! Then you blink your eyes for a second and the photograph reverts (returns) to its original resolution. In this imaginary scenario (story), in order to see this level of detail:

- What kind of lenses would need to be employed?
- How large would the photograph need to be?
- How close to the Earth would the camera have to be held?
- How close to the photograph would you have to be?

Imagine that you could have any kind of camera, at any cost, with any computer, any printing equipment, and any means of displaying this photograph. How would you go about meeting the challenge of creating the image with tremendous resolution? Instead of using a standard photograph, you would also have the option of using any kind of laser, holographic, or projection technology. Don't limit yourself to what is currently available. Lay down your requirements for what you need and you will instantly have these resources presented to you (this is because you have all the world's research labs at your service and calling). An aside: What would happen if you turned the Hubble telescope toward Earth and started to snap pictures? You better look up something about the limitations of the minimal focal length of a particular lens. Remember that since you are the boss of this idea, you can move the Hubble telescope out to any distance you want it to be, relative to the Earth. What would happen if you focused the Chandra x-ray telescope on the Earth? What kind of graphics would we get? Might we get a whole bunch of little x-ray shots from every hospital and dentist's and doctor's office?

CAN'T DO IT

Two thousand years ago, people thought that we'd never be able to fly to the moon. Airplanes hadn't been invented by that time, so it was an impossible notion (an imagined fiction) to think of flying through the air. To think about flying to the moon required a double leap of imagination: one, flying in the Earth's atmosphere; two, flying into outer space. Now we can "fly" to the moon and beyond. What are other things that people in the past believed were impossible? What are some equivalent kinds of things that people today think are impossible that might be possible in the future? What are some of these "impossible things" that require one, two, three, and more leaps of imagination? Is this a natural (expected because we're familiar with something) way of thinking? If so, why isn't it more common? If you answered no, why not? Some of the most interesting stuff in life emerges from unexpected realms.

Extensions

Look up persons throughout history who have had insights and ingenious leaps of imagination and intellect related to things that eventually did become possible. These people leap beyond the current understandings and conventions of the time. These people mystify most folks. This is not just a matter of intelligence alone. Don't stop with technological things. Who are people who understand that the way we create our cultures and social institutions can be different? Look up Leonardo da Vinci, Sojourner Truth, and Jules Verne.

CARS THAT ARE NOT JUST CARS

Look around at the variety of cars. We expect that cars are not just cars for us. They become symbols of other things. For some people, they are symbols of power, success, mobility, freedom, superiority, fashion statements, lifestyles, who we are as human beings, or class. When is a car not just a car? When is a car only a car? What have you noticed about the way people talk about cars or about their behavior as they are driving cars?

Extensions

What are other things that become symbols of importance to us? How do we relate to other people on a similar basis—making symbols out of them rather than seeing them for who they really are? Try to think of the ways in which we use things to represent or symbolize something we wish that others would see. How many people buy jeans that cost great sums of money because they have a little tag on them from some currently hot "designer" company? The jeans are practically all the same quality. The tags vary. Symbols are important. What are the ways that you need to have others interpret who you are based on the symbolic things you own or project as being part of your identity?

CARS AND GREEN LIGHTS

Have you noticed how long it takes for an entire line of cars to start moving after the light has turned green? Try timing this process. Compare the length of time necessary to get two cars moving, then four, eight, and sixteen. As the number of cars doubles, does the time double? What is the difference between arithmetic and exponential growth?

Extensions

Might there be a way to have all the cars waiting at a red light to proceed at the same time when the green light comes on? What would this do to the time necessary to get an entire row of cars moving? Imagine the consequences of this change for a large city like New York City. Would this be more efficient?

What are some other behaviors you observe that could be changed? Notice how we organize gathering places such as lunchrooms, classrooms, worksites and playgrounds, as well as recess times, places of worship, the hours for school, and the pattern of having two days that we call weekends. In your imagination, can you alter the patterns a little or a lot? See what happens when you make these changes in your head. Take one, two, three or more leaps of imagination in transposing (changing) an environment. Alter one or more variables and see what happens to the situation or circumstances. Often when you change one factor, the entire system changes significantly.

Practice the art of having many ingenious ideas in your head. Some of them may make a real difference in the world. All of them add richness to your life. Before breakfast everyday, ingest, dwell upon, create, remember, or conjure up at least one ingenious idea. See what happens to your life.

CELLS OF THE BODY—ALIVE AND THINKING

One of the bases for biological life is the cell. Plants, animals, and other forms of life that are microscopic (very small) all have cells as the basis for life. A cell is a living unit of life.

How many different kinds of cells are there in the human body? Look up and learn about some of the wonderful cells we have in our bodies. Some of the cells of the heart can control how often the heart beats. Some of the cells of the brain help with memory. Might there be some cells that are not located in the brain that assist in memory? Some cells create new life. Some cells fight disease organisms. All of them consume energy and create heat as a by-product (an effect of living). Can you imagine a cell that absorbs heat only? Imagine a cell that metabolizes energy in such a manner that there is no heat loss. Imagine a cell that does not require the excretion of metabolic by-products (stuff left over from ingesting and transforming sources of energy).

Imagine a cell that does not require water. Must all cells be microscopic? Could some of them (or have some of them) been large enough for us to see with the naked eye?

One of the more curious questions about cells is, if they are all alive, are they something like an independent living organism? How is it that any and all of these semi-independent organisms coordinate and communicate their many needs and functions? What allows them to act in synchrony (harmony)? Imagine if they were all running off in different directions trying to get everything they could for themselves. The entire bodily process would then collapse. We would soon die. Is there any nonmental process at play that coordinates, reorganizes, reorients, and thinks about emergent needs of the body's system as a whole? Think about the massive amount of information processing that is taking place every second of your life of which you are not consciously aware. What would it be like if you were consciously aware of all these processes all the time? It might be rather interesting to listen in to cells communicating with each other. Imagine what they say whenever we eat junk food.

When you are investigating any complex phenomena, create models or pictures to aid in your understanding of the process. In addition, another tool that you have available to you is to draw parallels (make comparisons of similar things in the same system). In this instance, you might use your imagination to look at other processes where there are cells living in synchrony meeting the mutual (shared) needs of the larger community of life.

Where we observe this mutual interchange (sharing) of life, we can assume that there is some kind of coordination and communication at play. If we expand our thinking and envisioning (seeing) wide enough, we can see that all life is interdependent (sharing a mutual relationship for common needs). The cells of the human body (or any other animal or plant) are not unique in the fact that there needs to be some form of coordination and communication between the cells.

Extensions

Another tool of comprehension (understanding) that can be used in exploring large questions is to take a close look at a piece of the puzzle. How does a single cell communicate the fact that it is deficient (in need) of the energy, water, or chemicals needed for transforming energy? Another way of saying this is that the cell is hungry. How is it that if a cell is being attacked by a disease organism it can communicate the need for special cells to come and eliminate this attacking organism? The focus has been on cells living in synchrony. Examine a beehive, ant home, or termite nest. These individuals live in synchrony with other individuals, each doing a specific job that contributes to the life of the whole colony. How do they communicate?

CHEMICALS ARE OUR FRIENDS?

Our bodies are made of different chemicals—so, of course, chemicals are our friends. How many naturally occurring chemical elements are there? From this base of chemicals, locate some resources that tell you how many synthetic (human-created) chemical compounds there are. Every year, we are developing more of these compounds. How many of them are being recycled through our bodies (put out into the environment and then absorbed into our bodies)? What are the various means by which chemical compounds get into our bodies? How are these chemicals being recycled through the environment of the Earth? Are they being broken down into their relatively harmless natural state? Do we have the technology to neutralize dangerous chemical compounds and return our leftovers back to nature in a benign (safe) manner? Do we have the technology to create certain compounds that get distributed out into the environments (and into our bodies and the bodies of other living organisms) but we fail in knowing what to do with them once they're out there in the environment? If this is so, what can we do about the situation?

What is creating the demand for so many new chemicals? Who is responsible? What could happen to the Earth and all life on it if our demands for technology don't change? Shouldn't there be some kind of social controls on what kinds of chemicals are produced and distributed? Do you agree with this proposition? If so, what kinds of controls do you think would benefit life and the Earth?

Should the needs of business and the economy take precedent (priority) over the environment? Ought environmental concerns take precedent over the needs and concerns of business and the economy? Is this a less-than-useful way to configure (set up) the question? Is it possible to frame the questions of what chemicals are produced, distributed, and used on the basis of ecological sustainability and the larger good of the society, which is dependent upon all other life of the entire world? While viewing business as an integral (unified) part of the way we choose to conduct life in common, can we make a more direct connection between economic viability and ecological sustainability? If this becomes the norm (the normal thing), all of us would have to examine our lifestyles and be responsible for what we consume. We would have to redefine how we value money. We would have to redefine what it is that we really need to live well. We would have to reexamine what it means to live in community. All this, just from the topic of chemicals? Yes, look at the backside of a bottle of almost any household good (stuff) and see how many different chemicals you have in your home. Try to list the number of chemicals that are contained in the things in your single home. Are there any chemicals in your home that are completely environmentally benign (nontoxic)?

Extensions

Are human beings a natural part of the ecology of the Earth? If so, then are the products of those things we create also natural? Does it make any sense when people say that we ought to try to get back to nature? Aren't we natural also? Do we have the power to alter nature so much with our synthetic chemical compounds and our other technological inventions and creations that nature will eventually be recast or reinvented as a thing of our own making? If so, what are the ramifications of this possibility? There is the phrase, "Don't mess with Mother Nature." What does this mean to you?

CHESS—COMBINATIONS

How many different combinations of moves are possible in chess? How could you begin to figure out the answer?

The general plan would be make one move, like moving your king's pawn forward one space. Then you would have to figure out all the other combinations of moves possible. This is an extremely complicated problem. When you are faced with a complex challenge, one way to approach the issues is to imagine a much simpler version of a similar pattern. Start on the simple side so that you realize from the beginning some of the core challenges you are facing.

For instance, assume that you had four squares across and four squares forward. Pretend further that it is a game like checkers. If you move one single piece, what are the other possible combinations of moves possible? You may want to talk to somebody who has studied the mathematics of combinations and permutations.

Another way of approaching a very complex challenge is to learn as much about it as possible in the present and then wait until further resources become available to you (like taking a class in which you study the mathematics of combinations and permutations). You may enjoy starting on the challenge of the number of combinations in chess. See the complexity and leave it at that—an appreciation for the complexity. This is a perfectly fine goal. For one thing, the next time a newspaper article appears describing a superstar chess player taking on the latest supercomputer chess program, you will appreciate the greatness of the challenge from both the computer programmer's perspective and the view of the human player. You will have a deeper appreciation for the interplay of logic and intuition.

Now back to the issue of chess combinations. When things get complicated, draw a picture. Each picture of a complex process becomes an available frame of reference for you. Given different sets of very complex challenges, your intuitions can guide you as to which picture or frame of reference is applicable. Recognition of emergent patterns is extremely important when dealing with complex evolving systems.

Using formal chess notation for moves or using graphical pictures of each piece, represent on sheet one the pieces in their original position. On sheet two, represent one single move. How many different combinations of moves are legal and possible in the opponent's response? The first move and first response are generation one. Now white takes another move. How many combinations of moves are possible for black in generation two? For every move that you make, you commit yourself to certain consequences. Instantly, the possible number of combinations is huge. How many generations of moves do you think you could graphically portray in this method? Try to imagine as many different methods to solve the problem as possible. Keep yourself happy and be satisfied with portraying one or two generations of moves.

The number of combinations is astounding. Try estimating in advance how many combinations you think there will be. This is called getting the right order of magnitude (inside the right universe of scale, inside the right baseball field, getting to an approximation that is kind of close). You are interested in getting the approximate right number of zeroes. Once you have made your best estimate, then go ahead and consult resources until you find the answer.

Is it possible that the particular moves that generate the greatest number of possible combinations in subsequent generations of moves also are the precise moves that are most effective and efficient? Learn the difference between being efficient and effective relative to working toward a particular goal. Another way of asking this same question is: What are the moves that allow you to occupy and control the most strategic positions on the board in the least number of moves?

This question related to the number of combinations in a game of chess is so big a challenge that you should limit yourself to a certain period of time. Then go to some experts to help you. Remember, when you consult with others, don't just seek "the answer." Study the many and varied methods by which answers are derived (figured out). Seek some information about how popular computer games work. Then try to get information on how supercomputers play chess. How are humans doing against computers? Are there computer programs available for the public that can calculate all the possible chess combinations?

If the combinations are so numerous and so complex, how can chess masters plan their games? Hint: it has to do with the rich interplay between intuition, experience, logic, and comprehension to the basic dynamics of the game.

Extensions

Are there other questions that you wonder about that are really too complex for you? Find somebody who is willing to help you develop simpler models that you can work on. Always avoid the temptation of simply getting an answer. You may observe an interesting thing happening. Talk to certain persons who are experts (or at least people who know more about a certain topic than you do) who have a gift for helping others gain insights on methods for deriving (getting) answers. Many teachers and other knowledgeable persons in different fields respond very positively to those few persons who are really seeking ways to solve problems rather than just getting an answer. The answers vary (differ) based on your assumptions used in your way of getting a solution. Bright, curious, and secure people really enjoy the persons who are willing to learn about creative options (alternatives) and who are willing to challenge basic and prior methods, assumptions, or beginning points for asking the framing (original) question. Find these people and you have found people worth more than gold. They (and you) are the pot of gold at the end of the rainbow.

What can start to happen in your life is that more persons respond to your curiosity in a positive way. You'll get more and more people wanting to assist you in your personal growth. Dare to be different. Look carefully at how any question is framed (worded), assumptions being made, the potential alternative methods, and the final outcome or answer. Challenge results! Not everybody—but some persons—will start to care for your growth. The brightest, most curious, and most secure persons will respond to you. Someone who is insecure may actually get upset with such questions. We all need friends of many different kinds. These kinds of friends can be like guides into new territory. Another little key for cultivating these kinds of friendships is to show persistent (regular) gratitude (appreciation) for what others do for you. The greatest gratitude is to pass on to others what others have done for you. This is the greatest compliment to a great teacher (passing on their wisdom and creativity).

CHESS MOVES

Do you think it would be possible to play a real game of chess against yourself? One move you play white. The next move you play black. Could you outplay yourself? Each time you'd switch sides, you'd try to figure out the strategy of the other side and play with all your willpower to beat the other "side." What you plan for one side would become what you suspect the same side would be doing when you switch sides and think about the possibilities for the other side. In the fine art of debating, the ones who are the very best are the individuals who can know the inside strategies of the opponents and who know how to exploit (take advantage of) this insight.

Learning how to play chess against yourself can come in handy if you plan to be involved in debating at any level. There are many benefits to you if you can sense the options and likely responses of others. The most important thing is not to learn to play chess against yourself (that could get rather lonely after awhile), but it can be helpful and useful to you if you can fluidly (easily) switch from one frame of reference to another.

Think of as many ways as possible to play with the possibilities of switching your frames of reference without losing sight of your identity. Too many people play different roles and then forget where their true self is. Not all people think alike, not all people hold similar values and sentiments, not all information systems neatly interlink (connect) with other information systems, and not all frames of reference fit coherently, logically, and easily together. Those who are able to switch their frames of reference easily, effectively, and efficiently in our age of closely woven and often contradictory communities, cultures, groups, and disciplines will be those with a form of intelligence and wisdom that will be of benefit to everybody.

Extensions

How easy or how difficult is it to change our frames of reference? Is it rather demanding and startling to see things from a very different point of view? You've been raised to believe that all people of a certain kind are bad. Then you meet one of them who is really good! How demanding would this be? Try a very practical experiment with yourself. Select some issue for which you have feeling, passion, values, and ideas. Take another view. See what it does to your feelings, passions, values, and ideas. Now take an issue that your nation has taken a very strong stand on. View it from another's perspective. See what happens to you. This is not forgetting your source of identity. It is not denying your upbringing. It is simply a way to see through the eyes and heart of somebody else or through the experience of another group. We desperately need people with this skill who can assist others in cultivating (encouraging) it.

CHICKEN AND THE EGG QUESTION

Which came first, the chicken or the egg? The manner in which questions are asked is of great importance because it sets the boundaries for which answers are possible. Those who choose to respond to a question will be more equipped to wisely respond if they are aware that they do not need to limit their response to the boundaries set by the question. Also, those who respond have a vastly greater array of options if they realize that they do not need to answer the question directly, but that they are able to reframe the question and respond in creative manners. Therefore, what you need to do is exercise your intelligence by applying your imagination to alter the basic logic underlying all questions. Expand and alter the basis upon which questions can be answered.

The presenting (apparent or surface) question is, "Which came first, the chicken or the egg?" With this question, look at the knowledge given to us by science related to evolution. The underlying question has to do with which came first, birds or reptiles and amphibians. Both reptiles and amphibians laid eggs outside there bodies that later hatched with babies. Therefore, the answer to the question about which came first, the chicken or the egg, can be altered and then the original question can have an answer! The answer becomes the egg came first because all birds evolved from reptiles and reptiles laid eggs before birds. Probably you've never heard that one before. It's simply an example of an original way of creatively dealing with a question that appears to be trapping you.

Extensions

We can take any question and reformat it so that other answers are possible. Whenever you feel caught between a rock and hard place in terms of not being able to answer a question, reformat the question. Put it into another context. Expand your horizons and then see the magic of other possible answers unfold right before you.

There are many questions of the chicken and egg form that cause us to presume that there is no answer because everybody knows there is no answer. What are some other questions or riddles that have this same form? Can you reformat them so that there actually might be an answer?

CILIA—BREAKING THE LAWS OF GRAVITY?

Cilia are tiny hairlike structures inside our bodies that move in harmony with each other. Some of these cilia move substances upward, against gravity. How could they be waving things upward? How do they know to do this? What would be the effect if we suddenly didn't have cilia? How could we ever have evolved with cilia? Could we have evolved without cilia?

Extensions

Do these hairlike structures ever need to be trimmed? Do they grow like the hair on the outside of our bodies? Have you ever closely examined the hairs on your body? Which one is your favorite one? Do you have any that really upset you?

CIRCADIAN RHYTHMS

There are many kinds of cycles in nature. Some last for a brief moment, like the flash of a camera. Some cycles in nature last for very long periods of time, like the expansion of the universe. Biological cycles affect our bodies in many ways. The most obvious cycles we all share in common are our breathing, the beating of the heart, the need for sleep, and the cycles related to our eating habits. There is the cycle of being born once and dying once. We are biological beings whose bodies are controlled by many rhythms and cycles within other rhythms and cycles. Look up circadian rhythms.

Extensions

List your various life cycles: birth, childhood, school years, etc. Think of as many cycles of your life as possible.

CLOUDS

What is it that makes clouds float? It sure isn't gravity. Are they defying gravity? How much does a cloud weigh?

Extensions

How do ships float or how does a leaf float in water? Define displacement. Do clouds float in the air and ships float in water because of the same principles? Under what conditions do ships not float in the water? Once you have learned about displacement, imagine the conditions under which a ship could float in the air. Who is the children's author who wrote about sailboats floating in the air?

COLOR OF LEAVES

What makes leaves turn various colors for the entire spring and summer? What causes them to turn other colors in the fall? Do the leaves of the same tree always turn the exact same shades every season?

Extensions

Do the trees in the tropics drop their leaves every year? Do they turn colors before they drop?

COLOR OF THE SKY

What makes the sky blue?

Extensions

Would the daylight sky be the same color from outer space?

COLORS—MIX THEM UP, SEE WHAT YOU GET

If you mix pigments of all the different colors, what color do you get?

Extensions

If you mix hues (colors of light), what color do you get?

COLORS OF A DIFFERENT KIND

The electromagnetic spectrum is the range of energy that is spread throughout our universe. Parts of it give us radio signals. Parts of it give us TV waves. Parts of it give us color. Our human eyes can only detect a small range of possible colors. Some animals can detect a wider range of colors. What could be the name of these colors? What would they look like? How do we know other animals can perceive other colors?

How many colors are there? There are the colors red, yellow, and blue (for the additive primary colors related to hues or light). There are the colors cyan, magenta, and yellow (for the subtractive primary colors related to pigments or paints). Then there are the psychological primary colors of red, blue, yellow, and green (those that affect us in certain psychological manners). Then there are all the colors that are derived from mixing these primary colors.

If we remember that colors are hues of light and that any tiny variation in the wavelength of light will cause a variation in the color, then we can assume that within a certain range of our human capacity to see color, there is an infinite number of colors. Take a certain wavelength of light measured out to the tenths of a wavelength (say 555.1 nanometers). Then we can find another color measured out to the one-thousandth decimal place of a wavelength. As long as we continue to add decimal points, we find different colors tucked in between other colors. Since there are no limits to the number of decimal points we can add, isn't there an infinite number of colors? How many names are there for colors? Can the human eye discriminate (tell the difference between) colors with a wavelength variance of one-tenth of one wavelength (one decimal point)? How fine is our capacity to tell the difference between two different and very close wavelengths of light?

Where in the world is color located? Is it out there in the universe? If there were no human beings or other life-forms with eyes and a brain (a body helps), would there be the experience of light? Remember the rods and cones in the eyes? If we didn't have them, would there be color? Isn't color the consequence of the neurological processing of photons that vibrate at certain rates? These waves of electromagnetic energy enter our eyes. They are interpreted by our brain as being light with the quality of certain colors. They do not enter our eyes as the color we perceive is out there in the universe. We don't create light. We do create the experience and perception of color based on the flow of particles and waves through space. What the universe is like, apart from our perceptions, cannot be known or directly experienced by us. This is a mystery and boundary line we cannot cross. It is one horizon that we cannot traverse.

The implications of this last point about not being able to cross this boundary line are tremendous. We need to use as many of our means of relating to our wider environment as possible. We need our intellect, feelings, intuitions, senses of all kinds, and imagination. We need the counsel (advice) of diverse people. We need to cultivate a sense of the most encompassing viewpoints on every topic of human importance. We need to view life situations from as many perspectives as possible. We need to pay attention to aberrant (unusual) and anomalous (out of the expected range of possibilities) experiences and pieces of information. We need to remember the deepest and best wisdom from the past. We need to listen to our own genius and to the genius of others.

When our intuitions say leap, sometimes we have to jump as though everything that matters is being risked. We also need good old-fashioned common sense and logical thinking. We must recall that logic by itself can be extremely misleading. Humility coupled with courage and wisdom mixed with the tincture (medicine) of compassion for all life is our best thing going.

Just because we cannot see the universe as it is doesn't mean that we are deficient. We are not in our right mind unless we realize that there is a tremendous mystery at play in our lives. This wonder and awe stemming from this mystery speak of the greatness of life. We never, never have it (life). We are always learning, growing, and evolving. This is our greatness and our lot in life. Risk the adventure of not knowing and not presuming that we are all-knowledgeable. We aren't all-knowing, and that can be the root of wisdom that liberates us.

Extensions

Look up information on the rods and cones in your eyes. These receptors allow us to interpret color. Do different people have a variance of the number and kinds of rods and cones in their eyes? Would this make a difference as to how well somebody is able to distinguish between fine variations in colors of light? Every human's body is different; therefore, the colors we see have a slight variation (given normal sight). Maybe there are people who can see colors more deeply and perhaps see more colors at the edges or limits of the color range of the electromagnetic spectrum (red on one end and violet on the other). In your mind, go from the middle of the human color spectrum and move outward to the ends in either direction. Picture the colors in your mind: green, yellow, orange, red, or move from green, blue, indigo, and violet. Then try to imagine yet another color. Is it impossible to imagine what you've never experienced before? Do some reading about people or talk directly with people without sight and how they think about and sense the world of color, light, and objects. Also investigate what people who have been blind experienced when they suddenly receive sight (or hearing). Imagine if we were to suddenly develop the senses that would allow us to experience colors beyond what we normally see. Would this disorient and confuse us or might it create a greater context for living that would be richer and more complete?

COMETS AND BLOWHOLES

One of the functions of intelligence is to make connections between far-flung ideas, experiences, feelings, or insights. What would be the possible connection between comets out in space and venting shafts under the ocean?

Learn all you can about these venting shafts and learn all you can about comets. What are they composed of? Have they always been in this form? What kinds of forces are acting upon them to change them?

Remember, what is written in this book or what you discover may be only one possible answer. There may be many other valid (true, given certain assumptions) answers. Investigate and play with it.

Hint: comets, interstellar dust, meteorites, and the venting shafts are very rich in chemicals, but not only chemicals in the form of elements. They also are thought to carry certain combinations of chemicals called organic compounds that could produce life.

Possible solution: Comets, interstellar dust, or meteorites hitting the Earth are thought to play a possible role in the evolution of life on our planet. How? Venting shafts under the oceans are thought to play a roll in creating an environment in which new basic or simple forms of life may have evolved. Imagine the number of ways you could carry on this investigation into the mysteries of life. Make connections and watch how your knowledge expands as you ask new kinds of questions.

Extensions

Read an interesting mystery book. Observe how the author develops the connections and relationships between seemingly absolutely unrelated objects, events, and dynamics. Patterns begin to emerge that were not apparent at the beginning.

COMFORT ZONE

We each have different kinds of comfort zones. We like to be around our friends. We like to do things we are good at. We like being unchallenged and comfortable. Describe your various kinds of comfort zones.

Extensions

Can we limit ourselves if we are always attempting to be comfortable? Where are the edges of our comfort zones? What happens to us when we move toward those edges of comfort? For instance, when you go up to a person at a dance that you do not know but with whom you'd like to dance, how does it feel? What do you notice about your behavior when you are at the edges learning about a new topic that is not familiar to you? Are there ways to experiment with being at the edges while being safe and secure? Some edges can be harmful to us. I love climbing cliffs. One time, as a youngster, I was climbing alone and without safety equipment. I almost fell off the cliff. Nobody knew where I was. It was in a very remote area, and it was quite possible that nobody would have found me if I had fallen. We need to be careful about the edges, but we also need to approach some of them in order to grow. The one example I gave is not an example of wise behavior! Nor is it wise never to approach the edges of our comfort zones. Reflect on your emotional, intellectual, and social comfort zones.

COMMON PROPERTY?

Because two things hold some common properties, are they the same kind of thing? If two people like to stay out late at night and one of them likes to vandalize homes and hurt other people, is this the same kind of person as the one who likes to stay out late and sit beside a tree on a moonlit night reading poetry with friends? Of course not! This is a ridiculous contention. In our real lives, we conflate (put two different things into one category) all the time. Someone is a lawyer; therefore, in the minds of some persons, the lawyer is a crook because all lawyers are out to steal our money and make themselves rich. Because some lawyers are unethical, does this mean the whole group is unethical? What are other examples of this kind of labeling? In what ways do you place people into groups that are convenient for you but not fair to them?

Extensions

We all need pictures or models of reality to help us function in the real world. These are like scripts that we use. They are an abbreviated way of making complex tasks simpler. When do these tools get in our way and cease serving as useful ways to deal with life?

COMPUTER IMAGES

Do you think producers of movies will be able to make computer animations and graphics to look as real as life? If you think they already do, what are some examples? Computer-generated animations and graphics are images and streamed images (made to appear like a movie) that originated as digital data within a computer. Then there is the realm of images and streamed images that were taken from movies and photographs of real life and then digitized (put into a data format used in computers). These images then can be transformed in many ways. One of the ways they can be transformed is to make them look like they were originally created in the computer. So we have transformed digitized data that is difficult to sense, which was originally produced in a computer and which was originally from movies and photographs of real life. What are some examples of this material being inserted within shots of real life? Can you always tell instantly when this material has been inserted? Now imagine computers being so powerful and users being so skillful that they are able to present streamed images that look as genuine as real life. Would this be dazzling? Would it be a big seller in the movie houses? Would this kind of presentation format be more attractive to some people than going out themselves and sitting by a lake at sunset?

Extensions

If we can digitize data and reformat it any way we want and then produce pictures and movies out of this data, isn't this the same as making fiction look as real as factual stories? Will this affect how we value the pictures and movies that supposedly show what really happened? With digitized film footage, could we produce a movie that shows what appears to be a convincing "factual account" of how President John Kennedy was never really killed and show him alive and well in old age in a secret Florida retirement community? Would this create some problems for what are called factual films? Imagine being a historian in the future. You've uncovered a whole collection of films that are intact. How would you determine which ones are factual and which ones are fictional? Look up *morphing*. Will movies and still photographs be admissible in court as proof of anything in the future?

CONFABULATED, CONFLATED, INFLATED, AND GENUINE STORIES

Confabulation is turning fact to fiction. Some people do this to themselves and to others consistently (often unconsciously). Many people at times turn fact into fiction by stretching the truth a little:

- Honest, officer, I was going under the speed limit.
- I only ate a few cookies.
- I'll be there in just a second.
- I never did that when I was your age.
- I ate everything growing up.
- Honest, this food tastes great and it is good for you.

If you're honest with yourself, when and under what conditions do you stretch the truth just a tidbit (little)? There is a paradox (a statement that appears to be contradictory but it is true) at play here. How can we even know when we are honest with ourselves when we grow into behavior patterns that have caused us to become unaware of when we are telling the full truth and when we are confabulating (turning fact into fiction unconsciously)? To be unaware that we are unconsciously transposing reality into fiction is a real problem especially if we try to ignore it. There are many situations in which people could be challenged by others to describe whether they were just telling the truth or confabulating, and the person questioned would not be able to give a lucid (self-aware) and true answer. What are examples of situations that you've seen or been in that involve you or somebody else stretching the truth? Be honest with yourself. Complete honesty is the only way to expand one's awareness.

Do you think that you can train yourself to observe the emergence of your thoughts, impressions, feelings, and senses in real time (as they are arising into conscious attention)? You may not be aware of this capacity. There are specific means to discover this ability. When you do learn about this potential asset (resource), you will be able to see yourself in the process of confabulating. All the time we are shaping what we call real. This is a huge and fascinating topic. I've spent years of my life studying this topic. As an incidental (side attraction) interest, occasionally observe how you and others shape, configure, mold, or regard what is taken as factual reality. Once we discipline ourselves to see these dynamics at play, we may discover an astonishing thing: how often and how much we exclude or fail to notice vitally important facets (features) of life. We tend to see and affirm what we are focused upon and aware of. Confabulation is one term for the process of shaping reality. There are many other means of filtering what we take and project as reality.

Sometimes individuals and groups get themselves into deception (twisting the truth) so deeply that they have to have outsiders intervene (become involved) in order to define and clarify (make clear) some boundary lines between what is true and what is fiction. If you ever know anybody slipping into this realm in which he or she can no longer distinguish between fact and fiction on a fundamental level, assist him or her in getting help as soon as possible. Of course there are gray areas in life, but some persons lose sight of any boundary lines that clarify the distinctions between fact and fancy (fiction). If you are going to have some benign (innocent) fun with twisting the truth, either make it so obvious that others get the humor of it directly and quickly or make sure others know that it is fiction at the beginning or at the immediate end (maybe with a little dramatic pause). Be careful with the art of deception. It can grow on you in ways that you may not be able to control. Under what conditions would a group of friends not confront a person in a loving moment with the fact that they are sinking further into the realm of not being able to distinguish between fact and fiction? This is a very sad and tragic thing when friends do not take the risks to do this. Our culture, in many ways, encourages deception. What are some examples that you've experienced of this corrosive cultural pressure to conform and be like others?

When we conflate stories, we get elements of different stories mixed into the content of another story. This is not turning fact into fiction necessarily. It is certain that when this occurs, truth is being contorted (stretched out of its original form). When two true stories are conflated, we wind up with a weird mix of facts that don't quite fit with what actually happened. When a true story and a fictional account are conflated, we wind up with an artful deception that is acceptable as long as everybody knows in advance the nature of the content and format of the story. There is also the issue of whether one is deliberately conflating two stories or not. There is the element of intent: If the act of conflating two stories is deliberate, what is the goal of mixing the two accounts? If an individual is unaware that she or he is conflating two different stories or accounts, what are the effects on innocent and unsuspecting people?

Conflating stories can involve the dynamic of time: two or more stories can be conflated with elements taken from the past, present, or future. All conflated stories blur the lines of what is truth. Gullible, unsuspecting, or noncritical (not asking important questions) people swallow the story as being true.

To inflate a story is to start with something that is true and then dress it up to make it more appealing. Inflation distorts facts in some ways, but as long as we are clear with our audience that what is being presented in not entirely factual, then everybody gets to enjoy an inflated factual story that has extra color added to it.

A genuine story is factual but it is much more than a merely true account. Genuine and authentic accounts bear (carry) the quality of being from the heart. They are self-disclosing (self-revealing). They always open up something in our own lives to a wider set of truths, a greater sensitivity for beauty, or a deeper appreciation of the value of life. Authentic and genuine stories are much more than factual accounts. They win the hearts and attention of readers or listeners because something rings true in the heart of others who experience the story in some deep manner.

Do some self-examination about the ways you relate to yourself and others. Under what conditions do you confabulate, conflate, inflate, and present yourself with candor (sincerity)? Once you have described to yourself what these conditions are, go a step further and discipline yourself to examine why you do these things. Learning to be honest with ourselves is the key to being honest with others. This is especially true when you don't have friends who are willing to take the risks of true friendship and confront you lovingly when you are consciously or unconsciously confabulating, conflating, or inflating stories. Every community and the entire social structure is dependent upon people being able to make these distinctions (tell the difference). Once the distinctions have been made clear and audiences know what kind of story they are experiencing, then confabulating, conflating, and inflating stories are several means to artfully spin a good yarn (tale).

Extensions

One of the group techniques I've used with others is the art of telling stories that the group knew in advance could be entirely true, partially true, or fictional throughout. After the story was finished, I would ask for a show of hands as to how many people believed the story was true, partially true, or entirely fiction. I discovered some interesting things.

Many people love suspending their own best judgment and tend to believe an untrue story if it is artfully and heartily relayed in a genuine and touching way (as long as it is not too fantastic). Others will not believe anything that even remotely appears to stray from everyday events and expectations. A false story with a ring of some authenticity can be passed off as truth if it is preceded with an unbelievable story that stuns the audience with being true. Usually, the most difficult kind of story to judge is the one that uses a combination of confabulation, conflation, and inflation with a major infusion (addition) of the spice of authenticity. It always helps to look people right in the eyes so that there are no signs that are taken to be evidence that you can't face the audience members because you are deceiving them.

My personal favorites are the true stories that are unbelievable. They are most effective when told with such wild abandon and passion that almost everybody believes that it is a good example of a well-enacted fictional story. Tell them the truths that seem like embellishments (inflating and dressing up what really occurred). Go all out. Once I was lying on the floor enacting a story of a personal account in which my brother and I were totally convinced that we were being attacked by two large grizzly bears in the middle of the night, trapped in a little backpacking tent, at high altitude, in a far off wilderness area, during a snow squall (quick-moving weather system that can be ferocious but usually does not last long), under the full moon, and with no defense because there were no trees tall enough to climb. From the perspective of the actual event, it truly did seem that the bears were magically transformed right outside our tent into a group of mountain goats bedding down for the night (a mother and her kids). Therefore, it became a story of true magic (from the lived experience of the actual event). While I was lying on the floor, a very important person walked past the room who had no idea what I was doing. The entire audience saw the person long before I did, and they all knew this individual. While I was focused on the audience, the other person was standing behind me out of my sight observing my antics (something that appears to be ridiculous). Of course, my audience got a huge hoot and holler out of the turn of events. When people love a good story and enjoy the storyteller, one has to expect that sometimes laughter will arise and you are the source of the humor. Whenever we tell a story with the fullness of heart and wild abandon (taking all the risks of going all out), unexpected things can happen. That's when the fun begins.

Try this technique of testing an audience with stories that can be true, a mixture of fact and fiction, or entirely fiction. See what it teaches you about the art of storytelling, human nature, and group interaction. Just be careful when you are lying on your back and you assume that you have only one audience. Be prepared for some unexpected and heartfelt laughs. Find out how many people correctly judge the style of the story.

CONSTELLATIONS ASKEW

From ancient times, observant and imaginative persons have created pictures in their mind related to the star patterns. We call them constellations. Do you think it is possible to get a star chart of what the universe would look like from the closest star to us or from the closest galaxy to us? If we were to look at constellations askance (from an angle that is askew—off angle—from our own common angle of viewing), wouldn't we see a vastly different configuration of constellations?

Extensions

Do constellations exist out in space or in our minds? Define precisely what is a constellation. For any kind of creative problem solving, it is extremely helpful to reexamine essential terms that make up the problem set. You are doing precisely this when you reexamine the definition of the term *constellation*. We form constellations of images and judgments all the time. They are highly dependent on our point of view.

CONTRARIAN

Have you ever noticed certain persons who have a habit of responding to other persons' words with the opposite opinion? What drives these persons?

Extensions

Have you ever noticed certain persons who love to try to control conversations? Some people are very sophisticated in their ways of controlling the conversation, while others try to control conversations but fail to do so. What makes these people tick? Why is this behavior so common and why do people feel that they need to do it? Is it always wrong to attempt to control certain features of our environment (like assuring that your car is in working condition, double-checking with people upon whom you depend, or creating a list of things you're going to need for a camping trip)? When do people go amok (off course) when they try to control certain things and people in their environment? How do you react to people who think of the shared social environment as being their own turf? What is the healthiest response to such people? Are you aware of it when you are doing this to others?

CONVENIENCE OF HOT WATER

Our water heaters are grossly inefficient. They waste a tremendous amount of energy. How does this loss occur? Try to determine how much energy is lost every year in a single household because of our water heater's current designs. Then try to find out how many water heaters there are in the country. What is the total loss per year?

Extensions

What are some alternatives? For one alternative, look up an on-demand water heater. Extend this research to include refrigerators. Does it make sense to manufacture refrigerators with the motors on the bottom? As motors run, they create heat. Heat rises. Heat is absorbed into the refrigerated compartment. We use up electricity running the motors that are cooling off the refrigerator while the refrigerator is running extra hard to compensate (overcome the effect) for the heat generated by the motor. Are there others means of refrigeration? Why don't we simply put the motors on top of the refrigerators? Look up some information on the coolants used in refrigerators and in the air conditioning systems for buildings, homes, and cars. Is this material environmentally benign (not harmful)? Are there alternatives? If we are all using air conditioning units, we are using up valuable Earth resources while we are also heating up the outdoors because every one of these units exudes (gives off) heat. So we wind up cooling ourselves down to seek relief from temperatures that are too hot while we are heating up the outdoors that results in us needing air conditioning units even more! Look up an exothermic reaction versus an endothermic reaction. Do a little research on how cities affect weather systems. The geographic zones of our cities tend to be thermal anomalies (exceptional); thus, they affect the development of weather systems. What about the air pollution from our metro areas—does this material affect the weather? What are other common behaviors that are self-defeating?

COOL SUNGLASSES

Most of us like to wear comfortable sunglasses. A good pair of glasses takes away the glare of bright light that can be so irritating. What happens to the eyes if we procure (get) a pair of sunglasses that cuts way down on the brightness of the light but does very little to filter out the ultraviolet (UV) rays of the sun? Look at the center of your eye in dim light and see how the eye reacts to bright light. If the pupil contracts, it is protecting the eye from bright light. If we have very dark sunglasses, how do you expect the pupil to react? We have a bad situation with glasses that filter out the brightness of light but not the ultraviolet rays. Why? Look up information on how sunglasses are rated. What are the various kinds of UV protection available? What are the various kinds of ultraviolet rays? When the pair of sunglasses you are thinking of buying has a little tag on it saying "100% UV protection," who has independently tested those glasses? Look at the label carefully. Do these glasses protect against all kinds of ultraviolet light? What about UV-C? Why not? Are there other things that a good pair of sunglasses ought to be protecting our eyes against? Look up polarized materials. What is the perfect pair of sunglasses? What kind of materials and what shapes would you like to see in your perfect pair of sunglasses?

Extensions

Can you trust the labels on sunglasses when they say they are "100% UV protected?" If sunglasses don't have any labels related to UV protection, should you be buying them? Under what conditions would you not want to have sunglasses with polarized lenses?

CREATING A NEW SPIN?

Assume:

- There is a bridge connecting all the landmasses at the equator;
- All the people and all the animals on the Earth were lined up at the equator; and
- They all began running at once in the direction that is opposite to the spin of the Earth.

Which direction would they be running in? How do you determine the direction of the spin of the Earth? One clue might be the direction the weather patterns flow. Another way would have to do with the rising and setting sun. Are there other ways?

Would these people and other animals affect the spin of the Earth? If you decide to do this experiment, be sure not to place yourself in a running position immediately near the elephants, because they really don't like running in crowds.

Extensions

What are examples of little things affecting large things?

CROSSING OVER

If you were to follow one single compass bearing, what would be the longest course in the world on water without intersecting a major landmass? Could there be a point of origin and a bearing that would yield a course all the way around the world? Remember that it's OK to trace a course through the northern polar ice cap, because it is all frozen ocean water.

Extensions

What would be the longest land course following one single bearing?

DATA AND INFORMATION

What are the differences and commonalties between data and information? What is raw data? What is formatted data? What is useful information?

Extensions

If someone is considered very knowledgeable because he or she knows a lot of information, what is the difference between being knowledgeable and being wise?

DATA, JUST DATA?

Data is the stuff people collect when they are seeking to learn more about any phenomena. For example, what is the data on the temperature of various places on the Earth over the course of time (a longitudinal study)? Does the data support the contention (belief) that global warming is happening? If the data supports this hypothesis (suggestion), does this data conclusively demonstrate (absolutely prove) that global warming is caused by human pollution? Look up the word *inference*. Can we infer global warming from the data of temperatures in various places around the Earth over the course of certain periods of time? If so, can we tell exactly why this is happening? What might be other explanations for significant temperature differentials (changes in average temperatures over the course of time)? Could there be significant human input to global warming that is intersecting with an entire host (great number of) natural factors whose period (time frame for the cycle of the phenomena) is indeterminant?

Extensions

An odd thing about data is that often we can deceive (fool) ourselves with data. The kind of stuff we are looking for affects what we see and experience. For instance, in one kind of experiment the subjects were asked to report the kind of playing card they observed. They quickly flashed in front of the eyes of the subjects a regular deck of playing cards in which diamond and hearts are red and spades and clubs are black. After a while, when the subjects got really used to the process, the experimenters slipped into the deck some red clubs, red spades, black diamonds, and black hearts. The subjects missed these cards entirely. They didn't see them because of their expectations of what they would see.

What are some other examples of people seeing what they expect to see and miss what they don't expect to see? How about the example of people who are prejudiced against persons of another race? When they run into a polite, very bright, highly motivated, and successful person of another race, do you think that the prejudiced person would change their opinions? Assume the experimenter is looking at the number of living organisms per volume of water in the ocean, and the experimenter only looked at different samples taken during the day, summertime only, at 12:00 noon only, and at only one depth. Assume further that the samples were taken with nets that only scooped up living organisms larger than one-quarter of an inch. The experiment was designed this way because the experimenter did not expect to find any life smaller than one-quarter inch across. The experimenter did not think to collect data during the night, at different times of the day, over the course of the seasons, or at different depths. What we expect to find in data greatly affects what we look for and observe. What are some other examples of biases and presuppositions (ideas that are set before we look at what is in front of us) that affect what we observe?

DEFINING MOMENTS

Certain events and realizations occur that define, in a very basic way, who we are becoming. Sometimes these defining moments occur without a direct relationship to outer circumstances. Rather, the defining moment occurs in terms of a deep realization of:

- who we are
- what our most basic values and principles are
- why it is that we are alive
- what our purpose in this world is
- what we are meant to accomplish in this life

One late night in a southern rural town, I was walking to the home at which I was staying. I had finished my night's work on a civil right's campaign. Just as I crossed the highway dividing the neighborhoods in which most of the African Americans lived and the neighborhood in which most of the European Americans lived, I was stopped cold in my tracks by a voice that I'll never forget. It was a Mississippi state trooper saying that I needed to stop and turn around. Inside, I already knew that there was a gun involved. Sure enough, I was looking right down the barrel of a large pistol. Essentially, he told me to get out of town as quickly as I could. In that moment at a young age, I knew that my life was going to be lived at the edges. The reason I was in that place was because of my ideals. I realized that being an advocate for change would cause not only transformation but also reactions on the part of very diverse people. There I was on a dividing highway, all alone except for this one very unfriendly and threatening individual. He saw me as the enemy. What he never knew was that he helped me gain a core insight about my life. That was a true turning point for me.

Often, our turning points are in less dramatic circumstances. These important decisions or insights guide us. We have all made such decisions. We have all gained such insights. Write down as many of these turning-point experiences of your life as you can think of.

Extensions

Some of our turning-point experiences and insights turn out to be detrimental (harmful) for us and for others. List these also. When we realize that certain turning points haven't been good for us and for others, what do you do about this realization? The deeper the impact of these key decisions and insights, the more difficult it is to change them. Ironically, it becomes massively more important to change them once we realize with some degree of clarity that the effects of some action or belief have been detrimental to us and to others. Take a careful look at yourself. See what your key turning points have been. We can't ever go back, but we can alter our course. This is one source of hope. We are responsible for our presence, actions, effects of our behaviors, and for our continuing growth and learning.

DEGREE

What is a degree in reference to temperature and thermal energy? How is a degree of temperature defined? What difference does one degree make? A degree of thermal energy varies according to the scale used. The particular value of one degree is relative to the number of total units the measurement scale has been assigned. What are the various scales used to measure temperature? How have the total number of degrees in the various systems of measuring thermal energy been determined?

Extensions

What is absolute zero? Is there an opposite end of the spectrum of heat (maximum heat)? If we raise the temperature too high, does this affect the structure of atoms (affect the state of matter)? What are various ways of raising the temperature of something?

DIACRITICAL MARKS

In most dictionaries, certain marks help in the task of pronunciation of words. At the beginning of the dictionary, there is usually a guide as to exactly what each of the diacritical marks means. The simplest are the marks for long and short vowel pronunciation. There are many more. If these marks are so explicit (precise and exact), why do people across the country pronounce words so differently? If the diacritical marks were followed precisely, would we all be pronouncing our words the same? Are the diacritical marks assuming one proper pronunciation of language?

Extensions

Is it common for us to feel that the people who live in our own geographic area (or the one we most closely identify with) pronounce things correctly and that their ways of pronouncing words specifically and using language in general are the norms for others? There was a major broadcasting school near where I was raised that trained radio and TV announcers. The story was commonly told (an urban myth) that the school is located here because our way of pronouncing words is the norm for the country. People are trained to talk that way because others need to understand what they are saying. Later, I met somebody else from another part of the country who gave me the exact same story about their area. This person's pronunciation and use of language was significantly different from mine. Do you think that others from elsewhere have an accent? Do you feel as though you are the only one without any real accent? What about the proper use of the English language? Is there one group that speaks correctly while others continually misuse and abuse the language? If you believe this is true, what are the various explanations for such variety? Many times, these explanations for one's own proper use of language and the abuse of language by others are very elitist. "They aren't educated like us." "They never had the opportunities we've experienced." Could it be that there are many forms of the same language, each complete with its own pronunciations and syntax (rules of speaking and/or writing)? Do we believe that there is one correct and proper culture while all the other cultural expressions are aberrant (straying from the norm) deviations? Could we accept that there is a formal use of American English alongside many variations that are reflections of rich and proud cultures?

DIAMONDS

Diamonds are one of the harder things in nature. Why? Is there anything else as hard or harder than diamonds? Is everything that is very hard brittle? Are there very hard things that are very flexible?

Extensions

Study crystalline structures. How do they fit together? There are two forms of crystallized carbon—diamonds and graphite. How do we get diamonds from carbon? What are some interesting properties of graphite? If diamonds are hard, can they be brittle? Can they be broken apart? How? Keep your eye out for the topic of cleavage points and how they relate to splitting hard crystalline objects. Could certain substances be turned into crystals in outer space that are harder than any crystals formed here on Earth? Hardness, toughness, and strength are related qualities. We think of steel as being hard, tough, and strong. We don't usually think of people or things that are hard, tough, and strong as being flexible and sensitive. Take a one-foot length of solid steel that is one inch square across its width. Try to bend it. It appears as though it is totally inflexible. If steel were totally inflexible, our tallest buildings would not sway. Find out how much the world's tallest buildings sway. If they didn't sway, what could be the consequences? People and things that are rigid and inflexible are also brittle.

Look up exactly what being brittle means. Airplanes are made of various kinds of metals for structural strength. When you are landing in some semiturbulent (rough) weather, look at the wings very carefully. They are very flexible. How could you bend a one-inch by one-inch solid steel bar with your bare hands? The only restriction is that the bar needs to be solid steel and one inch by one inch. It is very possible to do this with your bare hands. Assume that the steel bar and your arms can be any length you desire. Be careful! The only rule is that your arms will remain this length until the next month in which there is a blue moon.

DIMENSIONS—HOW MANY?

Portions of this section are complex and abstract. When you run into something that you don't fully understand, you do have some options:

- Go back to the basic theories and learn more about these basics for the discussion.
- Review the items that you do know about. Use these as a springboard for examining the other items you don't know about yet.
- Develop a clearer picture of the outline, flow, or pattern of the discussion.
- Get a clearer sense of what kind of discussion it is: a literal or figurative presentation; a tightly logical, straightforward linear sequence; a mixture of fact and fiction; a factual account that combines known facts with a projection of possible facts (inference); a totally nonlinear presentation style; or a relatively linear presentation style with digressions (side trips).
- Read it through one time. Don't get upset with yourself if you don't get it all. Get a sense for what the author is talking about. Get a general sense of the outline of the discussion. Then read it through again. It can be amazing how much you can understand the second time through complex or challenging material.
- Ask somebody else to coach you on the difficult sections, language, or concepts.
- Ask somebody else to give you the gist (essential points or condensed version) of the presentation.
- Skip it!

When we look at the universe, we can also talk about dimensions. We will begin with a concept that is not considered a dimension. It is a point. Take a pencil and make a dot on a piece of paper. In theory, this point is an imagined position in space and time. It has no length, width, or depth. It is a useful concept when dealing with space. Without the concept of a point, there would be no understanding of other geometric dimensions. Ironically, it is the other dimensions that give significance to the concept of a point. Is it the most peculiar of all geometric concepts? Is it really without dimension? There may be much more to a point than meets the eye.

The first dimension is that of length; for instance, the distance between two points. If a point has no dimension, how can you possibly measure the distance between two such points? Challenge the concept of points. See what you come up with. At the end of this section, I'll give you one means of challenging the current concept of points. An issue with the first dimension is that of the distance between two points. Is the shortest distance between two points a straight line? In one sense, of course, a straight line is the shortest distance between two points. In the real world, the answer is vastly different! With the supposedly simple dimension of length, we wind up with two conundrums: can there be any measurement of distance between two points if the points themselves have no dimensions? And is the shortest distance between two points is always a straight line?

The first dimension is length, and it is composed of at least two points. The second dimension is width. Theoretically, when width and length are present, we have a plane. A plane is a flat surface without depth and it must contain at least three points. This is why we have three-legged stools (the plane on which you sit is stable because of this basic law of geometry). Might this law of geometry be deemed (judged) to be valid (true) because there are things in the world like three-legged stools? We observe things in the universe and deduce (assume) that, because most things in the world corroborate (support) the fundamental pattern observed, there must be a law at play. If the domain (area) that we are observing is only a portion of the known universe, then we assume what we call a law really is a fundamental truth in reality. If we expand our domain of observed patterns, contradictory patterns may arise or patterns that are vastly more inclusive may arise that are the truer laws of the universe. Anything we call a law is relative to a certain domain of human observation and knowledge. In other words, the three-legged stool might be stable because of some other more-inclusive law about which we have no current knowledge.

Remember, the plane can contain these points because points have no dimension. A piece of paper is not two-dimensional, because it has another dimension to it (depth). Are there any entities (fancy terms for things) in the universe that do not have any matter or mass, thus lacking any extension in space? Might particles of energy (photons) be dimensionless? If so, is it imaginable to align a whole lot of these photons in a single plane (at least three of them) and thus we'd have a plane in the real universe that actually does exist without the third dimension of depth? When somebody says that something is an absolute basic axiom (rule) (for example, "a plane without the third dimension of width can't exist in the real world"), challenge the assumptions. Challenge all assumptions, because this is how you create some fantastic and sometimes very useful insights and inventions. All inventors look at the world askance (from as many different angles as possible, out of the ordinary). They've discovered two deeply interrelated secrets: things do not have to be the way they are now, and things aren't necessarily the way they appear to be. Memorize these two insights. They can change everything in your life.

The third dimension is that of depth. Finally, with all three dimensions, we are able to describe real objects that commonly exist in space that we can experience through our five senses. We're talking about donuts to toenails. Take a sheet of paper. It has length, width, and depth. How much depth? What kind of tool would you need to determine the depth of the piece of paper? The least expensive tool is a mechanical one. There are other much more expensive ones. See if you can find one of these mechanical tools and measure the depths of various kinds of paper and other thin things like the width of a needle or the width of a leaf, your finger or toenail, or the width of various kinds of keys. What is the thinnest piece of something that is lying around your neighborhood or home that you can measure? What is the thinnest three-dimensional object that you can imagine? Could it be composed of a depth of one atom? Could this superthin film be opaque, translucent, or transparent by the choice of atoms used? What kind of glue would you use to hold this superthin film together? The manner in which this question is asked presupposes that compounds or chemicals need to be added to this thin film of atoms in order for it to maintain its integrity. Imagine some force that, when applied to the thin film, would cause it to maintain its integrity. Could you make it in such a manner that it could contain information or gather in matter or energy in outer space? Could it be made in such a way that it would not only conduct electrical energy but also it would gather energy from other sources and transform it into electrical energy that could be transferred elsewhere?

The nondimensional concept of a point and the dimensions of length and width are theoretical constructs (ideas) that are useful tools we employ (use) in order to explain our universe. You cannot find a point in nature, that occupies space but that doesn't mean necessarily that points aren't there. This statement is literally true, but in a most paradoxical (unexpected and startling) way. (*See* "Spiraling into Infinity.") For instance, the geographic and magnetic poles of the planet (north and south) are mathematical concepts. I once met a woman who had ridden a Russian icebreaker many hundreds of miles to get to the North Pole. Once there, she and her husband danced around a large circle, and then she was let down nine feet through the ice. She went swimming at this mathematical point. Points matter. The swim would not have been the same a hundred miles away in any direction, and from this point there is only one direction—south. Anyplace else would have merely been a pointless cold dunk.

We give points meaning although we can't hold anything in the palm of our hand that is a point. Points are useful tools to help us explain and understand our universe. Length and width do not appear or are not visible anywhere in the universe. There was once a story published about an entire world that was composed exclusively of two-dimensional figures. Things got very confused when they met for the first time things that had more dimensions. See if you can locate this book. You have sufficient information in order to find it. It is quite sexist (unfair and dated in the use of gender references), but still it is worth at least a brief skimming due to its unique subject matter.

There is no piece of paper without depth. Something with width always has length if we are talking about objects in the universe. The next time you come across a length hanging around by itself, get a camera real quick. You'll have to shoot it at just the right angle. There are cameras that allow you to choose any focal plane (you can choose weird angles at will). If a plane has no depth, can you imagine a camera taking a picture of something infinitely thin to the point that it has no depth? (Remember the two-dimensional array of photons.) Cameras take pictures of objects illumined by light. Now try to imagine a camera that takes a picture of one particular plane (an angled shot of one particular area that is flat and has no depth). The focus is not on illumined objects, but the object of the photo is the light itself (a picture of the photons)!

Back to the three dimensions. The three dimensions and the nondimension of a point are very useful tools to help us explain space, but there is a little problem. We said that points, length, and width are useful tools. Then it appears as though once we add depth we have the real thing in our grasp. The problem is that there is another dimension that is necessary if we are to be talking about the real world. The missing element or dimension is that of time. This is the fourth dimension. Without it, many phenomena can't be explained (acceleration, movement, past, future, change, life, and transformation).

One thing that can't be explained with only three dimensions is why light bends from its straight path when passing massive objects such as the sun. Given a three-dimensional outlook of the universe, one would say that the planet or star bends the light because of gravity. The denser the material, the greater would be the expected warping of light passing the object. Albert Einstein proved that this is not the fullest and most accurate description. In order to explain how light appears to be bent requires another dimension. Once time was discovered to be the fourth dimension, then there arose another richer and more encompassing explanation as to why it appears that light is bent. It turns out that light is not bent relative to a fixed three-dimensional grid of the universe. The actual space-time continuum (grid) is warped by the presence of mass.

Mass is not how much something weighs. Something with great mass in outer space would not weigh anything. If you were in outer space on a space walk and something slammed into you that didn't weigh anything, but did have great mass, could you get hurt? Might the collision bump you into another path? If you weigh nothing and the object hitting you weighs nothing (zero), you weigh the same. If something weighs zero, it has no weight; therefore, how could it influence you? The answer lies with this weird stuff called mass. Although the weight of two objects may be the same, the mass can be greatly different. Something very big could have less mass, and something very small could have indescribably greater mass. Compare the mass of a black hole with a Styrofoam ball of exactly the same volume. Now back to light and the four dimensions.

Light is merely following the shortest path between two points (the point of origin and the final measurement point). Relative to our rectangular way of picturing things, we think of the light as being curved by a force acting upon it. Could this mean that the basic information our senses give us could be severely distorted? Perhaps what we see is not the actual thing in and of itself! Light being bent is following the shortest course between two points, just like you when you follow the shortest path of least resistance between you and the fresh, warm, good-smelling, home-baked cookies with no one standing around to tell you not to eat them. This is a basic law of the universe—cookies are meant to be eaten. You'll take the shortest path to those cookies possible—the proverbial beeline. Now you can clearly see that Einstein is correct about light, right?

Back to light, mass, space-time, and gravity. Light travels through curved space. It is following what is called a geodesic. Space is not rectilinear. It is curvilinear (from our perspective). Straight lines fold into curves (unless there is nothing there with mass). It matters that there is the presence of this quality called mass. If there were no mass, we would wind up with a rectilinear universe with all energy flowing in straight lines. (Actually, I just imagined this last idea, but keep studying this subject to see if physicists confirm this idea someday.) Imagining the universe without mass is like conjecturing about objects without time, length, width, or depth. It's impossible, but then little twists in comprehension have yielded some pretty incredible discoveries—like blue M&M's, Velcro, fire, the wheel, and food that is devoid of nutritional value, but which looks and tastes real good.

Only when we use the fourth dimension do three-dimensional objects make sense. If nothing in the universe were dynamic or in process, we would have no need of time; but then again, if everything were in a state of stasis (no growth, motion, disequilibrium, heat, atomic motion, or fresh pumpkin pie), this would be absolute zero in temperature (heat death from entropy). That would be a rather lonely universe if we were the only living being or object in the universe with heat. That's a relationship gone cold! The paradoxes of three-dimensional space are resolved when we include the fourth dimension.

If we look at the universe in terms of it being encapsulated (contained within) in a box, we have a neat working model for connecting all the things inside the box with straight lines. Any two entities (things) can be connected with a straight line. Inside the box is the known universe. If we change our view and see the universe as being curvilinear, it folds back into itself. For one example of a figure that could be infinitely large yet folds back on itself, look up the geometric figure called the torus. For a little diversion, learn what a

Klein bottle is. Try enfolding this tube back into itself. You get a fancy tube without an inner or outer surface. Is this just a fanciful theory or can it really be constructed?

In rectilinear space, three questions, conundrums, or paradoxes are:

- Into what does the universe expand?
- What does it mean to be infinitely big?
- What is beyond the box?

In curvilinear space, three questions, conundrums, or paradoxes are:

- Into what does the space-time continuum enfold?
- What does it mean to be infinitely small?
- What is at the substratum, core, or center from which the curved limits of the space-time continuum emerge?

This gets us back to the dimension that, in traditional thinking, is not allowed to be a dimension. If space-time is curved, to what extent can it fold back on itself? In some places, could it fold back on itself infinitely? If Einstein is right and the space-time continuum is curved (and folds back on itself), a basic premise of Euclidean geometry needs to be revisited. Does a point truly have no dimension? This can get us back to the substratum (source) from which curvilinear space-time emerges. There is another way of asking the question. Does a point have any extensibility (extension, taking up room) in space? If it does not, it has, by definition, no dimension. It may just turn out that extension in observable space may have its analog (equivalent, partner) in a dimension related to infinite smallness. This would be the substratum (source). What is extroverted in infinitely large space may have its analog in what is introverted in infinitely small space. (*See* "Spiraling into Infinity.")

Just because Einstein happens to be one of the brightest geniuses of all time—the Babe Ruth of science—could there be theories that will displace Einstein's theory of relativity that will make our universe even more seriously and weirdly mysterious, counterintuitive, and different from what our five senses reveal? Not that Einstein's ideas would be wrong. It could be that there are more encompassing theories that account for a greater range of phenomena in the universe. If our Euclidean universe leaves us asking questions about infinity out there beyond us and if the Einsteinian universe leaves us asking questions about infinity within points that have no geometric dimensions, then maybe other theories will reverse the course of looking for the ultimate building blocks of the universe. Instead of looking at quarks and other known subatomic particles (maybe even subquarks or superstrings), scientists may point us in the direction of ultimate fields that are more primitive than individual things that are greatly small. Be careful of any statement of the form "either this one or that one." Be careful because there might be more than two possibilities or there may be some previously unknown interplay between the two opposed and seemingly exclusive choices. There is also the possibility that there is a completely different phenomenon at play that nobody suspects in the present time and, therefore, our intellectual frameworks cannot possibly reflect this greater picture.

Maybe we'll learn about ultimate constituents of the universe that are greatly small (like quarks, subquarks, superstrings, foam, or knots) and large fields that give shape and possibility for existence. (*See* "Spiraling into Infinity.") If fields are one of the ultimate and most primitive (basic) constituents of the universe, maybe we can have a better understanding of space-time itself. If the entire universe is expanding, when two objects seem to move away from each other, we might understand that space-time itself has expanded. There is more distance between objects not because they have moved away from each other in static, empty, uninteresting stuff called space, but because this fabulous mysterious quality of the universe we call space-time keeps expanding its field.

The universe is expanding from all points, but the effects of this expansion are only obvious on sufficiently large scales. Look up a parsec. Hint: a parsec is a unit of measure for determining really huge distances in space. A light year is too small a measurement for astrophysicists, so they use the parsec or the megaparsec. The scale at which it is obvious that space dilation (expansion) is obvious is greater than many megaparsecs. So you don't need to worry that your Cheerio, yo-yo, knitting needle, or cell phone is going to be so big that it won't fit into your house in the morning. The reason that space dilation doesn't occur on small scales like our back porch or my dog's nose is that gravity is a pretty tough competitor relative to the forces that are causing space dilation. Gravity is a very weak force over great distances, but in a small pocket of space, it wins. You really are—more or less—the same size in the morning as you were when you went to sleep the night before unless you sleep walk and sleep eat a lot.

Back to fields. We are part of the field, and we are made up of very tiny mysterious particles of many different kinds. Only twelve different known particles (along with their corresponding antiparticles) make up most of the entire universe (six quarks and six leptons). The twelfth particle was just proven to exist. A whole host (great number) of other particles in high-energy situations also exists. The interaction of all these particles is mediated (controlled) by four basic forces. The carriers of these forces are photons, gluons, carriers with the letters W and Z, and maybe something called gravitons. (*See* "Vacuum Fluctuations—Something Really Weird Is under My Bed and It's Real.") It is beginning to appear that the field in which all else exists creates the potential for the four forces of the universe. The field itself may not be limited to what we call space-time. (*See* "Spiraling into Infinity.") The carriers transport the known particles that make up everything we see, smell, taste, hear, and touch (look up photons, gluons, W and Z particles, and gravitons). These carrier particles are also the means of communication between all particles of matter in the universe. Fields, four forces, carrier particles, particles, and antiparticles give us everything from Jell-O to fish smells. What a wonderful life! Try to imagine something extraordinary before breakfast every morning and see what it does to your hair. It might wind up looking stranger than Einstein's hair. Look up a picture sometime of a marvelous symphony conductor named Arturo Toscanini. When he was older, he also had unique long, silver, flowing hair. He was a genius with music. If you become too attracted to the extraordinary in life, look out for your hair. What a distinction! Is it the unique hair that makes you become a genius?

Now that you've had your breakfast, let's face an interesting little conundrum. The four dimensions of the space-time continuum actually need other dimensions in order to have integrity. Why worry about integrity in this day and age? We all need it. It is the glue of society and it's the underpinnings for the universe. Coherence is a rather nice quality in life. One of the many basic functions of intelligence is to detect patterns amidst seeming chaos and to discern (sense) connections between seemingly disparate (nonrelated) phenomena. With the use of our intelligence, we can determine that there is a coherence and integrity to the universe. Its unity is rooted in contexts that are greater than our knowledge. We deceive ourselves if we think that we can know everything. When we portray our current knowledge as the summation of all that is possible, this is hubris (really big ego). We detect that there is coherence to the known universe. We assume that whatever exists in the unknown universe (places, laws, dynamics) also possesses integrity. We may not be able to comprehend these places, laws, and dynamics due to our limitations. Riddles of the mind are a great source of strength and creativity. It's OK not to comprehend everything intellectually. Intellectual understanding is one kind of knowledge. It has its domain and its limits. There are other ways of knowing, and they are all interrelated.

It is a blast to go beyond the edges of the boxes many others live in twenty-four hours a day. Then again, if the universe is curvilinear, it is always interesting to explore our substratum and source. There is a massive number of very bright, highly educated people living within tightly controlled boxes. Learn to observe the deep inner workings of people at play, and you will begin to notice the existence of these confining and self-chosen boxes. Only a few persons dare to push the edges. Security is a powerful motivator. For a few persons, pursuing the great adventure and seeking great discoveries are a greater enticement than the allure of finding security in those things that most others accept from the past.

Try to define your boxes. Discover why you maintain them. If there were no boxes, would there be any order and stability? Do the creative few really threaten order and stability, or do they offer new kinds of order and stability on radically different foundations? Remember to always question the format when anybody says everything is always this or that. Toss in a third possibility and see how people respond. Transitions are very difficult for many people. If we are willing to examine options outside our normal boxes, we will see with astonished eyes and amazed spirits. This is being fully alive! Look outside the box, and you might see the need for other dimensions beyond the four standard commonly accepted ones. This is where the fun really begins.

If you would like to take a very big breath, you may wish to explore the possibility of an imagined fifth dimension. (Once I have demonstrated the necessity or possibility of these additional dimensions, we can return to the original nondimension of a point and perhaps discover that it is a dimension after all. This helps us with the problem of infinitely small points of singularity that exist in the center of black holes.) This will also assist in our comprehension that, in a curvilinear universe, a core paradox and rich source of wisdom is the substratum or source that by definition is not describable in terms of the other dimensions. The rationale (purpose) for the exploration into other possible dimensions is to emphasize that as we utilize (use) our imagination, varying forms of intelligence, intuition, diverse kinds of logic, sensitivities, feelings, and wisdom, we will encourage a broader way of looking at life. Breadth and depth of comprehension have a way of enriching us in ways that can increase our appreciation of being alive. We can learn to sense the presence of more dimensions to life issues than have been conceived or imagined. This is one root of creativity and wisdom.

If you are absolutely committed to the confines of one emotional, cultural, intellectual, academic, or social box, you and those with whom you choose to associate will choose to legitimize and make valid one certain kind of logic, one definition of intelligence, feelings, wisdom, and set of sensitivities. The preservation of power and privilege will be your primary focus. This is like living in a black-and-white world when there is also available to us the splendor of many colors of the rainbow. What it means to be alive will be enriched if we are willing to explore with the diverse resources of various kinds of intelligence, intuition, logic, sensitivity, feeling, and wisdom.

Diversity is our friend. How is it that so many people fear and are aggravated by the presence of diversity? You'll always have your core set of resources that are most natural for you, but it can never hurt to have additional resources in your satchel of life along life's path. Diverse ways of understanding life enable us to meet different kinds of life challenges with a marked quality of flexibility, adaptability, and creativity (not bad resources to have available). Also, it is my hope and purpose to encourage the emergence of genius that lies submerged and suppressed (held down) within every human being. As genius is liberated, new options and alternatives enter our individual lives and our shared lives. One way of defining genius is to portray it as leaping outside known and accepted boxes. Another way of depicting (portraying) genius is to view it in terms of a quality that is part of all our lives that becomes apparent and manifest only when we discover our true source, substratum, true identity.

There are ways of conceiving our universe that do not carry the burden of wondering what lies beyond the end of the limits, periphery, edges, or box of the known. You have probably heard of black holes in the universe. These stars have grown old and have ceased to be producing enough energy to stay alive. Gravity wins the game. The bell rings at the end of the day and the star is no longer there. It is now a cute little black hole. The star dies and eventually collapses. These special cosmic repositories of matter and energy called black holes are also at the core of at least some galaxies. Maybe black holes have something to do with the birth and maintenance of the galaxies and with the death of stars. As they fall in upon themselves, they create tremendous gravitational fields that pull in other matter and energy. If we look at the process in terms of space-time, it is not a tremendous gravitational field being made, but the space-time continuum (the whole thing) is warped by the presence of highly concentrated mass (according to Einstein). None of the black holes have been observed directly, but we infer their existence both from the body of advanced knowledge in mathematics, and physics, and from direct observations of matter being affected by what must be black holes. We can't see them because the escape velocity from a black hole is greater than the speed of light.

Black holes are concentrated regions of mass and energy. Mass is a very mysterious quality present in the universe. We can all too easily think we have a sufficient definition for mass, but if we take a closer look at the term, it becomes deeply problematical. Its first cousins, matter and energy, are equally problematical at a deeper level. (Everything becomes problematical at a deeper level because we are approaching the limits of our knowledge and we are approaching the domain of the substratum or source from which all else flows.) When we examine these terms in a deeper manner, we start to sense suggestive possibilities that imply the existence of a wider understanding or greater number of dimensions.

Our language is filled with terms that beg you to go deeper and wider in your understanding and vision. One way to locate these key terms in our language is to find root terms that can only be defined in terms of other things (like matter, energy, and mass needing to be explained in terms of each other but none can be explained by itself). Other words are defined in terms of multiple consistent words. However, there are certain core words that have to be defined relative to other terms that are not similar and the same. Mass is not matter. Matter is not energy. Energy is not mass. It took Einstein to figure the relation between them, but we still can't define one of them without reference to the others. Mass and energy are equivalent, but they are not the same. As soon as we start to talk about the equivalence of basic building blocks of human knowledge, we realize that we are at the very edges of our comprehension.

Energy-matter and space-time are warped in the presence of these black holes. Space-time is so warped that it is sucked into this point of singularity (an infinitely small space) at the core of the black holes. Does this point of singularity sound familiar? It sounds very much like a mathematical point.

Now remember the big bang theory. All of the energy and matter in the universe was supposedly contained in this primordial (original) lump of matter and energy. Was it a super-duper point of singularity like what exists at the center of black holes? Was it a great whopper-sized black hole? If so, what size would it have to be in order to contain all the matter and energy in the entire present universe? If space-time were warped infinitely, would it have any extension (size) at all? Can something come from nothing? Now we are at the edge of comprehension itself. We are facing the issue of the very real existence and importance of our substratum or source.

Black holes do take up space. They have a radius (distance from the edge to the center). The center of these mysterious objects is the point of singularity that has no extension in space, but which possesses infinite mass. The edge of the black hole is called the event horizon. Very strange properties exist at the event horizon. Light is allowed in but not out. The escape velocity within the event horizon is greater than the speed of light. The escape velocity at the event horizon equals the speed of light. The escape velocity outside the event horizon is less than the speed of light. You could get very close to a black hole, but the closer you got to an event horizon it would require massively greater amounts of energy to get away. An event horizon's effect on space-time is limited. It is the point of singularity that possesses infinite mass. Once inside the event horizon, you've just bought a one-way ticket to the point of singularity. Whether you like it or not, you're on the great adventure of discovering what it means that something infinitely small can contain infinite mass. This event horizon can be taken to be an analogy for the limits of our human comprehension. Might it be possible that, once we are beyond the event horizon, we've opened ourselves so widely and deeply that the substratum or source is revealed? If this ever were to happen, could you go back? You don't have to worry about a black hole zapping the Earth by sucking it into its own inner point of singularity. Nor do you need to worry about accidentally stumbling out of our limits of comprehension into another realm. The universe has some kind of structure that may be static, renewing, evolving, or alternating. Whatever the case, we are part of the process. Everything is deeply interrelated; therefore, whatever this substratum or source is, it is part of our lives in an intimate and essential way that defies all words. If it is part of reality, then wisdom would dictate that we continue to open ourselves up to what is real. So please continue on the journey.

Instead of saying that there is one point of origin, there might be many points of emergence for this self-renewing and evolving universe. Perhaps the expansion of space-time bubbles is much more complex than ever thought. Instead of defining the origins of space-time being rooted in the big bang, we might define the origins of the big bang as being rooted in a field that induced the big bang to occur. This field could reflect the presence of yet undetected dimensions. Maybe some deeper, more primordial force is at play in which there is a continual process of emergence—continual renewal everywhere, all the time. What is infinitely small is infinitely rich and full. This is much the same as saying that a point of singularity is a mathematical point without dimension. If this is so, we are left with the possibility that an infinitely large universe comes from at least one point with no dimensions that is infinitely small. (*See* "Golf—The Greatest Shot in History.") This deeper layer of metaphors suggests the possibility for a wider understanding of the universe replete (accompanied by) with more dimensions. As with the case of the three dimensions needing a larger frame of reference, we need a larger frame of reference relative to a point of singularity. More on this later.

If black holes pull in space-time and all relatively close matter and energy, this primordial point of singularity must have warped space-time into itself. If this is true, does it make any sense to speak of something being outside this point of singularity? Assume that the primordial point of singularity is right in front of you. Does it make any sense to talk of being one mile, one light-year, or one inch away from it? In one sense, there is nothing outside the box, because there is no box, but this is only one sense. Multiple perspectives are useful. If I really got that close to a black hole, I'd try to hide behind the biggest and closest tree as quickly as possible. If space-time were completely absorbed within this point of singularity, there was neither time before the big bang nor any space outside of the primordial entity. How long would it take you to get to the tree? Look up the term *ex nihilo*. This was used in the past to explain the unexplainable. (*See* "Vacuum Fluctuations—Something Really Weird Is under My Bed and It's Real.")

When we are talking about the infinitely great matter-energy that is also infinitely small, there is neither space beyond it nor any time before it. If there's no time before the big bang, and if it didn't happen within our space-time continuum, it didn't ever happen anywhere. This prior statement is literally true, but its truth content is relative to the limited domain to which the statement refers. From our perspective, there is nothing outside the box (that we presume to exist). There may be more encompassing realities. Actually, the initiating process that resulted in the big bang created the effect of what we call space-time. If it didn't begin as space-time, how could it wind up being space-time? Can a chicken give birth to a goose? I don't think so! There are many examples of things in nature beginning one way and ending up another. A chrysalis results in a butterfly. The very first animal of a particular species did not have parents of the same species (*See* "First Human Being"). However, all life comes from other life except in the instance of the first forms of life emerging from nonliving matter-energy. Even in this case, the potential for life existed in the underlying matter-energy that subsequently resulted in life. By extension and analogy, the stuff from which the big bang emerged carried the potential for the subsequent emergence of the space-time continuum, matter-energy, life, and french fries. This slight conundrum (conundra—yes, they're multiplying on us) might just be enough to cause us to seriously entertain the possibility of other dimensions. Next time you are beholding a perfect french fry, witness the grease liberally slimed throughout its entire fine length, width, and depth. Maybe the grease will remind you of the primordial goo oozing from the big bang. It's all the same marvelous process!

Could there be an infinitely small point of singularity containing all the space-time there is in the universe? All of this in something without dimensions? It makes no sense to talk of an interior, exterior, or surface of this point of singularity. When we talk about black holes that now exist, they do not possess infinite mass; therefore, they do not infinitely warp space-time. Their domain is limited within the space-time continuum. Are we stuck with an irresolvable conundrum that the point of singularity within black holes do contain infinite mass, but yet the black holes themselves are inferred not to contain infinite mass because they do not warp space-time completely throughout all of the universe? Might it be that all black holes do contain infinite mass but the reason they do not warp space-time infinitely is that there are countervailing forces at play in the universe that balance each other out? Maybe there is a creative and dynamic imbalance at play that is the foundation for the emergence of the universe and life! If everything were static, there would be no evolution and no emergence of anything new. Perhaps it is the case that there are innumerable emergence points that are like big bangs acting on each other all the time. Maybe the least complex process is the warping of space-time. Maybe there is a greater fabric at play that renews itself in ways that our current knowledge cannot begin to grasp. This is not all conjecture. It may be tomorrow's knowledge. Maybe is a powerful word!

Look up anything you can find on quark-gluon plasma. At Brookhaven National Laboratories, there is the Relativistic Heavy Ion Collider that is creating for the first time a new form of matter, relative to our experience, that may be similar to the matter of the point of singularity from which this entire universe emerged. This new form of matter might provide us with interesting insights into our origins. These assumptions about the point of singularity having no dimension presume that we are dealing with a rectilinear Euclidean or a curvilinear Einsteinian universe. They were merely humans who were geniuses outside the current boxes of comprehension. They had seen deeper and wider contexts for our cultural frameworks and intellectual constructs of the era.

The rectilinear and curvilinear universe concepts are not antithetical (opposites). On one level, Euclid's geometry still holds great explanatory power for things in the world such as basketballs, cars, plates, forks, and Frisbees. When you surreptitiously (secretly) smuggle your least favorite food to a safe and secure drop site under the table and let it go out of your hand, you are trusting that Euclid's geometry and Newton's physics still apply to our known universe. Newton's basic formula, f = ma, deals with force, mass, and acceleration. It still applies today, even under the table. Because this formula works in the everyday world, the food we drop under the table will be safely and secretly delivered to the gaping and salivating mouth of your dog (maybe your unusual cat). All thanks to the fact that gravity works—in spite of the fact that Einstein says that in one sense gravity doesn't exist. Did he ever try to drop food under the table out of sight from others at the table? Dropping your least favorite food is not ill-mannered after all! It is the highest form of intellectual inquiry. You are merely testing that certain known laws of the universe are still operable despite the fact that you've dabbled and lingered outside of some known box.

On another level (perspective is all-important), Einstein's picture of the universe holds tremendous explanatory power for such things as the macro universe. Quantum mechanics views existence from a very different perspective of the greatly small world of particles and waves. Superstring theory goes even further in the expansion of the picture of what is real. Next time you're sitting at the table wondering what to do with your least favorite food, devise a test to see if Euclid's, Newton's, and Einstein's worldviews and the worldviews of relativity, quantum mechanics, and superstring theory all hold true at the same time for the same piece of undesirable food! Keep your test simple. Be careful; something unusual might happen to your dog. Don't tell anybody where you got this idea for such a test.

Are past boundaries necessarily future limits? If we leap beyond the boundaries of conceptions rooted in a rectilinear or curvilinear space and imagine another picture of the universe rooted in fields, then suddenly it is possible to think of something not contained within the primordial or original point of singularity. These fields aren't something out there in the universe to which we can point (just like we can't point to an independently existing object called a point, length, and width in the real world).

In a sense, this primordial point of singularity is beyond our capacity to comprehend. None of our ideas or concepts is encompassing enough to allow us to picture it in our minds. There is no inside or outside to it. There is no time. It is infinitely dense and small. Our science cannot explain it. The point of singularity, which is assumed not to be a dimension at all, and the possibility of fields that are basic fundamental aspects of the universe lead us to the possibility of a fifth dimension.

Let's imagine that the fifth dimension is the dimension into which the universe is expanding. Remember that you can't point to some place out in space and say beyond that point is the fifth dimension. It's not out there beyond the box. That box or sphere only exists in our minds. The fifth dimension is a quality sewn into the fabric of everything that exists. After the big bang, not only is matter and energy spreading out into the universe from its point of origin, but also space-time continuum is expanding as well. Where is the point of origin? Are there multiple points of origin? Are there many big bangs going on all at once, each one of which creates a different universe that is related to the other universes only in ways that we can't detect? Run these questions by your dentist in a quiet moment. Remember that all patterns everywhere could be doing a combination of the following: repeating, renewing, evolving, alternating, or some other quirky and indescribable creative process. This has huge ramifications for our basic presumptions that there are fundamental laws that govern the universe. What appears to be a system that is coherent, interdependent, and marked by regularity may be a picture that is vastly too small and misleading. The use of the terms *fundamental* and *law* may be insufficient for processes vastly beyond our intellects and imaginations.

That into which matter, energy, and the space-time continuum are expanding is the fifth dimension. Without the fifth dimension, aren't the first four incomplete? Aren't you glad you read this far? The fifth dimension is what makes it possible for there to be any expansion upon old forms. The fifth dimension is not merely a spatial concept. It is also the potential for change, growth, novelty, and creativity. Your day could have been quite black and white and ordinary. Now you carry with you the hint of the fifth dimension. It is the dawning of a new age! Look out for what you are about to step into. Remember, you can't see in advance what's there.

Which is more difficult—trying to impart wisdom about love or trying to comprehend the goofy quirks of the universe? If Shakespeare couldn't fully explain love, we can be patient with ourselves for not being able to fully explain the incompleteness of our understanding of the universe. We're on a great adventure, and growth is the process of being fully alive. Let's keep going. Why stop right in the middle? Of course, by now you realize that in this kind of strange universe, there is no beginning, middle, or end. Ever wonder why most people really do stop without venturing to the edges in order to look over the horizon?

We can imagine that there is an expanding and enfolding universe that has no boundaries just as we conceive of a universe with limits and boundaries. Actually, in terms of space, the universe is not limited, but in terms of time, it is limited. This limitation is eliminated when we consider supertime later in this section and when we examine the domain inside a point of singularity in another part of the book. (*See* "Spiraling into Infinity.") There is no beyond; everything that exists is coherent and part of awesome unity and system, yet there is the potential for transformation into what has never existed before (relative to our limited framework of understanding). To the open, emergent, creative, and ever-renewing system (life, universe, cosmos), there are no conundrums, problems, or paradoxes. The mind is riddled. It is not riddled with something. The mind is riddled period. This means that our conceptions, feelings, intuitions, experiences, beliefs, and faiths must always and forever gaze upon what is greater than our capacities to comprehend. Therefore, riddles, paradoxes, conundrums, and problems are the gifts that impel us to wonder and be in a state of awe. They are not a failure of intellect. We are inquisitive and curious at the core of our being. To be alive is to be thunderstruck with the enormity, beauty, glory, mystery, and ultimate value of our home, this self, this body, this community of humans, this environment that has evolved so richly with such diverse life, our planet, and our universe. To be alive is to have heart (feeling, passion, intuition, and sensitivities). Heart and intellect combined lead to wonder and gratitude. This all inspires us to quest for a greater comprehension. Riddles are our friends impelling us to keep evolving and growing. Keep wondering. Remain in a state of awe. Now you know why geniuses have weird-looking hair—they're thunderstruck with wonder and awe. Next time you go to get your hair cut, see if there is a special shampoo or hair conditioner for people who are always thunderstruck with the greatness of Life! It'll be obvious once you locate it. Hint: they don't keep this stuff out on the shelf with the other products. Look around the room and ask the employee who has the most unusual hair—that's the secret.

One way to understand that our minds are riddled (in a very positive way) is to experience the insight that there is some source to what is. This source is not outside the perimeter of the box. Remember that the source cannot be beyond the box, because the box is only an illusion we create to locate ourselves in a safe niche. All that exists is unified and coherent. The source is close at hand. It is the dimension of existence that abides and is present within all. We can't point to it as an object anymore than we can indicate something is a point, length, width, time, or that dimension into which the enfolding-expanding universe pulses. The source is within because the entire whole or system interrelates to itself persistently. There is nothing outside of it. The fifth dimension is not outside the system. The manifest universe is a subsection of a much greater whole that is not directly apparent to us. We imagine there is an outside when we think we need some exterior structure or process to provide us a safe haven from our conundrums, paradoxes, problems, riddles, and self-limiting ways. The mind is riddled. The mind is riddled with holes in our comprehension. This is not a failure or shortcoming. Our rich resource signifies that we can forever grow and learn. The universe is magnificent art yet in the making. Life is a reflection of the universe and dynamics that are vastly greater than our intellects. Life itself is magnificent art yet in the making. How does the emergence of human awareness, intelligence, sensitivities, hopes, dreams, faiths, ideas, and feelings affect the emergence of the universe (if at all)? This is one of the great enigmas (mysteries) for which there are no easy answers.

This sixth dimension may be the source for what we may call the first five dimensions. If we believe that something comes from something, then creation ex nihilo (something from nothing) just doesn't cut it. In the past, people tried to posit (make an assertion) the necessity of God by proposing that the universe came from the imagination and creativity of God (out of nothing). This saved them from the problem of infinite regression in which it was believed that everything had to come from something, but also everything has to have a beginning. If one directly experiences the presence of God (a direct experience of the heart and soul) or cerebrally believes in the existence of God (a much more abstract notion), there are more immediate ways to feel secure about one's experience or beliefs than by having to resort to God creating ex nihilo (unless you discover that a point of singularity without obvious extension in space-time may actually reflect the presence of a far greater creative context).

When we say that something comes from nothing, we are really saying that something comes from something about which we can know nothing directly within the context of our worldview, in which we split our very consciousness into objects orbiting around us as being the subject. This is referred to as the subject-object split. This topic of the subject-object split could be a rich vein (area) of cultural, historical, scientific, and philosophical research. A chopped-up universe causes us to be unable to experience the wholeness of the fabric of life of which we are one small and important part. This basic split in our consciousness is the most fundamental filter upon which we become dependent. The filter creates a useful and convenient illusion of separateness. The sixth dimension is the repository of this unknowable source for matter, mass, energy, space-time, infinity, and life. What a rather interesting realm. Something is from nothing that we can't directly know, and this "nothing" is something. This helps us explain the existence of vacuum fluctuations in the universe. (*See* "Vacuum Fluctuations—Something Really Weird Is under My Bed and It's Real.") Life is complete with imagination, love, passion, intuition, intellect, faith, wisdom, awareness, and soap operas, all from such impersonal stuff like matter, mass, energy, space-time, and infinity that are themselves from a dimension that can be called the source or substratum! Try mentioning this to your next-door neighbor next time you're talking about the weather.

The seventh dimension may be inferred from the existence of apparent tendencies (patterns) in the universe. Trees, roses, the eye, the heart, the brain, cells—all arose from the big bang, or the big bang occurred because it was induced by a field. Either there was information out there into which the space-time continuum grew, or the space-time continuum contained tendencies, patterns, or potential for development within itself. One of the greatest questions of all time has to do with whether or not this pattern-producing presence is self-aware (mindful of its own presence). What is the source of consciousness itself?

The sixth dimension is the source of all things. The seventh dimension is the quality of existence that retains and evolves root patterns. The sixth dimension is latently present in that it is the dimension to which things return when a universe enfolds back upon itself and from which the universe emerges. The seventh dimension is the manifest dimension revealed in different kinds of patterns that give us life and gave the universe existence. The seventh dimension is a direct reflection of the sixth dimension.

The patterns we observe can appear not to be consistent. Birth and death may appear to be inconsistent on some level until we realize that they are both parts of more encompassing phenomena of ongoing life. The seventh dimension is the repository of all possible patterns. The fifth and seventh dimensions share some similar qualities. The analogy between space-time growing into the fifth dimension and humankind growing into a comprehension of the seventh dimension could lead us to the conclusion that there are no multiple dimensions whatsoever. What we experience as a multiplicity with segments is actually a unified whole or Oneness. It is seamless. What appear to be separate things are the results of our minds being riddled and the prevalence (commonly existing) of the subject-object split in our cultural conditioning. Just as the mind is riddled, so too is the mind a distorting means of peering into life. The mind distills, names, and formats what rises into consciousness. This is necessarily a distorting function because we presume ourselves to be separate subjects observing separate objects out there beyond ourselves (yet another box). We are not looking out at life. We are within it and a dynamic and interactive part of it. What we experience as a segmented multiplicity is actually a manifold (many-faceted) unity. For this comprehension to crystallize, our root consciousness needs to be altered. The subject-object split needs to be overcome. In the meantime, we'll assume that there are multiple dimensions as a metaphorical way of speaking of the multiple facets (faces) of the unified universe.

We could have emerged or evolved in many different ways. The way the system as a whole acts upon itself creates the potential for many different emergent (arising) forms. Many people make the big mistake of thinking that because something is in existence, the patterns or laws of the universe necessarily were forced to emerge in this manner. Another related mistake is to infer (assume) from the current state of things that this was the intention of the source. One of the most interesting forms of this assumption is called the anthropic principle. We humans exist; therefore, the universe was designed with us and our peculiar needs in mind. Of course, this puts human beings at the top of the food chain in the entire universe. Inferences are always interesting. Look up the difference between an inference and an implication. While you're at it, look up the distinctions between deductive and inductive reasoning.

What is in existence is the result of infinitely complex and creative emergent interactive processes that are forever changing. (A great enigma has to do with how certain things retain some form over time—like our bodies, sense of self, the Earth, our galaxy, or the unique shape of our ever-so-precious earlobe). Our earlobes and many other things remind us of the source of all patterns, which is the seventh dimension. Next time you look into the mirror, look at that funny flap of skin at the bottom of the ear and be reminded of the seventh dimension. If somebody asks you what you are looking at with such amazement, just tell her or him in three words or less and then walk away with a smile on your face.

What is it that binds emergent processes together and gives them the reality and appearance of coherence over time? If quarks have gluons (the stuff that holds the quarks together), then all emergent processes—like our own individual lives—must have something that binds the preceding and past material with the succeeding, future, and possible material. A larger picture is needed that allows greater explanatory power.

What exists in the current moment may not be in the future. What exists currently is not the only possible outcome for the universe. Things could have been quite different, and they are probably quite different from what we presume things to be. Such an interesting life! The source of all things is creative. Its patterns are ever changing. If all things emerge from the source, it is possible for this source to be present as a dimension within all emergent processes. We don't need to look for a separate thing that provides us with an answer as to what yields coherence, identity, form, and patterns in a universe in which all things are emergent processes. Rather, the source of patterns is within all things. The source is the matrix (womb) for all potential patterns, including any manifestation of life. The manifestation of these patterns is the seventh dimension. We can call this seventh dimension many things. There can be a faith, religious, scientific, philosophic, or artistic way of looking at it. None of them is fully correct and none of them is wrong. There is a paradox at play. The very act or inclination of looking upon any object distorts the picture of what reality is, because of our primary presumption of separateness.

As things have emerged, certain tendencies are put into play. These tendencies create patterns that replicate themselves. These patterns become known as laws. The seventh dimension is what provides identity, coherence, integrity, and form. It is the seventh dimension that holds in creative balance the forces of change, process, and emergence with the tendencies for stability, form, and identity. In terms of the traditional four dimensions, this seventh dimension is nothing. In this case, something does emerge from nothing, but then there is a whole lot of interesting nothingness in our universe that we are blind to within the box that contains our lives from within which we look out at this object we call the universe.

Our minds are riddled (limited in our descriptive powers of what is ultimately real). Awe and wonder are the responses of a person who is awake to the greatness of Life! and the universe. Peer outside the box and behold with wonder, joy, anticipation, astonishment, and always with curiosity. Snoop outside the periphery that is assumed to be set by most others. The irony is that as we look outside of our limited way of viewing life and the universe, we discover that all things are interrelated and there is no outside. The paradox is that we have to look beyond in order to comprehend that we never did have to look beyond for a source of all life that creativity generates order and coherence in fresh ways. From this greater point of view, you look back and see there is no box. Yikes! This means you can't go back inside the little walls we presumed gave us security. Swallow that morsel of wisdom food and see what happens to your diet.

Another way of describing this seventh dimension is to say it is what abides (remains) when everything else changes. Another way of describing the seventh dimension is to say it is the original (primal, root) pattern from which all other patterns emerged. This original pattern is infinitely rich and complex, allowing and encouraging infinite variability. There is no one particular end pattern or outcome intentioned from the beginning, nor is there one single path to get to that single endpoint. Rather, the end (purpose) is enjoying the splendor of existence. If there are beginning points, it is natural for us to assume that there are ending points. If the universe does conform to this common pattern, with each ending, the universe could lose all of its patterns and memory. If the entire universe is enfolded into a point of singularity, it would seem that all information, patterns, and memory would be lost. It's not lost. When we realize that there are alternative ways of grasping our life context other than the boundaries of singular beginning points and singular ending points, then we see that life is renewing and evolving itself from all points all the time. Actually, the creative process is beyond time, but that is another topic.

Nietzsche was another person with a unique hairdo. This unusual hair thing obviously occurs because the geniuses are attracted to unusual ideas, and the roots of their hairs that are rooted in an area close to the brain become attracted—a strange attraction—to the unusual dimensions of life upon which this person is focusing his or her life. This is a fancy way of saying the person is thunderstruck with wonder and awe. For more information, look up the areas of cosmetology or cosmology. Take your pick. Nietzsche assumed that everything repeated itself over and over again. He reported that this was the single greatest discovery of his entire life. He called this eternal recurrence. What he missed was the insight that the seventh dimension allows for infinite variability. There is no reason to assume that any possible future times, universes, and life processes would be identical to this one. In the greatest rendition of our universe, because there is no time, there incidentally is no future. It all occurs at once. Don't tell anybody because her or she might try to buy you a new watch.

The seventh dimension could be viewed as the dimension of supertime encompassing what we call the past and present. It includes all emergences of universes within the fifth dimension. In other words, black holes do not wipe out all information. (I bet you were just about to stumble upon this little known and underappreciated possible fact. This could be more important than where you put your shoes last night!) There is a residual memory of past patterns that influences future emergent processes. It is the vitally important seventh dimension that yields a possible answer to an ancient enigma related to how patterns and form appear and sustain themselves. Retention of information, patterns, form, or identity in a most primitive manner (in a basic way) is what allows there to be any manifestation of things that seem to abide over time. Nothing on the surface remains forever. All outward manifestations of everything pass through continual transformation. The seventh dimension's supertime presence is the substratum in which all processes interrelate. Some things catch on and take shape over time. All things pass away having lasted only a brief period of time. Some underlying impression abides. What has been matters. Once all matter ceases (if it ever does), something is retained. What will be matters. What we contribute in the present is of utmost (greatest) importance because we are all interrelated and no one being exists alone. Each of us shapes and affects our shared environment in ways that far surpass words. This is the basis for all life-honoring ethics. To be consumed with a self-centered existence is the greatest waste of the gift of life, and this manner of living projects unnecessary suffering that others must bear (carry, experience). The entire point of all existence is to be a full partner in sharing life. What we do with our lives ultimately does matter.

The trick is not to hold on to things that are by definition transient—as though our security and meaning can come from passing phenomenon (like being young, having a new red car, being married, being a parent, being a certain age). All things continue to be in process, but certain impressions linger. Giving ourselves to the process of life is the gift of finding peace. It's all changing. Hope is in our embrace of what is real. Hope is not in our imagined capacity to hold on to what we desire in the present moment or wish we had from the past or might have in the future. A great proportion of the violence people inflict on each other is rooted in misplaced and ill-defined hope. We create tremendous unnecessary suffering as the result. The greatest faith is giving ourselves endlessly to life, hoping only that we can contribute to the richness of the gift of being fully alive.

Given this dimension of supertime, it is possible to talk about prior and succeeding manifestations of emergent universes or about yesterday at the movies with our friends. Without this seventh dimension, there is no past or future beyond the event horizon of a big bang and big implosion. There would be no fourth dimension kind of time, either, in which we may realize that we're late for work or school because we've been reading about the seventh dimension. Now, at long last, you have the perfect excuse! Do you dare to use it? If there is a seventh dimension, there is memory and awareness that includes all actual and potential and all past and future universes. To talk about universes is cold and abstract. Remember that the universe is what makes life possible, and what applies to the universe is relevant to all life. Human beings like to imagine that we are metaphysical exceptions (absolutely unique) to everything else in the universe (including other forms of life). The universe is our home. It can teach us lessons about living. If all dimensions are one unified whole, life and the universe are a unified whole also.

This seventh dimension is not psychological memory and awareness. It is what makes psychological memory and awareness possible to emerge. It is the substratum becoming manifest in the form of Life! It's that simple! Now you've got it. Please don't try to package it. The seventh dimension is the retention of patterns that are more primitive and basic than brain functions, but this memory and awareness are the bases for our lives also. The terms *memory* and *awareness* are simply not synonymous with ego-based memory and awareness. It is very possible that there are residual manifestations of this primitive and primordial memory and awareness available to us as we go outside the box that we discover isn't there.

The sixth dimension is the quality of being the primordial source that is present in all things as a potential dimension that will emerge when there is an implosion or manifestation of space-time and matter-energy. It is the unrecognized home base for the first five dimensions. The seventh dimension is transtemporal (greater than the confines of time as it relates to the first three dimensions). Time is Janus-faced (two-faced, from Roman mythology).

As time relates to the first three dimensions, it appears to be limited to the space-time continuum. It appears to split the past and the future. In the formulas of physics, the arrow of time can run forward or backward. Given this kind of time, everything looks as though things are ordered in a linear sequence always proceeding according to the arrow of time that seems to inevitably run from the past to the future relative to our mind's interpretation of our five senses. (*See* "Senses—Imagine Some More.") The first face of time relates to the three dimensions.

The other face of time relates to the fifth, sixth, and seventh dimensions. One could realize this seven-dimensional reality as a simultaneous, interrelated, ever-emergent, and creative Oneness. In this seven-dimensional universe:

- Time is not chopped up into discrete (separate) units arbitrarily call the past, present, and future.
- Things are not rent (torn) apart as subjects and objects.
- There are no seams splitting apart, one dimension from another.
- Endings are not tragedies.
- Beginnings are replete (prepackaged from the life womb) with an unending and evolving set of possibilities that do not determine the precise form of emergent processes.
- There is no past and future, because all things occur with an ever-recurring seamless simultaneity.
- Every moment contains its own unique potential.
- In every moment, there is some degree of uncertainty and freedom.

- Multiple outcomes (results, effects, and consequences) are possible in every moment.
- Life is not a different order distinct from what has been called the inanimate universe.
- What we call learning, growth, and memory are reflections of this more basic impulse of the universe toward creativity and transformation.
- There is no radical bifurcation (two essentially different things being rooted in different kinds of dimensions of life) as to what is conscious and what is not (the system is not blind to its own existence).
- This Oneness labors and plays: the labor is toward greater orders of richness and possibility, while its play is related to delight, mirth, joy, and the sheer exuberance of life.

From our human perspective, the seventh dimension is the actual memory of all prior universes. The past matters are reflected in what currently exists. What has existed is not lost. What you do with your life is of greatest importance. What you feed Fido under the table and the reasons for the food drop bear the greatest consequences for all time and in supertime in the seventh dimension. Be nice. Strive to find your greatest sense of self before your body gives out.

This is truly stranger than science fiction and more wonderful than a three-year-old child running naked outside in a pouring rain in a blazing thunderstorm accompanied by howling winds! (I'm assuming everybody else did this when they were three, because every three-year-old knows that the seventh dimension of supertime bears patterns of other three-year-olds doing the same thing.) They even have figured out that the past and the future are one seamless simultaneous evolving miracle. That's why three-year-olds smile so wonderfully and jump up in the air with such glee (they know gravity, time, and space are an illusion). This is slightly beyond genetics and a nature-nurture discussion. Talk to your pediatrician or local librarian about this topic. At the doctor's office and at the library, they'll have a special section just for you. Hint: big people with white coats are standing at the door of these special sections.

The fifth dimension is that into which the universe expands and enfolds. The sixth dimension is that from which all else emerges—the source. It is present within all fields and things as a potential to which it will return and from which it emerged. The seventh dimension is quality of retention of patterns. This is relatively straightforward. Yikes! We "gotta get outta" this place, but there is no outside. We might as well stay put and make the best of it.

What takes a little more chutzpah (pizzazz, flare for originality) is to imagine the seventh dimension retaining the past's actual and potential patterns and the future's actual and potential emergent patterns! How? The sixth and seventh dimensions are not time-dependent. Time is something we invented to explain the three dimensions that did not have a larger context of the other dimensions.

Beyond the first three dimensions, most metaphors break down in being effective tools for communication. This is why symbols and metaphors of physics, poetry, religion, or mathematics are the tools most people use to communicate the ineffable (try ineluctable, and if that doesn't work, then substitute unspeakable). Call these musings anything, but please don't call them recondite or abstruse (really hard to grasp) and irrelevant.

A simultaneous past and future is a big bite. Ouch! That can hurt the jaws if we read the sentence aloud. Actually, you should never read this stuff out loud because somebody might hear you and wonder quite seriously if you are OK. It's not that weird. Why should the universe conform to what our culture and individual brains and minds think is necessary, given the box of the four dimensions? There is something living beyond the walls! Maurice Sendak in his book *Where the Wild Things Are* imagined another place beyond the walls with its own wild ways and life. The awareness of the other place began within the four walls of Max's own home. The wild rumpus for Max occurred because he was ready for such a journey. A more complete picture of life beyond the four walls of the four dimensions can cause an uproar and wild rumpus. We run across such strange creatures as simultaneous universes, virtual particles, and ideas that create revolutions in our current way of thinking. Don't try to keep these strange creatures locked in a zoo, or try to keep them hidden on a secret island. Life's creativity and intelligence won't be kept hidden on some secret island controlled by our conceptions and personal needs.

Broaden our perspective, and wild things begin to kick up a real rumpus with the old stuff contained in tight little boxes. The dust really flies. No zoo or park on any distant island could possibly control or contain this stuff. Life does find a way to express itself in ways that exceed our expectations.

In review: The fourth dimension really jerked things around for the people who had to stay within the bounds of the three dimensions. The fourth dimension was needed in order to explain paradoxes of the first three. Little did they realize that the fourth dimension is very strange because it is two-faced (one face relates to the first three dimensions and the other face relates to the fifth, sixth, and seventh dimensions). The fifth dimension is that into which the space-time continuum is expanding. The sixth dimension is the source of all the dimensions. The seventh dimension is supertime in which patterns are retained from all universes existing simultaneously. Our metaphors are extremely limited. Simultaneous here does not mean the future has already happened in the past. Nor does it mean that something could go from the present into the future to alter something that affects something in the past that creates severe disturbances for our present time. The seventh dimension is not confined by the limitations of the metaphors that obey the rules of language relative only to three dimensions. This round object is not going to fit into the square hole of the current metaphors. The fifth through seventh dimensions are slightly startling. Watch out for anything that is slightly startling, because this is the material of life we generally push to the periphery (edge) of our awareness. It is here at the boundaries that different renditions (versions) of reality meet and interplay. These boundary experiences are the interface (place of two faces—where we can see and experience at least two different realities that add depth, novelty, and richness to our lives).

When Dorothy in *The Wizard of Oz* was swept away by the tornado, her house slammed down into another place. She appeared to have been living in a black-and-white world. As she opened her door and looked outside, she said to her favorite little dog, "Toto—I've a feeling we're not in Kansas anymore. We must be over the rainbow!" She might as well have been speaking for all of us. She flew outside her black-and-white box. She opened the door and there was a world of marvelous color and sights. Once she discovered the world of color, she may have thought backward to realize that her previous life in Kansas (no slam on the real Kansas) was never just black and white. When we look back at her world in Kansas before the tornado came and whisked (took) her away, it never was merely black and white. It was shades of brown and white. In other words, our world of three dimensions or our world of any little box we've been confined to is never totally black and white. It is always at least sepia (a special rendition of brown that hints at the possibility of other colors, dimensions, thoughts, intuitions, dreams, feelings, wisdom, and compassion). Watch out for hints, glimmers, and things that intimate the presence of more-encompassing views, experiences, and comprehension. Go back and see the movie again. The beginning was not in black and white. Now once you've ventured beyond some kind of confining box, look back and see the many hints of greater things. These hints of extraordinary stuff are scattered throughout our lives. In our confined boxes that appear to be black and white, there is more than meets the eye. Always there are hints of greater things within our confines. Why do we miss these cues and clues of greater stuff? Go deeper and find your true identity that allows you to explore, grow, learn, and evolve without fear. With this discovery of your true identity as sojourner, you will discover the fullness of Life! You'll never go back to just using ketchup, salt, and pepper! Bring on the spices and hot sauce!

Now that we have the seven dimensions clearly in mind, we can go back to the first thing discussed—the nondimension of a point. What we call a point might actually be an infinitely dense focal point of dimensions that is not readily apparent to us. Sometime look up *superstring theory*, which can complement some of the things shared in this section. This point of singularity can be the eighth dimension. The eighth dimension is like the gateway serving as the entry to the fifth, sixth, and seventh dimensions. Some persons have theorized about the existence of white holes and wormholes—might these be the portals to other dimensions?

This infinitely small point of singularity would be the gateway to the source. Matter, energy, mass, space-time, and hot sauce are persistently (constantly) being reconstituted (transformed) because of the presence of this sixth and seventh dimension. Perhaps this eighth dimension is both a gateway to the sixth and seventh dimensions as well as the "place" into which any expanded form of a universe may collapse or enfold. All matter, energy, mass, and space-time would then be enfolded into this point of infinite singularity. It is infinitely singular only from our human perspective rooted in space-time.

We can only imagine what happens to matter, energy, mass, and space-time within this possible point of singularity. We can only have hints of this state of existence in what we theorize exists at the core black holes—the infinitely dense point of singularity. This is the Sepia Effect. Only after we gain a wider perspective (like Dorothy did; who knows if Toto ever noticed?) can we think backward and see the hints and clues of wider dimensions. We can't go beyond anything if we don't, in the current moment, sense the possibility of something greater. The other aspect of the Sepia Effect is that since our minds are riddled with holes of comprehension, we are able to sense the presence of these holes. Some expression of genius will leap through them. Recall that genius is the expression of the unique complex of gifts each individual carries within her or him. Discovery of this genius within ourselves is yet another example of the Sepia Effect at play in our lives. From within our current context there are the seeds of greater comprehension. The irony of the Sepia Effect is that we have to go beyond and look back to gain perspective, while at the same time the seeds of greater comprehension are sewn into the fabric of life in the form of holes that are opportunities for growth. In its simplest form, the Sepia Effect means that we always need a greater comprehension of our life situation and potential in order to savor the wisdom that is forever revealing itself to all of us in all our experiences.

From the perspective of the space-time continuum, the other dimensions are nothing—dimensionless, inexplicable, beyond the limits of human comprehension, and outside the box. From the perspective of the fifth, sixth, and seventh dimensions, all exists in supertime, there is nothing outside the box, nothing is wiped out, and all is whole. There you have it—eight handy dimensions. Don't worry about the ordinal position (order) of the named dimensions. In reality, all dimensions are a unity forming a perfect seamless whole. The described order of the dimensions is of no importance except as a way of comprehending something that is beyond our comprehension. Is comprehension of the incomprehensible a contradiction (inconsistency) or oxymoron (two opposites positioned next to each other)? The next time you need a conversation starter at a party, trot out an ordinary oxymoron and then transition neatly and adroitly into the topic of eight handy dimensions. See what happens!

A different view of more dimensions would be as follows. The first four dimensions are length, width, depth, and space-time. The fifth dimension is the point of contact with the sixth through ninth dimensions. This fifth dimension can be viewed as an infinitely dense point of singularity, a boundary, or as a quality seeded within all the other dimensions everywhere. The sixth through the ninth dimensions are the three geometric dimensions and time in an antiparticle universe. The tenth dimension is that into which these antithetical (opposite and potentially self-annihilating) universes expand. The eleventh dimension is the source of all dimensions. The twelfth dimension is the supertime dimension that retains impressions and patterns. Some people say that nature abhors a vacuum. (Look up a guy named Spinoza.) Perhaps nature loves perfect symmetry. Perhaps there is perfect symmetry and balance between the universe composed of matter and the other made of antimatter. Perhaps there is something inherent to the relationship between the two simultaneous universes that causes periodic big bangs and periodic processes of the universe enfolding upon itself.

Apply a similar magnitude of energy, imagination, observation, intelligence, feeling, sensitivity, and intuition to any other aspect of life. Go way beyond what others accept as being normal, real, and necessary. Apply this gift to art, mathematics, history, social issues, environmental issues, personal issues, and peace and justice issues. Don't just settle for what others describe as set things. See with your mind's eye and heart's intuition what might be possible. Have several such thoughts and visions every day before breakfast (so you can digest your food better) and definitely before you go to sleep (so that your sleeping energies can be very creative also). Just be careful what you feed your dog under the table.

Extensions

Any time somebody says something like, "There are three ways to understand this process or subject," start to think about alternative ways to picture or describe the process. Are there more dimensions than others are seeing? Remember that dimensions do not refer to separate things beyond the pale (what is known and accepted as legitimate). They refer to inherent (internal) qualities that may not be sensed, seen, intuited, imagined, thought, or felt. If you alter your picture of a thing or process, there are certain consequences. For instance, when somebody talks about thinking going on inside the head, start to play with the terms *in and out* of the *head*. Could there be anything that goes on inside one's own head that can be shared between two people? If you can picture this in your head, can you get out of the framework that says that everything about thought is inside of the head?

Play with words. Alter pictures of reality! You are the source of creativity! See things differently. Imagine some of the consequences. How many times have you had original thoughts and you didn't want to believe them? How many times have slightly strange insights been pushed to the periphery (edges) of your awareness as a means of not disturbing the predominant (main) way of thinking, feeling, or sensing? We most often neutralize and eliminate options that defy easy explanations and insights that require major transformations of all our life material. These original or novel insights or intuitions may have startled you. They do not fit neatly with your other sets of ordinary thoughts and impressions. You may have denied them because it takes too much work or play to entertain them. You may have excluded them because if you make a place for them you would have to rearrange the stage upon which your life is lived, or you may realize there is no stage to return to—all of life is not a stage, after all. You may not have wanted to share them with others because of what you think or feel they might think of you.

The process of the unfolding of these slightly startling insights and intuitions is a reflection of the realm of genius. Most often, genius is snuffed out, neutralized, eliminated, discounted, or ignored. Your genius is needed. Follow your heart and imagination along the trail that your genius reveals to you. The path is unique to you, and what is unique to you is needed by the world. Either we believe that there is nothing new under the sun (Nietzsche and the Book of Ecclesiastes) or we can believe that there is a dimension to life that is ever-fresh, creative, adventuresome, novel, and inventive (Alfred North Whitehead and Alfred E. Newman). Maybe what appears to be set is being examined in too small a context or frame of reference, and thus we miss the reality that all things are forever in flux (change). This book is an invitation to all readers: come out and play. The genius within you is something like a point of singularity. It can't be seen until something emerges from it. You are the source and you are the memory of such encounters with creativity, insight, and intuition. Don't just let them pass away.

DISCRIMINATION

If we discriminate (make fundamental distinctions or judgments about others) on the basis of gender, race, age, sexual orientation, or ethnic origins, this keeps certain persons excluded from the job market, from residence in certain neighborhoods, from attendance at certain schools, or from full participation in many groups. It makes life greatly more complex and projects massive unnecessary suffering. Many others believe that we need to discriminate in order to preserve the order of society.

In one sense, we need to discriminate. If we couldn't discriminate between a red and green light at intersections, our lives would be endangered. Imagine how the universe would rock if we couldn't discriminate between true, honest junk food and other stuff that only looks, tastes, and smells like junk food but turns out to be perfectly healthful and nutritious food. If you couldn't discriminate, you might accidentally eat something that is good for you and makes your body feel energetic. Some forms of discrimination are necessary and good. Describe them. What forms of discrimination harm other people? Are there some forms of discrimination that are morally wrong but are not illegal? Are we even aware of how powerful an influence it is to discriminate against others? Are we aware that some forms of discrimination can hurt people for the rest of their lives?

Extensions

Why do people so often discriminate in a way that hurts other people? Learn as much as you can about how people use power and privilege for their own gain. What stories have you read with themes relating to this topic? What have you seen in your own life? Wherever there is discrimination, some group excludes others. Have you ever been left out or excluded? How did it feel? Use your own experience to help foster (encourage) life-affirming values and behaviors.

DISTANCES IN SPACE

If we were to measure distances in space in terms of inches, we'd need many zeroes. Therefore, we have something called a light-year. What is a light year? Now scientists have come up with even bigger units of measurements for space because space is so big. Look up the term *parsec* to begin with.

Extensions

We have many different ways of measuring things. List the various kinds of things and processes we measure (rate of growth, life span, number of rotations of a planet per year).

Now with this list, look at any one of the items (for example, the volume of water flowing in a river per given unit of time) and try to imagine a different way of measuring the thing or process. In this case of the river, we might try to figure out the volume of water per year. Instead of looking at the phenomenon as a volume of water, try to figure out how much space the river occupies, and thus you might be able to estimate how much water is contained in a river at one moment in time. Change the picture or image of the problem in your mind, and then entirely different results become available to you.

DISTANT MOUNTAINS

If you were on the flat prairie at sea level, how close would you have to be to a ten-thousand-foot mountain in order to see its peak? Assume the flat prairie extends to the base of the mountain. If you were one hundred miles or five hundred miles away from a mountain, how high would it have to be in order to see its peak?

Extensions

Where on Earth or where in the universe is there a flat plane? Determine the kind of knowledge you'd need in order to figure out these answers. Is a one-square-yard plot of land curved? It would seem reasonable to expect that since the Earth is curved, then any section of its surface would be curved.

If this one square yard of Earth is curved, then you are higher if you stand in the middle of the one square yard as opposed to standing at the edge of the one square yard. If so, then what about the next one square yard of Earth's turf? Is that person just as high as you are if the other person is standing directly at the center of the other one square yard of Earth, assuming no hills or valleys and assuming the curvature of the Earth is uniform (regular)? If so, are persons standing at the edge that joins these two square yards together lower than the other two persons? If so, what happens if we choose to overlay (superimpose) a new one-square-yard half way over the first two (adding nothing except the markings for a third square yard of Earth)? Then suddenly, are the persons who are standing at the edges of the first two square yards higher, just as high, or lower than the other two persons standing at the center of the first two square yards? Wouldn't it be easier to believe that the Earth is flat? Ever hear the phrase: "Don't confuse me with the facts?" Frameworks matter greatly. We stage (arrange) what we focus on as being significant. This is why all of life really is a stage in a sense (*See* " Dimensions—How Many?"). Where the various stages or frameworks intersect, these are the places of conflict, confusion, growth, learning, and creative tension.

DIVERSITY IN NATURE AND HUMAN SENTIMENTS

As we look around at the various forms of life and the diverse inanimate objects in nature, it is obvious that nature loves diversity. Why is diversity a good thing for species, families, or groups as they are evolving? Why is it that so many people feel so uncomfortable with diverse kinds of people? Why do we tend to seek our own kind of characters with whom to associate? Why do so many people treat others outside of their immediate circles of loved ones and friends with so little acceptance?

Extensions

Another part of us likes and is attracted to others who are different from ourselves. What are some characteristics of other persons who are very different from yourself that you enjoy? Are there any cultures in which diversity is a core value?

DIVERTING ATTENTION

The shell game is one of the oldest games related to diverting the attention of observers. The practitioner takes three half-shells and puts something underneath one of them. The objective is to make it look as though the hidden object has disappeared or reappeared in an unexpected place as if by magic.

This is an artful way of diverting attention. What are other practices that people employ to divert people's attention? What are the various reasons people would want to divert other's attention? Look up the word *prestidigitation*.

Changing our point of view is a very important ability. When we shift our point of view, we may experience an entirely different situation. Becoming aware that we are currently experiencing life through the filter of a certain point of view can be surprising. As we learn how to be aware of our capacity for attention and concentration, we gain powerful creative resources. We can become aware that in every moment there is a focal point. It is amazing to learn how to shift our concentration from one object to the context in which any and all our thoughts and feelings emerge. This is shifting from a concentration that tunes out much of what is occurring around us to a deeply sensitive attentiveness that is aware of entire processes at play. As these capacities are developed, we are able to see deeply into the creative processes available to us and those that are being used by others.

Extensions

Great storytellers will be able to steer the listener's attention away from drawing conclusions that the storyteller doesn't want them focused on. One form of this is in debates or discussions. One method used at any point in the story or presentation is to state something that is obvious to any observer. Then the presenter implants elements of the story that ride along on the coattails of the obvious fact that has been shared. In this way, the story is shaped to fit the needs of the presenter. The perfect diversionary kernel at just the right place in a presentation will divert attention. When a teenager comes in the door hours late and begins by saying, "Don't worry, Dad and Mom, everybody is alive thanks to me"—fill in the blank with a good story. What are various tools you can use to test to see if you're being snowballed (blinded, diverted, being had)? Here are some basic tools:

- Test for internal consistency of the entire story.
- Test to see if the current story fits with the larger context of prior experience with this person.
- Carefully test to see where the organizing nuggets or kernels of the story are located.
- The nuggets or kernels that can direct attention in any story are not necessarily big and obvious turning points.
- Examine the effect of these nuggets or kernels on your judgment.
- Trust your feelings and intuitions in terms of the credibility of the story.
- Test to see if you trust the basic story but certain elements being presented as facts are askew (off-kilter, not ringing true).

- Test to see the goals, purposes, and objectives of the story.
- If the story seems to be confused, it may be because the storyteller is confused and is telling the truth to the best of her or his abilities at the time.
- Test to see who benefits and who loses anything from the story.
- Test to see if you feel compelled to accept it; if so, understand the dynamics that compel you.
- In the present moment (real time), we often miss cues, signals, and hints that later become obvious.
- Go back to the story later when you are fresh and distanced from the original exposure to the story.
- If you feel yourself getting impassioned or involved in the story, slow down and concentrate; listen as objectively as you can.
- If you have great stakes (involved in some significant way) in the story, be extraordinarily vigilant in listening.
- Test to see if you are falling prey (victim) to the dynamic that "everybody else believes it, so, of course, I will."
- What will be the consequences for you if you believe the story?
- What will be the consequences for others if you believe and share the story?
- Is the teller of the story speaking from the heart?
- Test to see if somebody is speaking from the heart but is so deluded that they believe an untruth wholeheartedly.
- Be mindful that some elements of a story may appear to be repugnant (disgusting) or extremely contrary to what you value but may still be true.
- Just because the person speaking or writing a story doesn't fit any of your personal criteria for being trustworthy doesn't mean that the person is diverting attention from what is true, in this one single instance.
- Just because a storyteller or author fits all of your criteria (profile) of a person who is trustworthy does not mean that you are hearing the truth.
- Use the tried-and-true method of suspending your judgment, and carefully listen to the story.

Always be mindful of whose point of view is being expressed in any story, accounting, or report. Be aware of who is controlling (or attempting to control) the point of whatever is being expressed. Carefully observe how there are critical juncture points at which the point of view can be changed in many different ways. Explore this topic of how people change the point of view in any presentation.

DOWN TO THE WIRE

When you pull on a light chain attached to an overhead light socket (often located in the basements of our homes), try to figure out if the little balls strung on the wire were created by hand or by a machine. How are these pull chains created? What are other common things around your home that make you wonder how they are made?

Extensions

How do they make wire? Look up *extrusion*.

DRAINING WATER

Next time you can observe water draining down a tube, see which way it swirls. If you are letting out the water in your kitchen sink, repeat this process three times. Does it always drain out the same way? On the fourth experiment, try taking your finger, a large stiff spatula, or large stirring spoon and just as you let out the water, stir the water in the opposite direction. Do you think it will continue to drain in the same direction?

Extensions

If you live in the Northern Hemisphere, what would you expect to happen if you were in the Southern Hemisphere? Would the water drain swirling down in the same direction? Why doesn't the water just drain straight down the drain? What might happen if you were on the equator? What might happen if you were at the North or South Pole (besides freezing very quickly)? Next time you meet an astronaut, ask her or him which way water drains on the moon (assuming the astronaut has artificial gravity environment). If he or she is on the ball (or at least has been to the moon), he or she would ask you to which part of the moon are you referring (Northern or Southern Hemisphere).

DREAMING—KNOWING YOU ARE AWAKE

When you are asleep and dreaming, how do you know that you are only dreaming and that what you are experiencing is not really happening?

Extensions

Is there a sense in which a person is awake yet dreaming? Could this be happening when a person makes something they desire very intensely seem real? Since we are dependent upon our five senses in order to communicate with the outside world, we never experience things in and of themselves. We constantly interpret what we see. What we have ever taken to be real, we also reinvent or reshape constantly. What is the sense in which we are dreaming while awake?

DREAMS—AND SOME COME TRUE

Is it a waste of time to have dreams? Is it wasteful to daydream how things could be if human beings would imagine new ways of existing?

If you like exploring the realms of human wisdom and insight, you might try keeping track of your dreams. Often they teach us things about ourselves. Sometimes they help us figure out complex challenges. Look up the chemical benzene. Who discovered it? More important, read about how the person discovered the benzene molecule structure. Dreaming will never be the same again! There is something special about early in the morning. The mind is alert and relaxed. It is fully focused in very creative ways. Many people report awakening to startling insights and great wisdom early in the morning.

There is another kind of dream. We go through life in many different ways. Some people are consumed with dreams of being independent of others. Others dream of power, while others dream of how things might be if human beings were to become alert to the possibilities of a different way of organizing our lives. Keep dreaming dreams of:

- how more people can be fed
- how more children could live and not die from starvation and malnutrition
- how people would not have to live in fear of violence
- how we could live and not pollute the Earth so much
- how we could settle our conflicts without warfare
- how men and women could find ways of communicating and relating on a more equal common ground
- how we could live in a world in which race was not used as a weapon against others
- how our schools could be better places

Dream and work for a better world. Some of these may come true. We need them all to come true if we are to have a viable future.

Extensions

List the things you'd like to see improved in the world. Do you really think these things could be changed? How? What can you do?

DUST BOWL

In the 1930s, a severe drought affected a large region of the central portion of our country. It lasted many years. This area was called the dust bowl. Find out some of the contributing factors to this drought.

Extensions

Could this kind of thing happen again? Where did all the dust go? Did farming practices in those times contribute to the severity of the dust storms and loss of topsoil? Are our current farming practices causing erosion of topsoil?

If we know better ways of farming, why don't we change our farming practices? Look up how many different kinds of pesticides, fungicides, and other toxic chemicals are being sprayed on our food. Which of these chemicals have been identified as being potentially harmful to human beings? Is there a totally safe exposure limit for these chemicals? Do we know what kinds of exposures cause cancers of different kinds? Are there alternatives? What is organic farming? Is it right and fair to ask people to harvest our food when they are exposed on a regular basis to toxic chemicals?

EARTH—ITS WEIGHT

Find out how to compute an arithmetic mean (average). The simplest form is to take two people, add their weights together, and divide the total by two. This is the average weight of the two people. For ten people, add all their weights together and divide the sum by ten.

For the sake of estimation, how much would you say an average child weighs? If childhood and adolescence run from birth through eighteen years, take the middle age of nine years. Alternatively, you could take the average weight of six-, twelve-, and eighteen-year-olds and then average these figures together. In order to assign some weight figures, you need to look up some data on the topic or you could use a group of persons in this age group. If the group of persons you select is going to represent all the other persons in this age group, what kinds of things do you need to do in order to assure (or at least raise the probability) that the selected group actually does represent the entire population of persons from birth through eighteen years? This is called criteria for research. One hint is that the group needs to have enough people in it that you avoid getting skewed (bent, biased, inaccurate) data. Derive (get) your average figure.

How much would you assume an average adult woman weighs? Repeat the process of selecting a representative group or get some data from a trustworthy data source. Assign some number.

How much would you assume an average adult male weighs? Repeat the process that you used for the other two groups. Assign some number.

Assume that there are about 5½ billion people on the face of the Earth. Slightly over 50 percent of the people are women. Assign some proportion of the total population to children, and adult females and adult males. There are figures available that will help you determine what proportion of the population is eighteen and under versus what proportion is over eighteen years of age. Derive a total figure for weight for all the people on the face of the Earth.

Imagine how much all the trees on the Earth weigh. Would all the animals on Earth weigh as much as the total weight for human beings? Now what about the total weight for all the microorganisms on the Earth? Be careful here; these microorganisms are very small but they're great in number. Next, try to figure out the weight of the air. Remember that the air pressure at sea level is 14.2 pounds per square inch. How many square inches in a square foot? How many square feet are in a square mile? How many square miles are on the surface of the Earth? Multiply the number of square miles times the amount of air pressure in one square mile.

Add all of these weights together. This is a huge number! Now try to guess how much the Earth weighs.

How much would you say the entire Earth weighs? Don't read any further until you've determined a method to figure out the answer. Get your approximation of the answer. Write down your answer.

Would you believe that the Earth with all the life forms, its own matter, and all the air pressure weighs almost zero? Why almost zero?

Extensions

Other than the sun, what else has a gravitational influence on the Earth? Have several different people do this same research project. At the end, compare your methods for deriving (getting) the answer and what answers you all came up with.

EARTHSHINE

Where can you find Earthshine? What is it? Hint: you may not be able to find it on Earth at all. If you were to observe the Earth from the moon, would the Earth have phases like the moon does (new, full, and in-between)? A major hint as to Earthshine is that the Earth's phase is complementary to the moon's phases (meaning that when the new moon is at its darkest (relative from the view from the Earth), the Earth's phase is full (relative from the perspective from the moon). Earthshine has to do with a double reflection of sunshine, and it is most obvious when the moon is in a new phase. It is a real phenomenon.

Extensions

What are the most unusual lighting conditions you've ever experienced?

EARTH SPIN

Do the other planets spin in the same direction as the Earth?

Extensions

Do they all spin? Do the moons spin? Does the solar system spin? How could we know if the solar system spins? Does the galaxy spin? Do the galaxy clusters and superclusters spin? Does the entire universe spin? Where does spin come from? When politicians are trying to minimize negative public reaction to something they've done, they hire spin doctors to come in and put a spin on the interpretation of events. Where did this use of the term *spin* come from?

EAST AND WEST

What is the easternmost point in the United States of America? If you want the answer, read on. If you want a hint, here it is. Where does east and west begin? Where do they end? Does this give you any clues? Another mind boggler: Where in North America is the closest point to the easternmost point in South America?

Extensions

Alter the manner in which challenges, problems, or life issues are presented to you. Often when they are recast in new ways, surprising solutions arise. The easternmost point in the United States is an island that is not off the coast of Maine. The closest point in North America to the eastern tip of South America is not the Florida Keys, the southern tip of Texas, or the southern tip of California. Look at a flat map first and then look at a globe. Does this change your perspective on the question? Hint: as you pass your finger over the curvilinear surface of a globe remember the great circle route. If you have not heard about this idea before, look it up. This turns to be the shortest distance between two points in curvilinear space or on curvilinear surfaces.

EFFECT AND AFFECT

What is the difference between these two words, effect and affect?

Extensions

What are other words that sound alike or are similar in some way but have very different meanings? Develop a list of such words. Try starting with some of the following word combinations: corroborate and collaborate, effect and affect, prescribe and proscribe, confidence and competence, healthy and healthful, immersed and emersed, loose and lose, inflect and reflect, refract and reflect, and its and it's. If you feel like it, you could develop quite a long list of interesting similar-sounding words with quite different meanings.

EFFICIENT VERSUS EFFECTIVE

Do some research and find out the difference between being efficient and being effective. This difference (distinction) is very important. Pretend that you are a manager in a manufacturing plant producing automobiles. What would it mean to be efficient versus being effective? If you are approaching a due date for a report in school, how do efficiency and effectiveness help you? (*See* "Light, Heat, and Electrons.")

Extensions

In any assignment, are you clear on the main expectations? Are the expectations consistent or contradictory? Are all the expectations expressed? When you look at the sum total of all the expectations, are they realistic? Are you meeting these expectations? Also, are you wasting a lot of energy moving toward the completion of the task? Name four tasks around the house. How are you doing on them? Define your success at the tasks in terms of efficiency and effectiveness.

EINSTEIN—E = mc^2

A penny weighs about three grams. If you take one-third of a penny and convert its matter entirely into energy, how much water do you think it will boil? Would you believe about forty-three million gallons? How many bathtubs would this fill? How many gallons does your bathtub hold? The famous formula $E = mc^2$ tells us that energy and mass are equivalent. How does this transformation occur?

Extensions

With this same one-third of a penny converted to energy, what else would you be able to do? What material on Earth is the most resistant to melting (which has the highest melting point)? Which has the lowest melting point? As long as you're at it, which material becomes a gas at the highest temperature? Which becomes a gas at the lowest point? When energy is applied or taken away from any given material, what other qualities of the material may be changed? One example might be its capacity to conduct electricity. Think of other examples of qualities that are altered by heat being applied or taken away from a material.

EINSTEIN—RADAR TIME-DELAYED CURVATURE OF SPACE-TIME CONTINUUM

There have been space program experiments conducted in which radar signals were sent over long distances from space to Earth. The length of time between transmission and reception of the signal on Earth was delayed in time for a longer period than was expected. The 1976–77 Viking space mission to Mars conducted these experiments. What caused this time delay? Hint: Einstein demonstrated that concentrations of matter curve the space-time continuum. The signal was sent through curved space and not the imaginary path of flat space.

Extensions

When we look out at space, we see three-dimensional linear space. We draw a line in our mind's eye from our source (point of view) to a destination (some planet or distant star that is observable). We imagine we see a straight line between the subject and us. What we see is reality, right? This is not the case. Space-time is curvilinear and not linear. What are other examples of seeing or experiencing things with our senses and minds that convince us things are a certain way, but upon further reflection, we learn that the subject under consideration is quite different? Try starting with an example related to your initial judgments about a particular person. Can groups of persons be inaccurate in their assessments (judgments) of other groups, or is this only something that happens to individuals? Think of some examples in your life and ask yourself how we learn and grow beyond our illusions and misunderstandings. What are the habits we cultivate that make it less likely that we'll learn and grow?

ENEMIES

Do people hate other people? Might they really be focused on a picture, image, stereotype, memory, anticipation, or definition that is hated, then this hate gets projected onto a person or group? If one hated insecurity and fear, when a person or group arises that causes this person to feel insecure, then might this person hate the other person or group? We see a person. We react to his or her presence based on our conditioning and prior habits. Our reaction is to project a certain interpretation, inference, or image of that person. We may be repelled by our projection, and strong emotional reactions may follow. Does any of this process necessarily have anything to do with the other person?

Extensions

Why is hate such an explosive feeling? What does it do to the one who hates? When we portray others to be a symbol of something we detest, hate, or loathe, then do we cease seeing this individual as a human being? Do we experience them in a very narrow and confining manner? Do we create a picture of the person or group that is like an object we can scorn (hate)? Have you ever caught yourself saying to yourself, "That person is nothing but . . ." Fill in the blank. Is hate justified when someone has been violent to you or somebody you love? Are there alternatives? What can you do in the presence of people who are speaking in a hateful way? When these utterances of hate encourage people to act in violent ways toward others, what is your response?

ENERGY—WHAT IS IT?

What is energy? You might give some examples of it like electricity, a nuclear bomb, and a flame from a fire, or the fertilizer people put on grass or gardens. These are all examples of kinds of energy. What is energy?

You may develop a very general definition like: energy is that stuff that allows work of some kind to be performed (gasoline allows somebody to drive the farm tractor to plow the field). What is this "stuff" called energy?

Develop as many examples of energy as you can. Then try to place them into similar kinds of categories. Then try to define what all of them have in common.

If you develop a big enough list, you will begin to see some patterns at play.

Extensions

Given any topic, there are certain basic building blocks of understanding that are helpful to understand if you are going to understand the discipline (like math, building a Lego set, or cooking supper). Try to define a basic list of fundamental building blocks for whatever it is you're doing. Keep your list as short as possible. In some of your examples, you may be challenged to define the building blocks.

Energy is one basic building block of understanding how our universe works. What are some other basic building blocks of understanding the universe? Keep them as few in number as possible. What happens to our understanding if our assumptions and definitions related to one or more of our building blocks turn out to be too narrow, inaccurate, or only partially correct? What happens to everything else if we alter our definition of some basic building block? Try this question out on such topics as love, the way people relate to change, the manner in which people react to each other, the way our schools are run, what we can expect from our government, how your family deals with certain kinds of issues, or how friendships can develop. Be mindful of what occurs when you alter some basic building block or assumption in any given system. Once a group becomes identified with a certain complex of understandings that make them feel safe and secure, what are the likely reactions when somebody from the outside or another member of the group suggests alternatives for some of these basic understandings? What are the ways of reducing the likelihood of strong negative reactions, and what are the ways to encourage an openness to the possibilities of change, growth, and transformation? Knowing the difference is wisdom.

ENERGY INTO MATTER

Matter can be turned into energy. One example of this is a nuclear explosion. Can energy be turned into matter? Are they equivalent to each other?

Extensions

Try to develop a clear understanding of matter and energy. The following example describes one method of converting energy into matter. In a hydrogen bubble chamber, matter can be created from energy when charged subatomic particles move through liquid hydrogen kept just below its boiling point. Now imagine being able to convert other forms of energy into matter. What comes to your mind? What might it be like to convert light to matter (in the form of paint pigments)? Could you take the light of a rainbow and put it directly into a painting? Imagine how vibrant and beautiful it would look. Let your imagination loose and try to picture other examples of converting energy into matter. Now do the reverse and see what kinds of examples and applications you can come up with for converting matter into energy.

Be mindful of what happens when we take any process and reverse it. Just because everybody talks about the major meal of the day taking place in the evening, what would happen if we all ate the major meal in the morning or at midday? Reverse any process that is taken for granted by most other people. You can get some very interesting results this way.

Another little tool for increasing your creativity (and fullness of life) is to extend the boundaries of what others assume to be necessary, logical, and natural. For instance, if others assume that persons of a certain race are inferior, what would happen to our human expectations if we draw the boundary lines much wider and start to examine the many manifestations of intelligence in diverse cultural and racial settings? For one thing, we would have to go outside the boundaries of our own group to examine the turf and experiences of others. Now imagine playing soccer where it is allowed to kick the ball out of bounds in order to hit a target that is not the goal. Imagine the fun if there were large boards against which you could shoot the ball. In this way, you could carom (bounce) the ball back into play at an angle that is advantageous to your team. This game could have boards of various sizes and shapes: curved ones and boards at many unusual angles! Imagine what would happen if you were involved in a group that had historically only elected men to the highest office and you convinced others to extend the boundary lines to include women, or persons of other races, religions, or cultural backgrounds. Wouldn't that be a fun afternoon project?

So far, we've talked about reversing the order or flow of commonly accepted realities and extending boundary lines. Another source for creativity can be inverting the meaning of anything in a situation. In a certain novel, it talked about a world in which there were no books. It was named after the burning temperature of books—see if you can find this book's title. You would have been considered an outcast and dangerous person if you were caught with books and worse if you were actually reading them. Even worse yet, you would really be a very bad person if you had books, had read them, had understood their wisdom, and were able to teach others about this wisdom. Given such a world, invert the value, belief, or sentiment that books are the source of evil. For you, books become the source of goodness. Suddenly, many things in your life and in the way you relate to life change. If people say the world is flat, could it be round? What are some examples of inverting some core value or assumption that would radically alter the circumstances, expectations, system, or group you are in?

Another tool of creativity is the process of taking up a radically different understanding of any process. A few people throughout history have been able to leap to a completely different system of understanding life. This is not extending the boundary lines of some given set of understandings. For instance, who was the person who is most famous for suggesting that the Earth is not the center of the universe? What are other major shifts in human thinking about ourselves and our place in the universe? Imagine yourself in a group that had assumed only very bright persons could be members of the group. Imagine yourself in a group that assumes that only people with sufficient income can belong (or a group based on having persons of only one religion).

Instead of extending the boundary line to include a person who is viewed as being a special exception, you convince the group to include all persons. You could successfully challenge the basic notion (idea) that there is no need for boundary lines, exclusion, and reinforcement of positive assertions (statements) about one's own self and group being rooted in negative assumptions about others. They are human beings; therefore, justice, a concern for the human family, and a dedication to our shared future suggest that we act with a sense of compassion!

Your trust is ultimately not in one person's or group's capacity to respond to fundamental truths espoused (spoken) or enacted by you. Trust is in the capacity of all human beings to eventually respond to examples of ways of living that provide us all with a more hopeful future. If enough people of goodwill and conscience speak up and enact ways of compassion and justice, then—minimally—others see living examples of truth in action. Minimally, this holds others responsible for their own continuing learning and growth.

Where no one else is doing it, directly talk about issues related to the existence of any boundary lines, the need to exclude others, and the need to define self-worth in terms of negative assumptions about others. Where there are individuals acting in mean and violent ways toward others, do not be one of the silent ones allowing the violence and meanness to continue. Truth telling is a desperately needed behavior. Being truthful means that we are acting with integrity while honoring the humanity of others. To invert fundamental assumptions causes revolutions in human understanding. An example to others has been provided.

In a final sense, all arguments predicated (based) on the assumption of "they" and "us" are less effective than the comprehension that "they" are "us"! See if you can find the cartoon in which the phrase "They is us" was first coined (written). We are one human family. We are all one family of living organisms. We are one community of living beings on Mother Earth. From this wisdom, cases for justice and compassion have a much firmer foundation. Without this insight of the unity of life, all—literally all—arguments for justice and peace can be twisted, mutated, and construed in ways that can turn something good into something destructive.

The three creative sources we've talked about are reversing the order, sequence, or flow of things; extending the boundary lines; and inverting the value or definition of basic things in our lives. The fourth and most radical creative option is to learn to relate to life on a different basis. Instead of looking at others as objects separate from ourselves, instead of looking at nature being separate from life, instead of looking at the universe as being separate from us, we can learn to experience ourselves, others, life, and the universe as one greatly diverse and unified whole. We are interdependent, and we are all made up of stardust. We are not essentially different from others. We share the same core energy and common fact that we are all alive in this mysterious and wonderful thing called Life!

Here you have four very basic creative ways to respond to life: reverse, extend, invert, and reexperience what is given to you in life. Apply them to your everyday circumstances and to the way that you experience yourself and others. You are a creative source of life. As you become well versed (practiced) in this way of living, you may come to realize that every time you refashion who you are and how you relate to the diverse people in your life, what is essential becomes renewed in a way that refreshes you. If everybody were to live in this creative manner, the world really could be a very different and kinder place. These gifts of creative living come into full bloom only when they are impelled (energized) by compassion and goodwill for others. We are not merely opening our own way of thinking. We are opening our core selves to what is possible in life for all others (not only for other human beings—but all life). When creativity of the heart is fully rooted in compassion and justice, then great things can begin to break out all over the world in surprising and encouraging ways.

Do you think everybody will welcome and value the fact that you don't respond to emerging events in perfectly predictable ways? Be careful with your expectations. I speak from experience that there will be great joy and challenges for you if you choose to be a creative source within any community. When you look back, you will say to yourself: I'd not have it different, but then again if I reverse, expand, invert, and reexperience some basic things, I wonder what if . . .

ENTROPY

One of the most curious phenomena in the universe is that of entropy. It is a basic law of physics. It was discovered by a genius named Isaac Newton. He discovered that the universe as a whole is cooling down. Energy is being dissipated (randomly distributed).Therefore, less energy is available. Another way of saying this is that, since the universe as a whole is cooling off, it will eventually experience heat death.

We don't know for sure that this is the case. Perhaps there are other dynamics at play in the universe that would provide an expanded picture of what will happen to the universe (and thus all life). Relative to the law of entropy is a mystery on how portions of the universe can trap and use so much energy. How is it that certain portions of the universe appear to be gaining energy? Examples are the human body and the Earth's environment. How is it that some little sections of the universe seem to escape the law of entropy? Are we in the end really escaping it?

Extensions

If the universe is entropic, can you imagine how a universe that has died from heat death could be reborn again with the emergence of energy? (*See* "Dimensions—How Many?") What are some other examples of systems that seem to trap energy and defy the laws of entropy? Do these systems really trap energy? Remember that any particular thing is part of many different fields.

EVOLVE AND DEVOLVE

How do we really evolve? Is all life evolving?

Extensions

Now take the opposite set of circumstances. What could cause us (or anything) to devolve?

EVOLUTION—A SLOW DANCE OF LIFE?

We often think of evolution as something that has occurred in the past. We also frequently think of evolution as a slow process. Certain bacteria evolve in one week as much as we humans evolve in twenty-five thousand years! What are other examples of evolution being on the fast track?

Extensions

Look up the term *punctuated equilibrium*. This concept helps us understand that evolution doesn't always proceed in regular linear movements.

EXPLOSIONS

What is the biggest human-made explosion that is nonnuclear? After you have listed every idea you have, look up and compare what happened at Seymour Narrows, British Columbia. There was an explosion that used a nitrogen compound as the source of energy. There was a shipping peril. It was an underwater mountain. Approximately 1,375 tons of nitrates were detonated, moving some 690,000 tons of rock. Might this be the biggest nonnuclear, human-made explosion in history? There was another explosion in Canada that is famous. Hint: it took place in a harbor on the opposite end of the country.

Extensions

Compare the estimated energy of these nature-produced explosions and the biggest human-made explosions. (See "A Very Big Bang") Hint: you may wish to look at the comet over Siberia, the comet or asteroid that hit the Earth 64.9 million years ago, and the Krakatoa volcano. These may or may not be the biggest explosions in history. What do you think? Other than the big bang, what is the greatest explosion we know of in space? Hint: it was observed as a gamma ray explosion.

EYE—FLOATING MICROORGANISMS

Have you ever seen floating microorganisms moving around apparently on the surface of your moist eye? They look like little snakes with tiny lines on the inside. How could the eye focus on something so close and so small? Are there other explanations? Ask a medical doctor or an optometrist about some possible connections to the retina of the eye. I can see little creatures floating by when I look up at the sky. See if you can detect these little critters. How many different ways can you figure out how to see them?

Extensions

When these little organisms show up in our field of vision, we're usually looking at something else. What are some other circumstances in which you've been looking at something and then you noticed something totally unexpected? Whether we are dreaming, awake, or somewhere in between the two states of consciousness, we most often have a point of view. We are usually aware that we are someone looking at something. Changing our point of view is always interesting.

Have you ever wondered if you were under hypnosis, could you change your point of view? When you are in a hypnotic state, might you be able to start with your point of view that you initially experienced and then start to notice other things you didn't notice the first time? Under hypnosis, might we be able to see something in much greater detail? If we answer yes to any of the above questions, might these new things that we notice be the result of suggestions or cues (intentional or unintentional) from the hypnotist? Might anything we become more aware of be a thing that we want or desire to be there? If changing one's point of view is possible under hypnosis, might we be able to change our point of view in dreams? How easily can we change our point of view while we are awake? When is it easy to change our point of view and when is it terribly difficult to change our point of view? Might it be possible to experience a state of consciousness in which you are not focused on your own sense of being the controlling presence and instead experience simple clarity and depth of comprehension that is startling and surprising?

EYEBALL SEEN SIDEWAYS

Have you ever looked at somebody's eye sideways? Try it. Can you see the clear part? Now take a more careful look. Can you see how the light is entering the clear part? Can you see objects on the other side of the clear part of the eye? When you do this, be careful to let the other person know what you are doing. Otherwise, he or she may think you're a little strange.

Extensions

Look at any number of things from unusual angles. You will see things that you've never seen before. Have you experienced the difference between seeing something and beholding something (experiencing something in its full depth)? This can be an extremely startling experience. In the second way of experiencing something, we come to understand it in a new manner. For instance, after having studied some things about Spanish history, I went to New York City and saw a painting called *Guernica*. I was stunned by its power and depth. I had seen pictures of it many times before, but this time I saw it differently. Sometimes, this switch in the manner of experiencing can occur in very beautiful circumstances such as sunsets or in sorrow-touched circumstances such as funerals. Take careful note when this kind of experience occurs to you the next time. Take care to allow this pause in your schedule to run its course. It is a precious moment of life. If you have no idea what I'm talking about, go see the movie *Dr. Zhivago*. It can still be rented in most video rental shops. There are many scenes in which Dr. Zhivago experiences this way of sensing and seeing. These are moments of realization, appreciation, comprehension, and truly getting something. My sister was recently sharing something about a role my father played in a very difficult set of circumstances when I was a child. I recently went through a similar set of circumstances myself. I now honor my father's memory and presence with even more value because I have seen him in yet another great role that he did not have to take on, but he chose to meet the challenge of the time. This kind of seeing and sensing changes our hearts and makes us richer.

EYEBALLING THE EYE

Look deep into your eyes in the mirror. What do you see? What do you feel? Have you ever stopped to pause and look into your eyes? Might you be wondering about who is in there? Who am I? Who am I really? This is not an identity issue related to where you live, how old you are, your career, or which school you attend. Who we really are has to do with the core of our identity. It has to do with the center of our lives that stays with us. This central core doesn't change like the seasons. This core is what makes us who we are. It is our true identity. Whatever the quality that abides within us, does it also evolve?

Extensions

Do you like yourself? Do you accept yourself as you are? Do you get along with yourself? Are there things from your past that you are constantly struggling with? How much energy does this struggle take from you every day?

If you become able to know your core self, it becomes much easier to see the core of other person's lives. What you find can be very surprising and astounding.

F OR *PH*?

Why is the word *photograph* spelled with a *ph* instead of an *f*? (Why use the term "an *f*" instead of "a *f*"? Why do we use the *ph* letter combination at all in English?

Extensions

There are certain patterns in life that have evolved without a logic or reason. They are just there. Someone somewhere started something and it caught on. When we start to compare some of these patterns, inconsistencies start to show up. We begin to question why things are as they are. This is an important element of creativity. Some people feel comfortable with this questioning, while others do not share this comfort. Get into the practice of turning over stones and seeing what is underneath them. In this case, the patterns have to do with spelling and grammar. Try finding the answer to why there are double letters in words like common, vacuum, and accurate. Maybe there were initial reasons for these odd letter combinations, but are they necessary now? Are there certain traditions that get carried forward mindlessly? Once something is a tradition, does that mean that we cease being aware of alternatives that may be more practical? Be mindful of the allegiance that people cultivate when it comes to traditions. If you are questioning some tradition, be prepared to learn how to invite and encourage people to reexamine their own innermost attachments.

In this case of spelling issues, there are some very interesting questions about why we spell certain words in certain ways. Our spelling rules are riddled with many inconsistencies. Be careful, there are some patterns in spelling that are very reasonable and consistent that only look odd on the surface. Investigate. Turn over stones! Just because you've found some inconsistencies and patterns that do not have any logical reason, do not assume that similar kinds of things do not have a reasonable basis. For instance, it may appear to be weird or unnecessary to spell *when* with an *h*, but there is a good reason for this letter *h* being used.

Be careful not to overgeneralize something based on a limited number of instances. If you find certain things that are inconsistent, unnecessary, or unexplainable, this does not mean that all things in spelling that you do not immediately understand are inconsistent, unnecessary, or unexplainable. Be careful about generalizations. We need them, but they can also lead us astray (confuse us).

Apply some of these insights to patterns other than spelling. Why do we drive on the right side of the road? Why do others drive on the left side of the road? Why do we place the fork on the left side of the plate when most of us are right-handed and use the fork most often? Think about eating. Look around the table just as pieces of pie are placed in front of people. Which way do most people place the pointed end? Try placing the rounded end facing the person seated. Examine the patterns of our lives and ask why.

FACE FROM THE SOUND

Have you ever wondered what a person looks like that you've heard on the radio? I've been surprised more than once when I finally saw what the person looked like who had previously only been heard on the radio.

Extensions

What are other examples of experiences with a single sense (sound, smell, touch, taste, sight) suggesting to us a mental picture of something? Often music suggests certain pictures. I was just down by a small river with my two dogs. Many pictures were suggested to me when I heard the wind and saw the wonderful fall leaves plummet downward on the surface of river.

FANTASY

Is fantasy a waste of time? Are there productive effects stemming from fantasy? How do you fantasize?

Extensions

Look up the biographies of great persons. Keep an eye out for the capacity to envision a world that really can be different. Some of these persons understand that the world must be different in order for us to survive. Look for people who can use logic and fantasy to create ingenious new inventions and insights into our human situation.

FAST AT THE EQUATOR

If you were at the North Pole or South Pole, as the world turns, you would not be moving through space. You would be turning around in one place. If you were at 40 degrees north or south, you would be moving at 770 miles per hour through space. At the equator, you'd be moving about a thousand miles per hour. Do you think it would feel differently to be at one of the poles compared to standing at the equator moving over a thousand miles per hour?

Extensions

Could you jump up and come down in a different place because of the rotation of the Earth (especially if you were standing at the equator)?

FEELINGS—NOTICING THEM

Do you have feelings every moment? Right now, as you are reading this sentence, are you experiencing a feeling? We all have feelings all day long. What varies is the awareness, intensity, and kinds of feelings we are experiencing. If we are not aware of our feelings, is there a part of us that is experiencing them?

Do some experiments with yourself. As you awaken in the morning, train yourself to immediately ask yourself what you are feeling right then. When you are doing various kinds of things, keep track of your feelings. Describe them in any manner you can.

Many people make many assumptions about their feelings, ranging from "feelings are a gateway to our heartfelt deepest understandings" to "feelings are a danger, impediment (bother), and source of confusion." Some persons engage in persistent efforts to understand their feelings while others beat a fast retreat anytime a feeling comes to the surface of awareness. One idea that some people are convinced is true is this: if I am having a feeling, I must act on it, and the feelings of those around me determine how I will feel. Must we respond to circumstances in a set manner? For instance, if you meet somebody who is being hostile or very negative, must you respond with hostility or negative feelings? If people are nervous, fearful, angry, or anxious, must you be this way also?

Explore this possible connection in your life. When you are peaceful, relaxed, or serene, are these also the moments when you can most be focused, concentrated, thoughtful, and caring?

Extensions

When you are not at peace or serene, what happens to your abilities to concentrate and your capacities to accurately observe what is happening around you?

FIGURATIVE WORDS

The phrase "rising above the details" is a figurative way to describe the skill of seeing the framework, context, or larger picture given a set of circumstances. Does this mean that you were physically floating above your own life up in the air? Figurative language points beyond the immediate obvious circumstances to something deeper. Literal language uses words to describe the appearance of common things in life. For example, "The tree has green leaves." Explore the definition and relationship between figurative and literal language. List as many figurative word combinations. Some of these phrases are the richest examples of wonderful expressions. Grab the opportunity. Snatch the time.

Extensions

Learn the difference between connotation and denotation. Certain words conjure up (suggest) associated (related) experiences and meanings. These suggestions or associations illustrate some deeper structure or meaning. A dying person in a hospice looks out a window in the fall and asks his beloved partner to look out at the leaves turning colors and falling off the trees. The person then says, "The leaves that fall become the earth from which saplings emerge after the long cold winter." The leaves connote something much deeper than the literal leaves. Words have different associated meanings that add depth and value to our communication. Denotative meaning has to do with the surface, obvious, or literal meaning of the words. A parent says to a child, "It would be good to get the raking of the leaves done right away." The parent literally means the leaves and is not referring to any regeneration of life.

Learn about the distinction (differences) between an inference and an implication. To infer something is your interpretation of something somebody else has said or done. To imply something is something you do, suggest, or intend. We get into huge problems with each other when someone infers that somebody meant something in word or deed (action) when these words or deeds were never in any way intended, suggested, or done in the manner inferred by another. Great and unnecessary suffering could be avoided if we only understood the distinction between what others mean and what we infer from what has been said and done. This is especially true when there are so many connotations to our words.

Look up the difference between something signifying and symbolizing. There are some interesting nuances between a sign and symbol. Be careful—this may well take you into the domain (region) of philosophy. Philosophers have never been fully trusted by their local cultures. They continually look for broader associations, greater understandings, alternative interpretations, deeper meanings, and the simple and obvious features of life amid massive obfuscation (when things are mixed up and confused). Often they have unusual hair. Look up the meaning of the wonderful metaphor related to the philosopher's stone.

FINGERTIP ATTRACTION

One day at a beach, one of my dogs got real attracted to my fingertip. She thought I was making up another game for her. She kept thinking that the point of the game was to lick my fingertip. The entire time I was pointing my finger to divert her attention in another direction. I thought she wasn't getting it. She thought I wasn't getting it. She wanted to lick the fingertip. I wanted her to understand that an extended finger means that I am pointing in a certain direction. Within the context of that particular game, I was playing with her and she was playing with me. Maybe I was in the context of her game. I had all the confidence in the world, at the beginning, that she would understand, because the little minigame was so simple. In the end, she licked my fingertip. Game over. She went back to sniffing for dead fish, and I went back to reading. We each thought of each other, "What strange behavior from such a peculiar creature!"

What was ever so important was that it was all a game. When we commence (start) playing with others, everybody contributes their own creative energies. No one controls the event. If it really is a playful activity, what are some of the things you notice that occur? I've observed some things:

- It is fun for almost everybody most of the time (if they've freely chosen the activity).
- Often, the understanding of the game may change.
- Everybody has a word as to how the play is evolving.
- There is mutual delight.
- Often, there isn't a purpose other than enjoying the moment.
- The play is nondestructive and nonviolent.
- Often, there is a suspension of the usual rules that dictate our lives.
- Often, there is a change in our normal roles.
- When we are absorbed in play, our usual sense of time is of less importance. (This is why it can be viewed as being irresponsible if we take time out to play.)
- We find ourselves relaxing and laughing.
- We use things around us in ridiculous, wonderful, and creative ways (brooms become flying instruments, toilet paper rolls become scrolls upon which to write secret coded messages, tomatoes become substitute snowballs, and cooking utensils become magic wands used inside secret hideaways).

When people simply play together, how do they relate to each other compared to when they aren't simply playing together? How often do you allow yourself to simply play? What are other things you've noticed and remember about what happens when people of different ages get together to play? How often do people of different ages get together and play? When there are people of both genders playing together, are there differences in the play compared to when only people of the same gender are playing? How often and under what conditions do strangers play together? Imagine being an artist who inspires others, who are strangers to each other and who are busy with their own tasks, to engage in spontaneous play. This kind of art would never be displayed in a serious art museum. When the action is over, the residue of the art remains as memory held in a place of delight and joy. What would a life of all work and no play be like? What would a life of all play and no work be like?

Extensions

Play isn't perfect human behavior. Sometimes:

- It is not fun for everybody all the time.
- Often, the understanding of the game changes in the minds of a few of the participants, creating conflicts with others.
- New rules are sometimes forced or imposed on others.
- There isn't always mutual delight. Feelings do get hurt.
- There isn't a purpose other than enjoying the moment, but some persons have a purpose and agenda that are not directly expressed.
- Sometimes unexpressed motives cause people to act in ways that are anything but playful.
- Play can be insensitive to the needs, feelings, values, ideas, and sentiments of some of the participants, and it can be outright destructive and violent.
- Suspension of the usual rules that dictate our lives can result in dangerous or inappropriate play.
- When we are really absorbed in play, our usual sense of time is of less importance; some people never take time seriously and thus others are left waiting.
- Laughter can be a weapon against others used in many different, vicious, and mean ways.
- While we can use things around us in ridiculous, wonderful, and creative ways, things also can be used as weapons that physically and emotionally hurt others.

What have you observed in the realm of play and games that isn't healthy and good for all the participants? What are creative options when any of these dynamics arise?

FIREFLIES

When fireflies light up in the nighttime, do you think they are warm or hot? What makes them burn so brightly?

Extensions

Have you ever taken time out of your regular schedule and routines to go out into some field or some woods to experience fireflies under starlight or moonlight? Take some people you care about with you and see what it feels like. Anytime you have an opportunity to experience life lit up in a different kind of light, avail yourself of (take) the opportunity. I recall going out onto the thick ice on a large lake deep in the winter. We left the comfortable shelter of our lodge and trekked out into the subzero weather. What attracted us were the northern lights. I'll never forget the looks of delight on all the faces as we stood in the great darkness of the woods cast in odd shades of color from the vibrating shooting and waving northern lights. Literally and figuratively, get out and see life in new light.

FIRST HUMAN BEING

When was the first human being born? Was there a first emergence of one individual that was fully human? Could human beings have emerged in multiple places at once?

Extensions

Who were the parents of the first human beings? Were these parents human? If not, how could nonhuman parents give birth to a human? What are some issues at play in this question? Some persons might interpret these questions within a context of religion versus science, forcing the reader to take one opposite side or the other.

What is science? What is religion? In a sense, they both claim to describe how life works and what the meaning of life is. Some scientists claim that science has nothing to do with the meaning of life but everything to do with discovery of facts. Do you agree with this position? Might the manner in which we assemble our facts demonstrate that we possess certain points of view about life and reality, and the picture we help create of life and reality by the way we assemble our facts creates meaningful contexts for human understanding? Some people believe that religion only has to do with the meaning of ultimate things (like death, afterlife, the existence of God). Some people contend that science deals with facts of nature and religion deals with values. Do you agree with these positions? Are there other possibilities?

If we use our intelligence, imagination, and logic, we might see the two realms of religion and science as being contradictory, complementary, or not related in any essential or significant manner. What do you think and believe? Can you think of ways that these two important realms of science and religion can be related? Be creative.

Since we are dealing with the first human being and his or her parents in this section, this raises questions about the story of Adam and Eve for some people. Were they the first humans? Did we all descend from two persons? What are all the possible interpretations of this story? Talk to others about it. How does it relate to what we know scientifically about nature and life? Talk to a wide circle of people who hold divergent (different) views on this topic.

Given this question about the first human and her or his parents, some persons would make connections with the raging (hot) issue around our country related to schools teaching evolution. Some religious people believe that evolution threatens their faith that God created the world in six days. They are trying to get discussions of evolution removed from science curricula (studies) all around our country. Find out as much of this controversy as you can. Should private religious beliefs be allowed to dictate public educational policy? In what ways have religious beliefs affected the development of our Declaration of Independence, Constitution, and our common and core values? Should people in a democracy have the right to determine what is being taught to their children? How do majority values relate to minority values? Put one way, we get one kind of answer. Ought science be held captive by privately held religious beliefs? Put another way, we tend to get another kind of answer. Ought science with all of its technological influences (both extremely positive and extremely negative) be influenced by values such as the ultimate values of religions? Wouldn't this help assure that science and its technological derivatives (offspring) stay focused on serving life? This is a very complex constellation of issues.

Never settle for shallow answers to simplistic and misleading questions, and don't allow yourself to stagnate (get stuck) in confusion related to complexity. Distill, discern, tease out all the complexities and precious nuggets of understanding that guide you in dealing with complex issues. The greater the complexity of the issues you are dealing with, the greater the need for certain pearls of wisdom that remind you of basic commonsense things. If you cultivate a life in which you gather in these pearls of wisdom, you will be able to adapt, be flexible, grow, learn, adjust, and be a person who can engage in radically new circumstances without losing sight of what is real, needed, and essential. We desperately need people who can engage our plethora (many forms) of emerging challenging issues in creative ways that help us learn how to treasure this gift of life. We have some very basic choices:

- We can be reactive or proactive.
- We can be creative, flexible, and adaptive persons or we can be narrow-minded, rigid, and inflexible.

- We can be engaged or disengaged.
- We can participate in finding solutions or we can contribute to creating more problems.
- We can be hopeful or cynical beings.
- We can live with absolute division lines or we can live in such a manner that the world is not black and white only (there actually is a rainbow).
- We can open ourselves to life fully or we can live in mighty small, dark, walled-in rooms.
- We can make enemies of those with whom we share disagreements or we can learn to listen carefully to the wisdom of those who are in some significant ways different from us.
- We can feel invigorated (having energy) as we face challenges or we can feel enervated (lack of energy) as we face challenges.
- We can sense the presence of options, alternatives, and possibilities or we can collapse under the pressure of life and become depressed (feeling that there are no options, alternatives, or possibilities).
- We can participate in an unfolding future that is evolving in part because of our contributions or we can live for the moment (or in the past) hoping to avoid the future.
- We can contribute to the welfare (well-being) of others or we can be focused on our attachments, desires, and needs exclusively.

What do you believe about the origins of life? Once you have clarified for yourself when and how you believe human life may have emerged, when do you think this first human being was born, and were its parents human?

If we evolved, is it possible to assign a certain exact time as the beginning point? Even if we could say that in this particular fifteen thousand–year framework of our choosing, it is highly likely that in this certain place and time (in Africa) the first human evolved, then we are left with the question about the parents of the first human being human.

Expand the basis upon which the question is being asked. (*See* "Chicken and the Egg Question.") One possible way to proceed on this question is not to think in discrete terms but in process terms. Look up *discrete*. Anything that is described as being discrete is a separate identifiable thing. I have five rocks in my collection. Each rock is discrete. They can be counted. If things are not discrete, they tend to share and blend into each other. The colors of the rainbow are not discrete separate units. Each color blends into the other colors. Every color is defined by a certain wavelength of light. There are many shades of each color, and they all blend into each other.

Back to the main question about the parents of the first human being. If you approach the question scientifically, you need to resolve the issue of whether you are defining the event in discrete or process terms. If you are looking for the answer to be discrete, you are looking for a totally unique animal now named *Homo sapiens* (actually *Homo sapiens sapiens*) who is the one and only first-time human being absolutely distinct from any other living creature on the face of the Earth.

If you are looking for this creature in process terms, the question resolves itself. We can switch from thinking in terms of a single human being to terms of groups of human beings (or protohumans—human-like animals) evolving. This evolution could have been in a slow linear manner, or it could also have been in swift jumps of evolutionary time (punctuated equilibrium).

Now we are dealing with population groups and with characteristics that are something like the rainbow. The characteristics tend to blend into one another. They become pronounced (noticeable) over the course of time and the generations. Now there are fewer problems in understanding the question of "Were the parents of the first human being human?" because we think in terms of process and group terms and not discrete and individual terms. The features we call human were shared in some manner between the parents and the offspring. There was no sudden total shift from two nonhuman parents to one complete fully human offspring. There was no first rose, mammal, dinosaur, or bird.

The question about the first human being and whether his or her parents were human was originally asked in such a manner as to predispose the listener to assume that the first single human being emerged only in one place. Now that we are thinking in process and group terms, might it be possible that human life emerged in more than one place on the face of the Earth? Also, the question was originally asked in terms of discrete and individual units. Learn the art of reframing all questions. Whole new ways of understanding and experiencing life can open to us. Our frameworks of understanding both empower us and limit us. Wisdom is to know the differences between various frameworks. Wisdom is to know that all human knowledge comes bundled in some kind of framework and that whatever frameworks we choose to call real will affect what we assume about life.

FISH IN MOST PONDS

How is it that there are so many dissimilar and similar kinds of fish in most little lakes and even small ponds around the entire world? How did they get there? Assume that there were fish in these places before human beings stocked lakes, rivers, and ponds.

Whenever you are dealing with an issue that appears initially to have no solution, we might call it an irresolvable problem (a problem with no answer—or a conundrum). How does one proceed with such a challenge? You can do several things. One of them is to look at the question from a different perspective (framework). You can reverse the flow of the question, extend the framework of the question, invert some elements of the question, or see the question in a totally different context. (*See* "Energy into Matter.")

You might examine if the land formations, lakes, and ponds have always been the same over the course of history. Never assume just because things are one way now that they have been that way in the past. Never assume from the fact things are one way (seeming to be static) that they are not dynamic and evolving. Might there have been other formations in the past that had something to do with the distribution of the fish and other forms of life found in the lakes? For instance, were lakes once interconnected? Did fish once fly? Did fish once crawl on land as they were evolving? Could fish have lived where lakes were forming, and after the lakes were formed, the fish's ancestors evolved and were able to adapt to the lakes? Did the lakes get there after the ancestors of fish were already present? Could birds have dropped fish into a lake? These potential answers illustrate how we can change our frameworks and get different answers to the same question. Remember to reverse the flow of a question, expand the framework of a question, and invert elements of the question. New possibilities start to emerge in this way of working through challenges. At this part of a creative process, what appear to be utterly ridiculous possibilities may in fact contain some unseen facet or kernel of truth. Risk being a little ridiculous.

Play with the key words that emerge in your explorations. One of them might be *distribute*. Were the fish distributed from one central location or might they have emerged from several places at once? In addition, other forms of life in the lakes might have been distributed in the air. Are any of them light enough that strong winds could carry them aloft (up) and then distribute them? Have there been any recorded instances of fish flying through the air during hurricanes, tornadoes, or straight-line winds?

Look at other forms of life living on land. How were they distributed so widely? For instance, how did all the land animals, birds, insects, and flowers get on the Hawaiian Islands prior to (before) the arrival of the first human beings? These islands were never a part of a larger mass (like Australia). There was not a period when the waters were frozen over so those animals could walk over to the islands. Birds may have descended from dinosaurs, but the other land animals didn't descend from birds on these islands. Could these land animals in Hawaii simply have evolved there from sea creatures of the past?

The manner in which this last series of questions is asked assumes that there were animals on the islands before the arrival of human beings. Step back and examine the way in which a question is asked. If you get used to doing this, you will be exercising your intelligence and perhaps evidencing genius. Given complex questions, get used to playing with the questions. Remember to reverse the flow of the question, expand the context of the original question, and invert the usual meanings of key words. (*See* "Energy into Matter.")

While you're at it, find out how the ancient Polynesians found Hawaii. They didn't have any maps. They had no global positioning system, sextant, or astrolabe (all instruments used to locate one's position relative to satellite signals or the stars). How could they have traveled thousands of miles in uncharted oceans and found these relatively tiny islands? Did they take all the animals with them? Are there any remnant (vestigial or left over) references to these ancient wanderings on the part of present-day Hawaiian myths and lore (stories about one's culture)?

Back to the question on fish. Look up some resources on geology, lakes, and fish. Talk to people who love to fish. See if they have ever wondered about this same question. See what kinds of alternatives they come up with. Talk to game wardens. Talk to biologists. When you are dealing with such a complex question, sometimes clues come from people in fields (area of training) that you wouldn't expect would be able to contribute to your understanding of the challenge. Often, some unrelated remark is heard and it triggers a major understanding or reveals a pathway for exploration. As with any big challenge in life, when you are committed to reaching some goal or deriving (getting) some answer, you become very focused on many different levels. If you learn to be highly concentrated and attentive to wider contexts, you will be amazed at how your mind works on the issue even when you are asleep. You will be surprised at how many resources are available for delving (entering) into the depths of a really mysterious, interesting, and complex question. Most of all, enjoy the exploration process. Play with it! Play and enjoyment are major keys to discovering how to unlock our hidden treasures of intellectual, imaginative, intuitional, and emotional resources. Enjoy the play, and remember there is no one right way to get to your goal. As you discover more and more things along the way, you become changed. Your perspective on the important issues evolves. The goal may be altered. You may discover that the answer is not nearly as important as the journey.

Extensions

While you are thinking about people who fish, try to imagine how far a fish can smell things. Do some research on this topic. Can fish smell anything that is out in the air? Can fish hear very well? Can they sense electromagnetic fields? Since they migrate great distances, how can they do it so accurately? When they migrate, is there a leader to the pack?

FLAT EARTH, FLAT UNIVERSE

We have now disproved that the Earth is flat. Could the universe itself be flat?

Extensions

If the universe is not flat but is shaped more like a sphere stemming from the big bang, what might it look like if we were beyond the boundary related to how far the stars have dispersed? If we were looking in at the universe from the darkness of the void beyond the space-time continuum, would the entire surface of the universe be dotted with stars and star systems equally distributed on its "surface?" Would there be huge holes without stars? Is there space-time beyond the limits of the big bang? Are there any other ways that you can imagine yourself outside any system and visualize what it might look like? Try thinking of yourself outside of your family and cultural system. What does your "self" look like?

FLOATING IN SCHOOL

I went to an elementary school and was asked to help a group of the older students assemble a geodesic dome in the large, centrally located, circular library. We had all of the doweling sticks and plastic connectors. It was a relatively simple job, so we had plenty of time to talk. As we were assembling the geodesic dome, I started to ask the students if they could imagine using the same materials to create a riding chair in which a student could sit. Then I had them try to imagine what it would be like to attach helium weather balloons to the top of the chair. The unanimous group response was that the student would float to the ceiling and get trapped up there. I switched the orientation of their thinking just a little bit. I challenged them to find out what volume of helium would be required to float a student up in the air midway between the floor and the ceiling. This could be the magic reading chair. At the mention of a magic reading chair, they scrambled to find all available resources related to helium gas. Instead of being bored with school, they became so excited that the librarian was shocked that so many students were so inquisitive. The library quickly ran out of resources for the quick-thinking adventurers. They worked as teams to come up with an answer.

Think of the library in the school you attend or attended when you were younger. Picture yourself floating several feet off the ground and reading (no food fights allowed). How much helium would this take? Figure out the weight of your chair (don't forget to add your weight) and the volume of the balloons filled with helium. Now picture floating your favorite and least favorite teachers from the past or present up in the air. Under what conditions would you let the teacher down?

Extensions

Would you believe that a fellow took a lawn chair and attached weather balloons filled with helium? He floated right up into the air traffic corridor for an airport. Pilots began to report that a man in a lawn chair was sitting at their altitude drinking beer. Apparently, he had taken a six-pack of beer with him. What was the most dangerous thing about this very risky adventure? Are there safer ways to float into the air? How much does it cost to ride a commercial hot-air balloon? Are there some adventures that could be much safer than this one but just as fun?

FLOATING IN SPACE

Since our Earth has significant gravitational effects reaching out into space, why don't astronauts fall back to Earth when they are in orbit? Hint: you do not have to be in outer space to be weightless while in the air. How can people in airplanes become weightless? Astronauts become weightless when they begin falling back toward Earth. We've all seen the pictures of them free-floating in space, and it appears as though they are not falling back to Earth. Learn about the trajectory (path) they are following when we view them floating in outer space. Are they going in a straight line or a curve? How does the path relate to the surface of the Earth? They are not just floating out there in space; they are in a free fall of a special kind. Learn something about the importance of the speed of these astronauts in this special kind of free fall. What are the effects if they are going too fast or too slow?

Extensions

Name as many things as you can think of that may appear to be magic if we didn't know the underlying dynamics and forces. In our Western culture, we tend to believe that everything can be explained. Do you believe this? If we had enough knowledge, would we be able to have perfectly logical explanations for everything? Are there other cultures that practice ways of knowledge that are different from our own? If we look at what they know, does it appear to be magic to us? Does it appear to be superstition? Does it look stupid and uninformed to us? Might there be ways of knowing that are different from our ways while being valid with integrity? Might many of the things we do and believe in appear to be very stupid and uninformed to persons of different cultures?

FLOATING ROCKS

Can rocks float on water? Look up pumice. Are there other rocks with unusual characteristics (traits or unique qualities); for example, rocks that are soft?

Extensions

Are there other examples of things that absolutely do not fit neatly in any way with our categories of thinking? Think of contradictory kinds of things like:

- fish that live on land
- birds that do not fly
- things that might float up against gravity
- lightening that flows from the ground up
- ice that feels warm
- liquid water that feels as hard as rock

- parents who say yes to everything
- a life without any fear
- a triangle with four sides

Try to list as many unusual images as you can think of. Some of the examples will be true descriptions of things in nature that are merely highly unusual. Some of them will be ridiculous. Some of them may be ingenious insights and opportunities for humankind.

FLYING UPSIDE DOWN

If you were to fly from North America to Tasmania off the coast of Australia, when you landed in Tasmania, would you be upside down?

Extensions

Everything you know is relative to a framework of understanding. To any and every question, we benefit when we can ask ourselves, "Relative to what?" We have tremendously strong feelings and deeply held sentiments related to the preservation and validity (truthfulness) of our way of describing life on our terms. In what ways would we benefit from leaping beyond our core assumptions of what is real? Why bother?

FOOD STUFF

What do you know about the process and effects of irradiating food? What do you know about issues related to food coming from genetically altered animals and plants? Do a little research and determine for yourself how you feel about this topic. Try to discover some of the political and economic issues related to these topics. Where is the power? Whose power is being threatened if there are changes? How do some changes affect wealth and the potential to create new avenues to accumulate wealth?

Extensions

How are different countries dealing with these issues?

FOND OF OUR DEPENDENCIES

Most people enjoy eating. Some people use food to make themselves feel better about life. For these people, to eat is to erase unpleasant feelings. Some people love to wear certain clothes that give the appearance they want others to see. This is a way to be somebody. Can we become too dependent upon our outer appearances? Is some concern for our appearances a good thing while an overdependence is not good for us? Where is the line? Some people like to be seen with others who are successful. This helps them with their sense of self-identity. Do you depend on certain things to make you feel better? Some of these things are vitally important, like friends. Other things are not good for us. When does a behavior or feeling become a nasty habit upon which we depend?

Extensions

There are many forms of dependency in life. Name some of them. What do you know of them?

FORCED OPTION

Often we think that we are trapped in circumstances. There appear to be only so many options available to us. Some people call this a forced option situation. An example might be that we are in a cave with only two exit points that we know of, and suddenly one of them collapses and the other is filling up with water. It appears as though this is a forced option situation and you must (with great difficulty) get out of the cave quickly through one of the two exits.

In many circumstances, we feel that we are in a forced option situation. I remember as a youth somebody saying somebody had hit him so he *had* to hit him back. I wondered how the individual couldn't have known that he had other choices. What are other examples of what look like forced option situations when in fact there are other options?

Extensions

In a way, this is a problem-solving issue. have available to help rethink circumstances and create new contexts for understanding your options? (*See* "Energy into Matter.")

FOREIGN WORDS

List as many "foreign words" as you can that are used in our language. Are some of these words used so commonly that they are no longer considered "foreign" words? For example, before you look up the words *ketchup* and *shampoo*, try to guess which culture we got them from.

Extensions

What does it mean that something is a foreign word? Does it mean that it comes from another country and culture? If this is the case, try to determine which words we use that are originally from our country, culture, and land. Are there some words we use that come from our country or another current culture within our own country? Is there more than one culture in our country?

Look up what Standard English means. (*See* "Standard English.") Are there words we use that come from a culture of this continent from times long before people from Europe ever came to North America? If so, then is English a foreign language?

FORESTS OF NORTH AMERICA

Find a map that shows the areas where there were forests in North America before the time in which European American settlers headed west and cut down the forests to make room for farms and settlements. Where was the line separating the plains from the forests? Then compare a map showing existing forests in North America today. Figure out approximately how many acres or square miles of forest were destroyed. What kinds of forests were destroyed? See if you can find any article talking about the possible effect of the destruction of this vast forest on global or regional weather. If there has been a significant effect on the weather systems, do we as North Americans have the right to urge those in equatorial areas not to cut down their rain forests? If human beings were to disappear, would the forests return? If so, would they be the same kinds of forests?

Extensions

What are other major ways that human beings have altered the ecology of the planet? What would happen if we replanted all the trees that we've eliminated? Be careful to picture what would happen to the planet's ecology and to the human population.

FORMS OF MATTER

We all learned that there are three forms of matter—liquid, gas, solid states. Can you think of any unusual forms of matter? Here are some interesting examples of unusual matter. Colloids are substances dispersed in a substance that are too small to be seen by the naked eye. Some examples of colloids are colored glass (colored solids dispersed in a liquid that appears to be a solid), clay (a solid dispersed in a liquid—one that is very viscous—not easily pourable), smoke (a solid in a gas), mist (a liquid in gas), or foam (a gas in a liquid).

Another unusual fact related to the topic of matter is that lead flows over centuries and glass (a supercool liquid) flows over time.

Are there any other forms of matter other than liquid, gas, or solids?

Extensions

Look up plasma as a state of matter. Also, find out anything you can on a very recent development. A form of matter recently created in laboratory conditions is called Bose-Einstein condensate. Find out what you can about this form of matter. (*See* "Bose-Einstein Condensate.") Another theoretical form of matter is that stuff that existed before the big bang (quark-gluon plasma). It is thought that this matter was different from anything since the big bang. Do not expect to get quick easy descriptions of these possible states of matter. How about one more? Let your mind try to imagine other states of matter, such as states of matter composed of material made of out of antiparticles. We can produce antiparticles at the present time. Could we create different states of matter with stuff made up of antiparticles? Try to determine the state of matter in a black hole or a neutron star.

Let your imagination loose. Use the knowledge you do possess or can obtain related to the more common states of matter. Use this base of knowledge to commence your adventures. What is presently known and accepted is the beginning point for the adventure into the unknown and unexpected realms of human knowledge. Be clear on what we presently know. Test for possible alternative viewpoints related to that body of knowledge that most people accept as fact. Look at these facts differently. Question some assumptions. Proceed into new realms of possible answers with both logic and imagination. Because nobody else has asked such questions, don't be afraid that your ideas are too far out. Let your intellect and imagination go. Let your genius out!

FOUR BASIC SUBSTANCES OF LIFE

The four basic substances of biological life are carbon, oxygen, nitrogen, and hydrogen. Find out how these elements fit together and how they can create the base for all life on our planet.

Extensions

Could there be another base of elements that sustains life on other planets? Recently, scientists have discovered the remains of *Homo erectus* (an earlier form of human-like life—hominid) that existed at the same time and same general location as *Homo sapiens* (us). There is no evidence that they interacted in any way. Might we be coexisting with other forms of life on this planet and not even know it? If life on other planets would be called extraterrestrial, what would noncarbon, nitrogen, oxygen, hydrogen life be called if it existed on our planet? Might it be possible that in some microenvironment that human beings don't know about, there might be other forms of life that might be based on a different set of elements than our four? If this might be the case, where might these microenvironments (small) occur? Might this other form of life exist on our planet in a macroenvironment (a really big one)? The oceans are huge. Do we know everything about the oceans? How about under the surface of the Earth? We make many assumptions about what is down there, but do we really know? What are the tools that we have available to explore the materials under the surface of the Earth? Be careful; they are not all mechanical tools. Since we're looking for life, define life. What is a living thing versus a nonliving thing? (*See* "Life—What Makes the Difference?")

FOUR SEASONS—WHY?

Can you describe why we have four seasons? Hint: it has to do with the manner in which the Earth rotates around the sun. Are there four seasons everywhere on the planet?

Extensions

Do all the planets in our solar system have seasons? Are there any that have only one season?

FRESHWATER TO SALTWATER BY CANOE

Look up on a map the location of Lake Mille Lac in Minnesota (central part of the state). With a careful eye and a good map, figure out a number of ways to get to saltwater in a canoe from this lake. There are several unusual routes. Hint: some routes head toward the north, south, east, and west (eventually). Small portages (hikes over land) are permissible (OK). Hint: find a map in which the rivers and lakes are easy to see. A little town in Wisconsin named Solon Springs may help in your location of alternative routes. A lake on the South Dakota and Minnesota border will also be useful. Watch for places where two rivers have their headwaters located in an area very close together. How many states in the United States can you canoe from a freshwater lake or river and get to an ocean or gulf of an ocean (assuming some portages of relatively short distances)?

There is a movie about a child who carves a little boat. The story is about the boat floating its way from Lake Superior to the far-off sea. Have you ever thought of really sending a message in an ecologically and life-respecting manner to some far-off place and see if you get a reply? Do not use balloons (this is unsafe because many animals can swallow them and choke). What would be a way to send a message in the air or on the waters that would be ecologically sound (safe)?

Extensions

As you are looking at maps, imagine a map with no highways, state lines, or countries. Imagine one only showing pre–European American, Native American migration trails (related to the need to move because of the seasons and due to changing food sources), major trade routes among the Native Americans, and major animal migration routes. Imagine a map showing only old foot and horse paths before any roads were made on the continent. There might be such maps in existence. If these maps do not exist, might there be people alive and resources available to make such a map possible? Maybe there is the data available that would enable you to be the first one to make such a map. Go to a major research library and go to the map section. Ask for maps depicting such trails and paths. You might be surprised (the librarians may also be surprised).

Anywhere in the world, trace a line with your finger from an ocean along rivers. Follow various branches of tributaries. What is the furthest inland headwater that connects with the ocean?

FROM ANOTHER PERSPECTIVE

If you could be a dog or cat, what do you think you'd feel when certain kinds of things happen to you? How do you think you'd feel if people were mean to you? Imagine what kinds of thoughts dogs and cats have. How about a whale when it is being hunted? Alternatively, imagine a bird as it finds its certain home base after migrating thousands of miles.

Extensions

Do you believe that animals have feelings? Might they have ideas and be able to think? Can they plan complex forms of behaviors for given ends (porpoises responding to a school of sharks attacking them)? You might be quite surprised as to how animals give evidence that they do in fact think, plan, use tools, and act together in groups for a specific purpose. Look up recent discoveries on the use of tools by various animals.

FROZEN IN PLACE

Recently I saw an adolescent operating a kind of lawnmower that he had never used before. It was self-propelled and had two different release bars: one that shut off the engine when they are released and another that engaged the drive mechanism. I showed him how to use it. He set off to cut the grass. My friend and I were standing on the driveway observing him, making sure everything was OK. As he approached the street, a van was driving past. A bicyclist was on the other side, making it impossible for the van to swerve around him. The adolescent didn't release the neutral bar in time, and he hung onto the machine as it veered into the street. In a split second, he was in front of the vehicle. I could see it all happening, but it occurred so quickly that I couldn't do anything. The mower was loud and he was across the lawn. He was OK because the driver was alert. I felt horrible that I couldn't react faster. Have you ever been in circumstances that unfold so quickly right before your eyes that it seems like you are frozen in place?

Extensions

When you are responsible for explaining a new idea, concept, or operation to somebody, how do you double-check that he or she really understands what you think you've just taught him or her? Is it sufficient having someone describe the operation and show you that he or she knows how to do the operation? Even with repetition, how can we be reasonably assured the person really knows what he or she is doing?

FUTURE HOPE

Name ten to fifteen challenges that we face on this planet. What are the major things that threaten life? Are they natural and inevitable (nothing to do about them)? Are many of them caused by human beings? Once you have created a list, examine it very closely. See what kinds of groupings or patterns of life challenges you have listed.

If most of the major items are defined as being inevitable and natural, you have created a model or picture of the future that is not very hopeful. If something is inevitable, some people call this fate. Look up the ancient Greek definition of *fate*. If you view that certain human behaviors that result in damage to humans, other life-forms, or the planet are inevitable, this can be called cynicism (the view that we can't expect humanity to change for the better in the future in any significant manner). Combine the fatalism with cynicism and we have a rather bleak picture of the future. How are the terms *fatalism* and *cynicism* used today? Many different cultures have many different views of what is inevitable in life. Do a cross-cultural examination of ideas related to fate and cynicism. Is it possible that some things that appear to be inevitable really aren't inevitable? Might it be possible that the sum of all human decisions and actions creates certain situations that are inevitable as long as human beings continue to act the way they do (like air pollution)? If we change the way we act, is air pollution of the kind and on the order of magnitude (size) of today's air pollution inevitable? Might it be possible that any problems human beings have created can eventually be solved by human beings (hope)? What would have to happen to human beings in order to solve the issues we've created? Might certain problems created by human beings be solved (taken care of) by nature? What would be some examples of this kind of "solution"?

Is it our beliefs and values that need to change? Is it our behaviors that need to change? You could write an award-winning paper on the topic of what human beings need to discover or recover in order to have a hopeful future. Do you believe that we already have the inherent (inborn) gifts necessary for the creation of a better world? Do you believe that we can learn to acquire (get) these necessary traits (qualities) necessary for a hopeful future? Now that communication is easier between people in far places, think globally. Help create hope for the world. You are the needed spark of hope and light. Go for it! Please be careful when you meet resistance and insensitivity; do not become cynical and resigned (given in) to fate. Be the spark of hope and transformation! Your life will never be dull!

Extensions

All around the country, there are cabins with outhouses and old septic systems that are leaking pollutants into the lakes and rivers. The same people are pumping their drinking water out from the same body of water. What are some equivalent situations in which human beings are doing things that are directly detrimental (harmful) to our health and well-being? List as many examples of behaviors that are detrimental that ought to be extremely obvious to everybody. Now go to the list and try to determine some common factors as to why these behaviors are so common.

GALAXIES IN COLLISION

What would happen if two galaxies moved toward each other and occupied the same space?

Extensions

Have you ever thought that maybe there could be more than one universe? Maybe the space-time continuum in which we exist has exploded and imploded an infinite number of times. Or there may have been more than one big bang forming multiple discrete (separate) space-time continua (plural form of continuum). If there are different loci (plural form of locus—location) of big bangs, would the space-time continua be self-referential only (each system can only refer to itself)? Given this possibility, can we only imagine the existence of other space-time continua? Could there be another big bang that results in antimatter being the basic form of matter? Beings in that universe would call our universe an antimatter universe. What would happen if this other universe and ours came into contact? What would happen if three of them collided all at one point in time and space (whose time and whose space)?

Have you ever seen something appear as if out of nowhere—something that is approaching you very fast? I was talking with one young woman in the hospital who was telling me how she pulled out from a parking lot onto a busy street. She carefully looked both ways. As she pulled out, a pickup truck suddenly appeared coming right at her driver's doors very quickly. Right out of nowhere! This has happened to all of us. If one or more universes were to collide, would they appear suddenly as if out of nowhere? If they were to occupy the same time and space, would there be a collision necessarily? What are some other possibilities? If there were a black hole at the core of every galaxy, what would all of these black holes do to each other? If one were an antimatter universe, what could occur? If space-time continua are self-referential only (warp back into themselves with no reference to other possible space-time continua), might these two or more continua coexist without converting each other to 100 percent pure radiant energy?

Might there be a broader and more encompassing set of laws of physics that has yet to be invented (discovered) that could allow us to test out this hypothesis of the existence of different space-time continua? We started this line of questions with an imaginary picture of two galaxies colliding. They might coexist in the same realm, but in a different order of space-time continua. If they did coexist, we'd need to conceive what it means to coexist in a way that describes some order of existence greater than simply space and time.

Another possibility is that the different space-time continua do not or cannot occupy the same realm. If this is so, what is it that separates these discrete space-time continua? Could it be simply empty space? Think of this possibility: a kind of super space-time being infinitely large. Big bangs take place in different sectors of the universe, but they are so distant from each other that it would take an infinity of time to reach each other because they are separated by an infinity of this super space-time. We already know that our normal kind of space-time is expanding when we view a large enough scale. (*See* "Dimensions—How Many?") Maybe there are such things as supertime and superspace that are not dependent on any big bang releasing normal space-time. Maybe this supertime and superspace are just there forever and infinite in span (distance across—no end). This is another possible dimension. If they are entirely self-referential, it may be because they are too distant in this supertime and superspace.

When you couple your intelligence with your imagination, wisdom, intuition, and deep sensing, then genius can be unleashed. Never settle for the known and the generally accepted ways of behavior and kinds of knowledge. What is the difference between invention and discovery when it comes to the realms of possible human knowledge that we are discussing?

The only times I was sent to the principal's office in elementary school were for suggesting another set of rules for baseball during gym time and for organizing an ecologically sound (good) alternative for the use of rotting tomatoes in the late fall. I thought everybody would be grateful that their fall-season, frozen, thawed, and rotting tomatoes could be used for useful and playful ends. A friend and I organized the biggest tomato fight in the history of this known universe. The tomatoes really enjoyed the game. All the participants really grew in their knowledge of physics. It was good for the earth because many tomato seeds got scattered in unexpected ecological niches (microenvironments). The only problem was that it occurred on school time. I guess it might have been a little minor issue that our two groups were positioned on opposite sides of a major four-lane thoroughfare. Maybe we ought to have asked permission to borrow the tomatoes. So, when you start getting very creative in your thinking, don't expect everybody to love you or your ideas just because it is on school or work time.

GENES AND OTHER STUFF

Jeans are what we wear on the outside. Genes are what make us who we are on the inside. Look up pictures of a gene, chromosome, and the DNA chain. What is the difference between a chromosome and a gene? What's an allele? How do you suppose that long chains of chemicals can deeply affect qualities of our lives, such as unique voices, instincts, fingerprints, reflexes, talents, characters, bodies, emotions, tendencies toward certain reactions, and behaviors?

There are a massive number of genes that appear to be doing absolutely nothing. If we learn how to turn them on or if we discover what they actually do, can you imagine the results? Should we be altering our genes? Is this messing with "Mother Nature," or is this using our human intelligence for the good of humankind?

Extensions

A really *big* question is: how does a string of chemicals, no matter how complex, that results in the brain being formed, cause us to have consciousness or awareness? Could there be other sources or contributors to human consciousness? Does consciousness necessarily stem from this chemical sequence of our DNA? Are there alternative explanations? What are instincts? How can it be that a newborn baby when placed on its mother's chest will begin a sucking motion with its lips and move toward its mother's closest nipple to get some nutritious food while the mother's nipple reacts to the presence of the suckling baby? Are these examples of instincts in humans? Look up flight-or-fight reactions. If these are instincts, what are some other examples of instincts in human beings? What are some examples of instincts in other animals? Are all instincts recorded in our genetic material? What kinds of instincts (if any) do we share with other animals? Might simple cells also have instincts?

GENIUS

Is genius something only found in extremely rare individuals? Have you ever had insights, visions, or deep or lucid dreams (more vivid than normal)? Have you made connections, determined patterns, grasped difficult or complex material or challenges, or comprehended how to draw something that was extremely difficult? Have you figured out how to perform a physical movement with special grace, beauty, complexity, or simplicity? Have you had smells, sensations, and experiences that trigger associations or remembrances of specific detailed events and processes? In your dreams, have you created stories, music, poetry, math formulae, and derived explanations to baffling unexplained phenomena? Have you experienced a way of resolving conflict with a group of people that nobody else thought of? Have you seen others express some insight that is startling, comprehensive, elegant, simple, or profound? Have you been in a group in which there is the startling confluence (coming together) of understanding and insight? In such instances, the curious question always arises, "Where did that come from?" Some new light of understanding is shed on our lives when genius emerges. Some new and indescribable fresh breath of life becomes evident, at least to some persons.

This is all genius. It is within us all. It needs to be cultivated, but it also needs to be given permission to be expressed. Genius means that we go beyond the present and the known. We transcend what is culturally given.

Many people view genius as occurring when we are outside the current norms or box of accepted definition. Being outside the box simply means that we are being different from others or some expectation. Genius is something that is focused and distilled (concentrated, purified). Genius has to do with seeing a composite picture of some issue or problem that previously has been a riddle or enigma (something baffling us). It is something more than a direct experience of a larger context, which resolves a wider range of problems. Genius has to do with the experience of a radically different context that yields very different questions, answers, views, and ways of comprehension. It has to do with some leap of human activity that others presumed was impossible. It is the genius who leaps into the impossible, while others only dabble (safely pick at) the improbable in such a way that they take no significant risks and venture no great discovery.

Genius has to do with our unique contributions to life. Every one of us is capable of risking great things and venturing great discoveries of some kind. The contribution of genius has to do with the expression of some insight or action that sheds new light on preexisting presumptions. We are all capable of this contribution. What we concentrate upon, pay attention to, value, regard, create, make real, amplify, and magnify through our lives becomes the base from which genius can emerge. Genius is called forth by necessity of circumstances or the sheer impulse of our passion, concentration, and dedication. Its causes are a subtle (not real obvious) interplay between outer pressures and necessities and inward passion and gifts. Necessity may be the mother of invention, but it is an inner focusing of loosely related insights or gifts that fuse together, igniting and giving birth to the moment of genius. This is not for the lazy. Moments of genius only occur for those who have completely given themselves to some issue, problem, challenge, venture, goal, or way of living at the edges of comprehension. Individuals or groups that express genius demonstrate a faith that there is something greater at play in our lives.

Genius has to do with the expression of a focused and distilled perspective, a unique combination of gifts, and the presence of people leaping into a context of understanding that requires a letting go of past ways, views, values, and attachments. Each of us has a unique collection of gifts. There are moments of genius. In order to express this moment's insight, we must take risks. Society and our local communities desperately need the expression of genius. Courage is a prime note in genius. Imagine what the world would be like if we all allowed our genius to be expressed.

Genius is not necessarily abstract. There are moments of genius for the inventor, mechanic, engineer, dancer, sculptor, cook, counselor, teacher, religious leaders, political leaders, businessperson, writers, administrators, and yes, even accountants! Employees flipping hamburgers down at the local burger stand can be seized by moments of seeing so deeply into some situation or facet of our shared lives that they leap into a greater comprehension. Next time you're at a burger joint see if you can spot the one who is experiencing a moment of inexpressible genius.

Every one of us can have moments in which we see and comprehend that things can be very different from the norm that is accepted as being natural and necessary by most people. If everyone were liberated to express their genius, the many and diverse contributions would change the possibilities for how we live on this planet.

Why doesn't this happen more often? What do we risk if we allow our genius to be expressed? Might one of the great impediments (something that holds us back) be fear that if we let our genius out, we'd have to change how we live? Would others react differently toward us? How would our schools be organized and how would classroom teaching be different if we all gave ourselves permission to let our genius be expressed? Would there be classrooms? Would there be "teachers?" Would education be something that happens to us by other persons in separate buildings during daylight hours only? What would our work sites be like if genius were encouraged and allowed to flourish? Look out—there may be tofu burgers offered at your very own favorite burger stand next week. If so, maybe somebody read this book and the inevitable chain reaction of mutual encouragement for the expression of genius may be accelerating. If so, either go out in the street and dance or go inside the house, close the windows, pull down the shades, lock the doors, and go hide in the closet. Either way, there are some risks.

Make a concerted effort to study the topic of learning and growth in a system (any grouping of people) that values, honors, and recognizes the presence of genius. Would there ever be a boring day again?

Extensions

Is there a connection between the words *genie* (as in the bottle that needs some rubbing and coaxing to allow it to come out) and *genius*? While you're at it, look up *genius loci*.

GENTLENESS IN A WORLD THAT CAN BE HARSH

There are many reasons why certain persons are harsh or mean toward others. When we've made a commitment to be gentle and loving, we can become vulnerable to others who do not have the same commitment. How do we take care of ourselves in such circumstances?

Extensions

When others use you to meet their own needs, how can you react in a nonviolent manner? Violence comes in many forms. The easiest form to spot is physical violence. One of the most common kinds of violence is when people use others as a means of feeling better about themselves. This form of behavior usually puts someone else down. Others are used as a symbol of something that is hated, loathed, or feared. There is a double challenge at play for us. One of them is how to respond to people who act in such hurtful manners. The other has to do with discovering why people act this way. What are forms of violence that are acceptable to many persons in our culture? Where is the line between acceptable and unacceptable violence? What are the subtler and less obvious forms of violence in our culture? Learn all you can about nonviolence. How can we learn to act in ways that honor the presence of others while not being violated ourselves?

GEOGRAPHIC CENTER

What is the geographic center of the country? How could this point be determined? If you included only the contiguous (next to each other) forty-eight states, what would be the geographic center? If you included Alaska and Hawaii, what would be the geographic center? Try to figure out these center points just with the use of a map. What is the geographic center of the Euro-Asian landmass? Mark a center point for each of the continents. Connect each of these points with a line. What are the patterns you observe? What assumptions must you make in order to derive (get) an answer? Whenever anybody is doing any kind of research, it is essential and extremely helpful to know the biases and assumptions the researcher is using. For one thing, this helps us to understand how intelligent informed people can arrive at different answers to the same challenge. This also illustrates that, in more complex questions, the process of deriving an answer is often more interesting (and more important) than the specific conclusions.

Extensions

What are some other kinds of centers that you could think of relative to landmass? What is the center for the least populated sections of the country?

If there are multiple centers, they are called epicenters. For any of these centers, are there multiple epicenters? What is the center point of the densest metro area in the country (or the world)? Does this point or points of greatest population density change during the course of a day?

GETTING CREDIT

Do you always like to get credit for what you have done? Do some people depend too much on getting credit? Do some people get too little credit for what they do?

Extensions

Have you ever done something good for somebody else and not claimed any credit? Try it sometime.

GIFTS TO YOU

When wonderful things have been given to you and people have acted kindly toward you, do you try to turn around and return these same kinds of gestures of kindness to others? For instance, if someone were to go out of her or his way to teach you how to be a master reader, do you think you'd like to teach someone else to read?

Extensions

When less than desirable things happen to others, why do some people do to others what has been done to them? Some persons do not return hostility in reaction to other hostile or violent acts. Why? How? Who are the people you know who give back to life compassion and understanding?

GIVING AWAY AND GETTING

Is it true that if you give away something, you have less than what you started with?

Extensions

I'm sitting with my friend at a chess tournament. He is going to teach us everything he knows about chess, and my son will teach him everything he knows about chess. The friend says to me, "Wow, the more you give away, the more you get." What are some other examples of giving away something and getting more in the end? Does it matter that something good comes back to you personally? Can you be satisfied that this good thing will be passed on to others whom you may never meet? There is an old phrase, "What goes around, comes around." What you share with the world will come around to others. It is distributed and shared. Can you be satisfied with this dynamic of life?

GLACIERS

Glaciers once covered major portions of North America. Did they cover large masses of Asia at the same time? There have been many glacial periods. As Asia was covered with glaciers, was it covered with glaciers to the extent that North America was covered in the same period? Did major glaciers ever move from the south to the north? Hint: there are maps available that show how fast certain landmasses are still rising, due to the fact that the tremendous pressures exerted on the surface of the Earth by the glaciers is now gone. Where are the areas of most significant rise? Why do you think these areas are so concentrated in one region of the Earth's surface?

Extensions

There are certain areas of the Earth that are sinking. Is this related to the glaciers? What can you imagine? Glaciers existed in places that you might not think of because of the present-day climate. Search for these odd and unexpected locations.

GLASS—WHAT IS IT?

Glass is not a solid, it is a supercooled liquid. Do some research on this topic, and you may be surprised at the kinds of things that appear to be solids but are liquids. Glass is actually a liquid that is slowly in motion. Do some more research on liquids that appear to be solids.

Extensions

If glass is liquid and if all liquids evaporate, does glass evaporate? Next time you lose your glasses, you may now know what happened to them.

GLOBAL POSITIONING SYSTEM

List as many ways the global positioning system (GPS) is used by different people. Find out how it works.

Extensions

If you thought that Einstein's general theory of relativity only dealt with unusual places on the other side of the universe, guess how many miles your GPS would be off if it were not corrected for clocks running at different speeds at different distances from the Earth? (*See* "Relativity—Time Clocks.")

GLOBES OF A DIFFERENT KIND

What are the different kinds of globes you've seen? Geopolitical globes with some physical relief (physical features displayed) features are the most common. What are some other possible kinds of globes of the Earth? Could you imagine one that is of the Earth's interior? The oceans might be tinted slightly green and the dry land could be tinted light blue. The core would be solid metal, then there would be various layers of magma, chutes of magma extending right to the surface, chutes of hot water, areas where the magma swells to the surface along long cracks (tectonic plate lines), and places where surface materials are literally gobbled up by the depths (the other side of the tectonic plate lines). How could you get the viscous liquid that simulates the magma to glow and be slightly warm? What would the magma look like in a dark room? If it were true to scale, how much would this globe weigh? What is the difference between magma and lava?

Extensions

There is a passage in a book called *War and Peace* by Leo Tolstoy that talks about a dream one of the main characters has about an old teacher holding a globe. Someday, see if you can find it.

GLUE LIMITS

Imagine you are conducting an experiment related to the effectiveness of glues. You have a wall that is smooth, various kinds of glue, and several cylinders of plastic of all different diameters (distance across the circular width). Could you glue a short, lightweight, small-diameter piece of plastic to the wall, sticking straight out (perpendicular to the wall—horizontal to the ground)? You can only put the glue on the ends of the plastic cylinder. No other supports are allowed.

You start out with a common kind of glue and a smaller plastic cylinder. What are the variables at play? Some of them are the weight of the plastic (related to density), diameter of the plastic tube, friction qualities on the wall and the ends of the tubes of plastic, and quality of the glue. There are some other important factors or variables in addition to those mentioned. Try to figure out the various combinations of these variables that will enable you to successfully glue the cylinder to the wall. If different glues were more effective, could you keep gluing on longer and longer pieces with greater diameters and densities? Is there a limit to the strength of glues? Might there be glue that is so powerful that you could glue on plastic rods ten feet long, fifty feet long, or one mile long? If the wall was strong enough and if the plastic was rigid enough, could you continue to increase the diameter of the plastic tube while you increase the length of the tube?

One way to think about this challenge is to assume that instead of starting with a straight rod of plastic you would start with a rod that is curved like a big crescent. If the glue is strong enough when the rod is glued to the wall, gravity would force the crescent shape into a straight rod. Is this possible? Imagine if this rounded piece bending into a straight piece were made of the kind of plastic that when it is bent it lights up and begins to shine in different colors. Then you could try this experiment at nighttime. Everybody in the entire city will thank you.

How do glues work? What do they do to the two opposing surfaces? If you thought superglue is tough stuff, look up *gluons*. What do they hold together? How do they do it? Can you buy them in a tube?

Extensions

Could the glue be so powerful that it enables you to glue the cylinder to the wall and hang some weights on various positions of the cylinder? What would be the different effects of hanging weights closer to the wall versus further from the wall? Are the most powerful glues safe to use? Are there limits to the effectiveness of the amount of glue you use (is more glue necessarily better)?

We talked about variables. There are two kinds of variables in an experiment—independent and dependent variables. In a simple experiment, you want to change one variable at a time. The outcome depends upon how you change this single variable. In this situation, you might hold constant (keep the same) everything except the kind of glue you are using. Then you use the various lengths of tubes that vary in diameters. You could vary the kind of surfaces that become joined, like the ends of the tubes and the wall. Everything depends on this kind of glue. What are some other things that you might choose to vary while keeping the other variables consistent or held constant? Try to define the other variables that need to be held constant (kinds of glues, diameters of the plastic cylinders, kinds of plastics, amount of glue, temperature, humidity, amount of sunlight, kind of lighting, or time of the day). Would the shape of the tube be a significant factor? You do the experiment in precisely the same manner with all the identified variables being held constant except for one. All the ones you hold constant are dependent variables. The one that you change is independent. The independent variable is what you change to test for the effect of this change on the dependent variable. When what is independent is altered, what is dependent is affected in observable and repeatable ways that can be replicated by others elsewhere. If you have more than one variable that is changing, it gets much more difficult to analyze what causes the outcome. In the real world, experiments have to be conducted with many variables changing. There are ways to conduct experiments in this manner. Talk to a teacher or scientist about these methods.

GOLF—THE GREATEST SHOT IN HISTORY

Who do you think made the longest golf shot in history? This is a bit of a trick question. It assumes that you are able to probe the question and ask it in a new way. The manner in which certain problems are posed or questions are asked predisposes most people to react to the challenge based on the presumed original context. Always be willing to transpose, convert, or extend the context and then discover the many creative options for responding. This response is vastly different in kind from an automatic reaction to the initial challenge embedded in the presenting and presumed context. Response is always an option; reaction is never a necessity.

The answer is that the American astronaut Alan Shepard took along a golf club with him on a trip to the moon. He got it out and whacked a ball. The ball probably flew many times as far as a similar shot taken here on Earth. What are the differences between hitting a golf ball on Earth compared to hitting one on the moon? How much farther might you estimate the ball flew on the moon compared to how far it would have flown here on Earth?

Could we assume that the ratio (comparison of two numbers or quantities) of the Earth's gravity compared to the gravity of the moon could be used to determine how much farther the golf ball would fly on the moon compared to how far it would fly on Earth? Are there any other significant factors (variables) that would affect how far a ball is hit?

Extensions

How far could you throw a baseball on the moon? Could you throw a baseball so hard that it might escape the moon's gravitational force and keep flying into outer space? If so, could you throw it to Earth? If it got to Earth, would it burn up entering Earth's atmosphere? What would it be like catching this ball in a baseball mitt? Might you be able to fling a Frisbee into space from the surface of the moon? What would be your first choice of things to chuck (throw) from the moon to the Earth? Look up the topic of escape velocity. Think of other ways of projecting objects. Start with methods with the least amount of energy and move toward things with increasing energy. For instance, you might start with throwing a ball. Move on to a slingshot. Then move on to a rifle. Try to find out how much energy it would take some object to escape from the surface of the moon. Now compare this result to the Earth. Compare these two results to one of the giant planets in our solar system. Compare all of these results to the energy needed for an object to escape the gravitational pull of a neutron star. Finally, compare these results to the energy needed to escape the gravitational pull of a black hole.

Will you ever look at a golf ball the same way? Every wonder what is in the inside of a golf ball? The deepest secret of all time is that the interior space of a golf ball may be a black hole that is exactly the same size as your little toenail!

GOOD AND BAD?

Good or *bad*, *weak* or *strong*, *beautiful* or *ugly* are terms we use so often. Do we really know what they mean? So many people rate the following terms as being good or bad, weak or strong, beautiful or ugly: liberal, conservative, women, men, African Americans, European Americans, North Americans, Mexicans, Canadians, Americans, the rich, the poor, the educated, the uneducated, people who live on this side of the railroad tracks, those who live on the other side of the lines of acceptability, straights and gays, married and singles, or young and old. What does it mean to be good or bad, strong or weak, ugly or beautiful? This is a topic that is not usually discussed, but since so many people in so many ways use these terms and practice a lifestyle based on judgments that flow from these terms, isn't it about time we start talking about these things? When you hear certain terms used for other people, how do you react? Do you automatically react based on your prior tendencies and cultural conditioning, or do you respond creatively with an open heart? Is our world really based in reality on everything being in two groups (either this or that—either/or).

Try to figure out as many reasons as possible that account for why so many times critical topics are squelched (snuffed out). Can polite conversation ever include critical topics that challenge the current behaviors and values? Why or why not?

Extensions

Is there another way to relate to each other? Do these terms always imply a hierarchy (an order of existence in which something or somebody is inferior while others are superior and some hold power over and against others)? Do you think that hierarchies such as these may be destructive to life?

GRAPEFRUIT OF A DIFFERENT KIND!

When the universe was one-trillionth of a second old, it was about the size of a grapefruit. How many years was it until grapefruits came into existence? How do we get grapefruits from the big bang? How did we get animals that enjoy eating grapefruit from the big bang? At that split second (one-trillionth of a second after the big bang), there was an even ratio of matter and antimatter particles. Every particle had another particle with an exact opposite charge (negative or positive). From what we can see and from what we theorize, the universe is made up of primarily matter and not antimatter. When antimatter and matter meet, they annihilate each other totally and everything is converted 100 percent to radiant energy. Why didn't this happen in the first trillionth of a second when the universe was the size of a grapefruit? Why didn't the universe evolve with antimatter grapefruits? How did matter win out? Next time you see a grapefruit, ask the closest person to you about these various connections and relationships related to grapefruit. Try finding something under the topic of CP violation (violation of the expectation of even distribution of matter and antimatter). Just because it appears that the known universe is primarily made up of matter, does this rule out the possibility that there are aspects of the universe we have not yet detected that may be fully made up of antimatter? Is what we see all that there is? Look up *dark matter*. Is what we theorize to be actually possible all that is possible? If people only think about what others tell them is possible, how do we grow in understanding and knowledge? Maybe all the dark matter is really a collection of antimatter grapefruits.

Extensions

How much would that grapefruit have weighed in the first trillionth of a second? If all the particles in the universe were contained in that grapefruit-sized mass, were they the same size as the same particles are today? Is there the same number of particles in today's universe as there was back in that one-trillionth of a second after the big bang? Were the particles during those early moments of the birth of the universe dissimilar (not like) to our particles in the known universe today? Maybe there weren't any particles but only predecessors of our current particles. If there is matter and antimatter, might there be space and antispace? What would this antispace be like? From our limited perspective of space/time/matter, what could we imagine antispace/antitime/antimatter to be like? There is such a thing as antimatter. Experiments are being conducted with antimatter right now. Might there be a future possibility of doing experiments with antispace and antitime? What are some stories that reflect these imagined possibilities? If there aren't any, make them up.

GREATEST CANYON IN THE WORLD

Where do you suppose is the greatest canyon in the world? Many people would contend that it is located in the western United States—namely the Grand Canyon. Might it be a canyon in Mexico? Look around for evidence of great canyons. Where are they?

When do you suspect it was discovered? Who discovered it? Continue to read after you do some investigation work.

The Russians in the late 1950s made a most fascinating discovery as they were preparing to construct the Aswan Dam in Egypt. As they bored their holes in the ground for the foundations of the great dam, they discovered that they were boring through a much greater depth of sediment than expected. They weren't hitting the expected bedrock (solid rock). Tests were performed and sure enough, there it was—the greatest canyon in the world under the sands and soils of the present-day Nile River.

Extensions

How did it get there? Apparently, it had to do with the Mediterranean Sea drying up at least at one point in history. As the seawater evaporated, the waters flowing out of the Nile River might have eroded into a massively deeper canyon. How could the Mediterranean Sea have dried up? The narrow inlet of water through the Strait of Gibraltar was blocked, and thus the water evaporation rate was greater than the water replacement rate. This was also corroborated (supported) by a discovery of huge salt deposits under the present-day Mediterranean Sea. Once the ocean came tumbling back into the Mediterranean basin (from the Atlantic Ocean), this water created what was probably the world's greatest waterfall throughout history. Try to imagine what the bottom of a dried-up sea would look like. If you want to see one, go to the Great Salt Flats in the western United States.

GREATEST INVENTIONS OF ALL TIME

What do you consider the greatest inventions of all time? Try arranging them chronologically, and then try to arrange them in order of importance. How do you define or measure greatness? Would the wheel be placed on your list? Would fire be toward the top? How about pizza?

Extensions

Think of as many kinds of inventions as possible—mechanical, artistic, electronic, social, medical, intellectual, biological, cultural, mental, etc. This is a third way of ordering your list—by kind of invention. Ask other people in different professions what they think. Ask them to list the inventions in these three ways (time, importance, and kind), and ask them if they can think of other ways to list inventions of importance. A possible fourth way is to list the inventions that never were noticed that could have made a huge difference in the way we live. Were there great inventions that didn't get credit? What could possibly account for such an occurrence? Hint:

- Somebody or some group in power didn't want something to emerge.
- It came too late relative to other inventions.
- It was too early relative to the readiness of society to comprehend or accept.
- Somebody chose to simply keep it private (it could have been discovered later).

What would be some other possible reasons for a great invention not to be given credit?

GROWING UP

Between which years are most people done growing taller? How about the issue of growing shorter? How much does an average person lose in height when she or he grows older? When does this growing shorter start to happen in most people? Why is it that people tend to grow shorter after a certain age?

Extensions

Is it natural and necessary that people put on more weight as they age? Do men and women put on weight differently? Is aging inevitable? Since we are all going to die, isn't it obvious to everybody that aging is inevitable? Convert the question to one that asks, Is aging in the manner in which we age now necessary? Could we alter the diet, the way we live, and our expectations related to aging? Could we alter our social and physical environment in order to alter the manner in which we age? Look up information on research related to aging. Is death inevitable? Can we clone ourselves into unending life? What about cryogenics? This is the science of studying phenomena in low-temperature situations. Some people use cryonics, to freeze the bodies of persons who have recently died in the hope of being able to revive them again someday when our technology has advanced. What are some ethical issues related to cloning human beings and cryonics? Look up some research on the relation between health, aging, and the shortening of our telomeres.

GROWTH OF DIFFERENT KINDS

There are many ways to describe growth patterns. Arithmetic growth can be described in a way that is similar to adding: 2+4+8+16+32+64+128+256+512. Each generation in the series doubles the preceding amount. Soon the numbers get large. This means that a population of things like insects would double in each generation. Now instead of doubling in each generation, how would the growth rate be affected if in each generation the increase would be like the following numbers: 2+4+16+256+65,536+4,294,967,296. This is one form of exponential growth. In a series, each generation doesn't just double, it grows by multiplying the preceding number by itself. By the sixth generation, we're into the billions. The sixth generation would be what? Try calculating this product (two numbers multiplied together). Can your calculator do it? Don't feel bad if it doesn't work for these large numbers. Change your batteries and see what happens. Go to a different room and see if changing the context alters the presenting issues. Try changing calculators. For such large numbers, we may try switching to another numbering notation system called scientific notation (only do this if changing the batteries, room, or calculator doesn't work). If you don't know scientific notation yet, either be patient or ask somebody who can teach you. What are some other possible growth patterns numerically described? (I sure hope it's not a virus!)

For a little extra challenge in numerical growth patterns, even if you have not studied something called exponents, it's OK. Imagine a sequence of numbers in which each generation is a product of multiplying itself in the following way. Take a simple example 2×2=4, 4×4×4×4=256, then the next generation would be 256×256×256 (you keep doing this 256 times). Is there anything in the universe that grows in this kind of pattern?

What are some other number patterns of growth that you can think of? Once you have identified different numerical growth patterns, try to imagine things in the real world that would grow in this manner as described by. Is there such a thing as a negative growth pattern? Depending on the number of negative numbers in each term (odd or even), you're going to get a term (generation) with either a negative or a positive number. These terms begin to cancel each other out. One generation may be a huge negative number while the next generation may be a much larger positive number. So each generation flip-flops between negative and positive realms. Try to imagine something in the real world that approximates this growth pattern in the real world. Hint: look up any wave pattern.

Are there any numbers you can multiply together and get zero while not using zero as one of the numbers being multiplied?

Extensions

Look up the surface area of the Earth. If things grew according to one of these numerical patterns, and if each thing were one square inch, how long would it take these things to cover the entire planet's surface?

GUNS AND BUTTER

In an economics course, I recall the professor talking about a fundamental choice countries must make. If they are putting their resources into making weapons for war, there will be fewer resources left for human needs related to everyday existence, such as schooling, health care, and food. Nations make choices related to guns and butter issues. How does this debate affect the life of our country today?

Today we are experiencing many shocking incidents of people using guns to hurt and kill others. Does every culture need to decide that there are limits to the number of guns that need to be sold and purchased? Is there a relationship between the number of guns being sold in our country and the murder rate? Should everybody have an unlimited right to buy as many automatic weapons as they want every month? Once entire industries tool up (set up) for the production of guns, is it in their self-interest to market these guns very effectively so that their machinery and factories can run as close to maximum production as possible, twenty-four hours a day? Once machines get going on a production run, it is highly efficient to produce as much as possible, as quickly as possible, for as long as possible. The gun industry creates the demand, and collects the industry the tremendous profits. Isn't it an interesting irony that one way to create demand is to emphasize the need to be safe. When there are guns everywhere, who is safe? Young children in their own homes and those in the home of a friend comprise one of the primary groups of victims. Children play with guns. Children play with real guns. Children play with real guns with real bullets or shells in them. Children die. Is it interesting that the gun industry has resisted putting effective safety locks on guns? In the past, we presume that our murder rate was not as high as it is today. Is this true? If we now have the highest murder rate in our country, what has changed in our culture?

Extensions

Is violence a necessary part of our culture? Why is violence glorified so much? Is it ironic that some actors and actresses who have made millions of dollars by portraying characters in movies illustrating stark, gory, and massive violence later speak up against violence (sometimes while they continue to produce and act in violent movies)? Do you believe there is a connection between the many forms of violence portrayed in movies, videos, and television shows and the subsequent acts of violence done by those who regularly have watched such stuff? What are counterarguments against the direct connection between passive observation of media programs and active engagement in violence? What is the case for making this direct connection? Research the number of professional organizations that have come out with public statements saying that there is a direct connection.

HAIR

Do you think that the hair on your head grows at the same rate as the hair composing your eyebrow? How fast does hair grow?

Extensions

Do you think that your arms, hands, feet, teeth, and legs grow at the same rate? What signals them to stop growing? If this signal could be blocked or a growth signal initiated, could we just keep growing? Look up information on our human growth hormone.

HAIRS ON YOUR HEAD

In the middle of the night, the question arose—what is the surface area of the hair on my head? I thought, "My, that is a useful question." Many people would laugh and say that this is a ridiculous question. They're no fun anyway. Might the surface area of your hair be greater than the surface area of your skin?

Now it all depends. If you want the genius inside of you to awaken and become a strong influence in your life, then you will have to learn how to look at the world sideways or differently.

Back to the hairs on your head. Before you actually begin, estimate the surface area. Try to guess in what order of magnitude (approximate amount of something compared to certain contexts), like a square foot, a square yard, or a football field. It is useful to make initial estimates, because later you can compare your original estimate with your calculated answer. Probably nobody you have ever met has figured this out or has even thought of trying to figure it out. Ask others what they think the answer will be. Get different groups of people working on the issue. They will have to invent their own method for deriving the answer. Remember to try to get others to estimate which orders of magnitude (one square inch, one square yard, one square mile, etc.). Wouldn't this make a great fund-raiser for your school or community group? You could have the entire community involved making guesses. Somebody would then have the most closely observed and studied hair in history. Select somebody to be the subject. Then get the groups started with some hints on how to proceed. Maybe you don't want to give any hints. Start to think of ways that you could figure out something that looks initially to be impossible.

When you have a complex issue in front of you, one way to solve the problem is to brainstorm with a group of people about possible methods to solve the problem. Who says you have to work through issues of life alone?

Some suggestions—you may wish to start with estimating the number of hairs on your head. One way to do this is to count the approximate number of hairs in a one square inch of scalp. It might help to have a friend helping you. To be more accurate, you may wish to repeat this process about two or three times in different areas of the scalp. Why? Might there be different densities of hair in different places upon your head? You could then figure out the mean (average) number of hairs per square inch. (*See* "Earth—Its Weight.") Once you have this approximation of the average numbers of hairs per square inch, then you need to figure out the total number of square inches of scalp area.

There is a big challenge at play here. Your head is curved and irregular; therefore, it is difficult to measure its surface area (only the surface area with hair on it).

One possible solution is to take pieces of paper and tape them together in such a manner that they cover your head. Make sure you use several different pieces. If the pieces overlap, be sure to color the part of the pieces that do overlap so that later when you disassemble them you do not count overlapped pieces, thus overestimating the total surface area. Don't let too many people see you doing this activity. If others ask anything, merely tell them, "I'm creating the next popular hair craze."

Now you have a nice piece of taped-together paper upon your head. You could at this point disassemble the pieces. You'll probably notice that all the nonshaded areas are irregular. Lay them out flat. Take chunks of one-inch squares and figure out approximately how many of these squares you can lay on top of the nonshaded areas. Do not overlap any of these squares. Pack as many of them as you can into the nonshaded areas. Now take other one-inch-square pieces and, one at a time, cut them into the irregular shapes that are not covered by your other one-inch squares. Keep track of how many of these cut-up one-inch squares you have applied to your nonshaded area. This method should cover up most of the nonshaded area of the original paper you had on your head. This method approximates the surface area of your head. It is not perfect because of the crinkles in the paper when you originally forced a flat object to bend into an irregular curved shaped. (When space-time is warped by the presence of mass, could there be crinkles that are odd places in the universe?) Count the number of square inches. Have several different groups trying to do the same thing. See who can come up with the best way to measure irregular surfaces.

Once you have the estimation of the total number of square inches of the person's head being measured, then what do you do next? It might be that you multiply the total number of square inches by the approximate number of hairs in an average square inch. Congratulations! You now have computed or approximated the number of hairs on somebody's head.

Now you might treat each hair as being a cylinder. Find a decent math book that teaches you how to compute the surface area of a cylinder. It is a simple formula.

Now that you have the formula for the surface area of a cylinder, what more do you need? You need the average length of the hairs on your head. You now know how to do averages. So take about ten hairs and measure them. Average the lengths. Next, you need to go consult some reference book that will give you the average widths of an average person's hair—or—you might ask around to discover what kind of instrument would allow you to directly measure the width of your hair. You would find this instrument in many well-equipped science labs. Measure about ten hairs. Compute the average width. Be sure to measure each hair at least in three different places (just in case it turns out that hairs have varying diameters). Be sure to measure the different hairs in approximately the same place so that your measuring methods are consistent. Now that you have the average length and average width of your hairs, go to the formula for computing the surface area of a cylinder. Multiply the numbers and, lo and behold, you have the average surface area of one hair on your head.

Go ahead and multiply this surface by the number of estimated hairs on your head. You've done it. Go back to your estimate before doing this creative act of genius. You've multiplied the surface area times the average number of hairs per unit of surface space times the average surface area of each hair. Were you close?

How many people have done this throughout history? If nobody has done it before, it would be because nobody ever thought of doing it before! Try this at least once before you get old enough to have your hair thin out. In your spare moments, cultivate (encourage) the process of having original thoughts or unique angles on old thoughts. Many of them are interesting, and some of them will stun you with their beauty. If you get into this practice of tracking your original or creative thoughts, you may notice that they tend to occur in certain times of the day, in certain circumstances, or in certain states of mind or moods. Note these differences. Keep a journal. These insights could be very useful to you. If you want to have some fun, read through and study the drawings in the journals of geniuses. Their doodling can be insightful beyond measure. Keep your eye out for what appears in the margins. Look for little side comments.

Reflect: there are many kinds of processes in nature and life. One kind is a linear process in which you begin at point A and wind up at point Z. One of the implications of this method is that it implies by force of its format that there is one right way to get the one right answer. For many mechanical procedures, this works. Like starting a car. It really does help things to turn the key to the on position before attempting to go someplace. It helps matters if you put gasoline in the tank before running out of gas.

Other processes in life and nature are not necessarily or predominantly (mainly) linear. Most biological and human processes are not linear. Look at a soccer game. It does begin and end and has a logic of internal rules, but it is extremely fluid, dynamic, and always changing swiftly. There are many possible ways to get to the same point.

Extensions

Take this example of a nonlinear process and apply it to the challenge of the hairs on your head. Imagine other ways to have reached the same end by using different methods or different sequences. Try to think of other things that you could figure out the surface area of—like a Koosh ball. Try measuring the surface area of someone's big ego.

HAIRY PROBLEMS

Ever noticed that some older persons have long curly hairs protruding out in all directions from their eyebrows? Ever noticed that the same thing happens at the edges of ears when some people reach a certain age? I used to think that was somewhat odd. Now, all of a sudden, I have these kinky hairs sticking out of my eyebrows and these same kinds of hairs on the edges of my ears. Why do you think this happens? Is it a mark of wisdom and distinction?

Extensions

What else happens to people as we age? Are all of these changes absolutely necessary and natural? Might some of these changes be related to diet, exercise, and the quality of our environment? Do you think that mental stimulation throughout life has any effect on our physical and mental health?

HANGING FROM THE TREE

It was springtime in the Midwest. The great snows had melted, and the early rains had arrived in great deluges. At my friend's house, suddenly a wonderful large lake spanned several different people's backyards. Four of us got into canoes and went canoeing in the backyards. It was great. My friend's mother was in the bow of the canoe I was in. Just as we passed under a large tree, I grabbed onto a branch and ever so gently lifted myself out of the canoe. When my friend's mom was several yards away, I began to shout like I was deserted and left behind. She turned around with the most amazed look on her face! She asked me, "How did you get caught up in the tree?" She actually did come back for me. She was a very kind person. There is a most special look on our faces in that instant in which we are very surprised about something. Try to mimic (match) that look on your face right now. Go look at a mirror. Can you make the same face? How would you verbally describe the look? Do you look into a mirror or at a mirror?

Extensions

What are other common facial expressions related to certain life experiences? Try to make these faces. Then go to a mirror and try it again. Is it different the second time in front of the mirror? Do we become self-conscious? The instant we become self-conscious, what happens to our spontaneity?

HAPPINESS—JUST A DREAM?

What would it take to make you happy? Don't be bothered by what you think you ought to be thinking. Take a few minutes and start writing as fast as your thoughts come to your mind. Keep going until there are no more ideas about what would make you happy. Put the list away for a period of time. Repeat the process. Put it away in a safe place. Again after a period of time, repeat the process. Now compare your lists.

What are the patterns that emerge? What are the differences in the three lists? Within each list, try grouping or color coding the things listed that are similar.

Talk to others about what they think would make them happy. Try talking to men and women, people of different ages, different socioeconomic strata, race, religions, temperaments, or personal histories. See what you find in common. Figure out ways to elicit (encourage) spontaneous, real, heartfelt responses.

Extensions

Are we basically contented with life? Happiness, contentment, joy, peace, and acceptance—are these all the same? What do they hold in common?

HAVING A MIND FOR CERTAIN THINGS

Some things come to us easily and effortlessly. Other things take much work to accomplish. There are certain kinds of facts, impressions, images, and senses that I only have to experience once in my life and they remain with me forever. They are indelibly (deeply and permanently) marked in my memory. Other things I don't remember so easily. What comes easily for you? What requires real concerted work?

Extensions

Try to determine the patterns of the kinds of things that are easy for you. Do the same for things that challenge you.

HEARTLAND SEAPORTS

Find the seaport (harbor accessible to ships from the ocean) that is farthest from the oceans. Hint: it could be anywhere in the world, but be careful to keep your eye out for interconnected freshwater lakes, rivers, canals, and seaways (large human-made systems combining locks, rivers, and lakes).

Once you have found this seaport, find out the world's second and third seaports farthest from the oceans. Now try to find out the world's highest seaport (elevation above sea level). Are there any seaports that are below sea level?

Extensions

Look at maps or a globe and simply wonder. See what kinds of questions come to your mind. Don't be goal-oriented. Simply let your mind wander from one thought to another while you are focused on the globe. If you hear a voice shouting up the stairs asking if you are wasting your time, answer back, "Yes!" Some of our side diversions turn out to be extremely useful and productive while others are just fun. Who says that simple fun isn't a good thing in life? Try doing this same activity while you are gazing at the stars, clouds, a group of people, or the depths of a lake. What occurs when we switch from concentrating on particular objects to the open context in which everything emerges into our attention?

HEAVY BOOKS

What do you think would be the world's heaviest book?

Extensions

What is the heaviest imaginable object that might be one cubic inch (one inch wide, long, and deep)? What material could make it so heavy? Could it be so heavy that it could fall right through the Earth? If it did, would it go all the way through or just to the center of the Earth? Is there material (matter) that could be one cubic inch, weigh nothing, and pass right through the Earth? Work on this one only after your normal jobs for the day are all finished.

HEMI

When I was still in junior high school, one of the most popular cars to purchase was a Dodge Ram Charger with a 426-hemi engine. At that time, it was popular for boys to wear blue or maroon sweaters, wingtip shoes, powder-blue shirts, and for casual wear, Adidas track shoes. The young women had their things they considered popular and necessary, like wearing their hair high on top the head (like a big bee nest), short dresses, and certain kinds of makeup. In your community, what is most popular right now? What is not popular? Are there certain persons who are beyond trying to impress others in any way with their outward appearances who have a certain self-confidence that allows them to do what they want to do and pursue the things they want to pursue without thinking what others will say? In terms of the things we want and in terms of our behaviors, to what degree are you controlled by what groups of people think is acceptable? Why? If you're an adult, are you beyond any of this group influence stuff?

Extensions

What do you notice about the way others react to you when you are self-confident? Try observing yourself or others when anyone is encouraging, sensitive, engaging, and honoring and valuing the presence and contributions of others, when you take delight in the presence of others, when you are able to stimulate curiosity in others, and when you are able to play well and help create a sense of joy.

HELLO, DOLLY!

Look up the definition of cloning. Scientists have cloned a sheep named Dolly (and other mammals). Now that scientists have successfully cloned mammals, do you think that we ought to be cloning human beings? If so, why? If not, why not? Are there any circumstances under which you think it would be permissible and ethical (OK) to clone human beings? If you had yourself cloned, would the new person be your offspring? How would she or he be related to your parents? Try to figure out the meaning of different relationships if we start to clone humans.

Extensions

Would your clone be identical in all ways to you? Should we ever allow human cloning? Might there be some good reasons to clone human beings? If we could clone human beings without heads, could the bodies be used to harvest (collect) organs to be used to save the lives of other living humans? If this sounds shocking, we need to be mindful that the technologies to do such procedures may be available in the future. We should start thinking about such things now. The genetic material in an insect that determines whether a head will develop has been discovered. Whether this can be applied to humans has not yet been determined. We are discovering things in the insect and animal world that may influence what we are able to do genetically to humans someday. Look up and study some of the fascinating things being discovered about genetics. How much of this new knowledge could be applied to cloning?

HOME, SWEET HOME

Assume that we divide the United States in sections labeled East, Southeast, Midwest, Southwest, Northwest, and West. What label or general section of the country would you use for people in southern Missouri, Indiana, or Illinois, people in western Oklahoma, people in northeastern Oklahoma, people in western Texas, people in western Pennsylvania, people in eastern Ohio, people in western Ohio, people in the extreme northern tip of Kentucky, people in northeastern Kansas, people in Western Kansas, people in eastern Colorado, people in western Minnesota, people in eastern North or South Dakota, people in western North or South Dakota, people in northern Virginia, people in southern Virginia, people in northeastern Nevada, people in northwestern Nevada? Make out a chart of these possible locations and ask different people what they think. Do you think that the people who actually live in these locations would be in basic agreement with the answers given by persons in others sections of the country? Where does Hawaii fit into this scheme (picture)? Where do Alaska and the Aleutian Islands fit into this scheme?

Extensions

Nomenclature (how we name something) and taxonomy (how we organize the elements of a system) matter a great deal. They affect what we are looking for and reflect what we know about a particular system. The names and structure we attribute (give) to any system are a result of our biases (assumptions). Sometimes the divisions we create (like the name for sections of the country) are just fine for one level of analysis. When we start to ask more detailed questions, the gross (macro or large) divisions might no longer be effective. In this case of the sections of the country, how many more sections would we need in order to cover all of these border and overlaid (being in two different sections at once) locations?

There was a five hundred–year flood (a flood of a certain magnitude that scientists estimate only occurs once in a five hundred–year period) in the Red River of the North (on the border of North Dakota and Minnesota). Might this kind of flood occur more often than once every five hundred years? Names matter. Structures we indicate as being real deeply affect the way we view any phenomenon.

HOT LOVE ON ICE

At age five, I was skating at the Phalen outdoor ice rink. It was a perfect starlit cool night. Dozens of people of all ages were skating around in a large circle. I was your average five-year-old. The last thing on my mind that night would have been girls. Suddenly, while the public address system was playing a song that I can remember very clearly, there she was—the most beautiful young girl skating through my life. It was pure love at first sight. I was absolutely stricken with passion for her. I could barely stand up. I recovered and raced after her. It was as though she was the only person that existed in the world beside me. Everything else was merely the setting or stage for the two of us. Since I was totally twitterpated (from the movie *Bambi*), I wonder if my skates were thumping on the ice. If so, it must have been quite the sight. Look up what it means to twitter. I hope I wasn't twittering that night, because sometimes when we twitter we can be twitchy. How do such feelings arise? How can our feelings be so strong for somebody we've never even met before? Is everything in life rational? As I raced toward her, in very best skating form, I realized I didn't know what to say. I was so struck with love that I couldn't say anything. Later in high school, I wondered who that wonderful skating, dreamlike person was.

Extensions

How many songs about love can you name? How many can you sing?

HOT SAUCES

There are many different kinds of hot sauces on the market. Most of them are labeled as being mild, medium, or hot. Some claim to be the hottest of all sauces. What is it that makes them hot? Look these ingredients up; once you have the answer, try to determine a way to test the relative hotness of various hot sauces. Is tasting sufficient? Are there other methods? Even if there are other simple methods that do not require expensive lab equipment, is tasting still necessary? Recently, I was at a farmers' market, and one of the sellers of fresh produce (vegetables and fruit right out of the garden) was selling these interesting-looking peppers. She warned me that due to the unusual weather the peppers that are usually mild to warm were quite hot. Having been around hot sauces for many years, I blew off her words and went right home to make some shish kebabs on the charcoal grill. A piece of one of these little fresh-picked, innocent-looking peppers fell off the skewers (sticks used to cook the food). So, of course, I popped it into my mouth (an irrepressible genetic instinct). It was so hot, I couldn't talk for five minutes . The first thing I thought was that I was going to die speechless. Ever since the skating rink when I was five years old, I've disliked being speechless at the most inopportune (the worst) moments. How can weather change the qualities of a warmish nice pepper into a roaring, burning, hot piece of food that probably shortened my life by five years?

Extensions

What are the four classes of things we can taste? One of them is sweetness. Given these four basic properties of foods that we can taste, all the foods and nonfood items in the world can be described in terms of these four properties. Where does hot fit into these four properties? Are there other tastes you can think of that do not clearly stem from one of the four taste properties?

HUGELY DIFFICULT TOPICS

Why are sex, politics, and religion so challenging to talk about for so many people? What is polite conversation? What are the strictures (imposed rules—spoken and unspoken) placed upon polite conversation? How are these strictures enforced verbally? How are they imposed nonverbally? Next time you are in a nice polite conversation, bring up this topic for discussion.

Extensions

Why do you suppose that, when I was in high school, a gym teacher who was supposed to teach us "sex education" talked for three straight days about acne? Zits and babies must have an underlying connection somewhere. Where did the word "zit" come from? Where do babies come from? I thought of going to college and majoring in physical education so that I could discover this connection between sexuality and acne. I'm sure this kind of perplexing talk has never been given anywhere else in the world. Why did it have to happen in my gym class?

HUMANS BREATHING LIKE FISH?

There was an announcement in the *New England Journal of Medicine* that doctors can rescue certain critically ill, premature babies from almost certain death by filling their feeble, underdeveloped lungs with oxygen-rich liquid for a few days to restore their breathing. This fluid takes the place of air. The same experimental technique is being tested on children and adults with a variety of other life-threatening illnesses and injuries, including infections, near drowning, and smoke inhalation. In Infant Respiratory Distress Syndrome, the lungs lack enough of a chemical that keeps the airs sacs open so oxygen and carbon dioxide are exchanged. Almost 3 percent of premature babies die of the condition. Does this sound weird, to have the lungs filled with liquid and live? Do some reading on emergency procedures that are being developed. What sounds most interesting to you?

Extensions

With the advances in medical research, what might be some great changes in the next few years? Might we solve the mystery of how to cure cancer, AIDS, and heart-related diseases? If so, will this come from advances in medical research alone, or might it also come from us changing our ways of using and ingesting chemicals and other stuff that is bad for our health?

HUNGRY FOR LIFE

Why are there so many people dying and suffering from hunger and malnutrition on this planet? Who or what is responsible?

Extensions

What can we do about hunger and malnutrition? Can you do anything locally? Are there persons benefiting from the current worldwide systems of organizing the way in which we live together on this planet? Look into the past also. Have there been groups that have benefited from the suffering of other groups? What are the common patterns? What can be done about such circumstances? Who is responsible? What responsibility does each of us have for this most difficult and challenging issue? Have you ever gone to sleep hungry?

HURRICANES AND MONSOONS DOING THE TWIST

Which way do hurricanes rotate when they are north of the equator? Which way do they rotate south of the equator? If a hurricane were to cross the equator, would this cause the direction of the rotation to change? What would happen if a hurricane were to live through its entire cycle (from birth to death) along a path precisely along the equator? Would it have any rotation? Might it rotate along a vertical axis that would look like a doughnut (a torus minus the fat) rotating around its own enclosed surface area? Next time you're flying over the ocean and you see a giant-sized doughnut forming down on the ocean's surface, you may not just be hungry—you may actually be seeing the world's first hurricane torus!

Extensions

What is the difference between a hurricane and a monsoon?

I DIDN'T DO IT!

Sometimes somebody is standing around when an event occurs. The person standing there had absolutely nothing to do with the event that occurred, but the individual is blamed for what occurred. This isn't logical, right? That is correct. It is not logical, but this kind of misplaced blame happens frequently.

Somebody says, "I saw her standing there right before the diamond was discovered to be missing off the countertop. Then I saw her walk away very quickly while she was putting something into her pocket. Yup, she's the one who did it all right!"

In the realm of court trials, this kind of thing occurs all the time. "He was walking down the hall toward the scene of the crime right before the crime took place. He's guilty as all get-out!"

In the realm of bigotry (where prejudice reigns supreme), these kinds of things occur. In Ireland: "She's Catholic" or "He's Protestant"; therefore, I can assume certain things about the individual. In the Middle East: "She's a Palestinian" or "He's a Jew," then people fill in the blank with their biases.

In the area of statistics, a person reads some data and observes that 95 percent of the time two phenomena occur one right after the other. The study clearly says that it is a correlational study (no causal relationships are implied). The reader infers (assumes) that event *x* causes event *y*. For instance, 95 percent of the persons in the study who play the violin smile much more than other people. Does playing the violin really cause people to smile more than the general population?

In the area of science, one might observe that whenever the sun rises, the streetlights go off. Someone might conclude that the rising of the sun causes the streetlights to go off. Actually, there are streetlights with photosensors that cause the lights to go off when there is sufficient sunlight. How are most streetlights turned off? The time in which the streetlights go off is, in fact, related to the time the sun rises, but the rising sun is not turning off the streetlights. How does this work? So many of our challenges are related to false attribution. Learn to be precise in describing what you mean by what you say.

Look up the form of argumentation called *post hoc, ergo propter hoc*. Because something occurs after something else, it is assumed that the prior event caused the subsequent event. What are some examples of assumptions people commonly make that are related to this kind of reasoning?

Extensions

When people make these kinds of mistakes, are they reasoning or arguing a case? Alternatively, do they just make assumptions without much thought?

When people make such assumptions, aren't they still responsible for the invalid reasoning behind the assumption? If you wish to examine other very common invalid "lines of reasoning," "arguments," or "assumptions," look at the distinctions between something that is necessary and something that is sufficient. Look up the difference between a valid and a sound argument. Find out something about arguments that are a form of *modus tollens* and *modus ponens*. While you're at it, learn the difference between presenting a case for a point of view versus arguing to defend some opinion. Compare how people respond to a careful and heartfelt presentation of a case for a point of view how people commonly react to a heated argument involving conflicting opinions in which people are obviously defending some kind of turf.

ICE MELTING

Scientists are talking about how the oceans could rise if the Earth warms up, due to the emissions of waste gases like carbon dioxide. These gases float into the atmosphere and remain suspended there. When the sunlight enters the atmosphere, its radiant energy bounces off the Earth, but this energy is not allowed to return to space because the gases mentioned above block this energy. What other gases do these greenhouse emissions interact with? Why do the scientists mostly refer to the melting of the Antarctic? What about the Arctic and its massive amount of ice that would melt if the temperature of the Earth were to rise? How much snow and ice are contained in the Antarctic versus the Arctic?

Extensions

Next, compare the volume of ice on Greenland to that in the Antarctic or Arctic. If Greenland is mostly covered with ice, why is it called Greenland? Are there other places on Earth that seem to be greatly misnamed?

IMPACT OF LIGHTNING

When lightning strikes people, it kills some of them; others who have been struck manage to live through the experience. One of the mysteries of those surviving has to do with the temperature of the lightning. Look up how hot lightning is. When you compare this temperature to the temperature at which food in the oven is cooked, you can see how it is rather a mysterious thing that anybody survives a direct lightning hit.

Extensions

What is the safest thing to do if you are caught outside in a severe lightning storm? One of the times I was caught in a lightning storm in an exposed area was on a large mountain with my son. We were approaching the top, or promontory, of the mountain when black clouds started to flood across the sky directly above us. Right then, a mountain climber came racing by us running down the mountain. He had seen the approaching storm. We saw the look on his face. We asked about what he was running from. We decided to race off the mountain also. Others kept hiking right into the face of the storm, even when lightning bolts were coming straight down upon us from the sky! By the time the lightning strikes got very close to us, we were in a much safer area. Lightning will follow the path of least resistance. There are specific things you are supposed to avoid. Learn what body position you are supposed to get into if lightning is ready to strike very close to you. Sometimes you may have a fraction of a second to respond. What are the signals of an impending (something about to happen) lightning strike? If you are with a group of people and you must sleep overnight on a mountain when lightning is expected, what kind of land features should you be looking for?

IMPLY AND INFER

Words really do matter. The words you are saying imply a certain meaning. For instance, when a parent says to a teenager, "Please be home around 10:00 P.M.," they are implying the meaning that a few minutes either way will not make a significant difference. Inference has to do with the meaning you interpret from the words of others. In this case, "around 10:00 P.M." may mean to you that it's OK to be home at 11:30 P.M. You arrive home according to your inferred time schedule right on time, but you find both parents up and upset with you. This is the difference between implication and inference. Notice that their hairs are actually standing on end on the back sides of their necks, and the little curly hairs on their eyebrows are suddenly straight also. Don't confuse them right when they're upset by attempting to look at the little hairs on the edges of their ears. Also, don't try to explain the difference between an inference and an implication in the heat of the moment.

In research, you look for evidence that supports some claim or hypothesis. The evidence implies certain things. You, the researcher, infer meaning (get, extract, or derive meaning) from the evidence or data. There is a huge difference. Be careful of this distinction. Inference in research of any kind is extremely important, but we must be careful to delineate (distinguish) between what is implied directly and what is inferred. For instance, scientists observe certain phenomena in weather patterns. The data suggest that changes are in fact occurring worldwide. Is it an implication directly from the data or is it an inference from the data that humankind is causing 100 percent of the observed changes? Ask a researcher sometime about the difference between knowledge that is indirectly implied and knowledge that is inferred. What are some examples of miscommunication that are rooted in the confusion between implication and inference?

Extensions

How do we know what others have inferred from the things we've communicated and implied? The most useful tool in communication is feedback. How do you get feedback when testing that others are inferring what you think they ought to be inferring from something you implied? A very common form of feedback is to say, "Will you please repeat back to me what I've just stated? Please put it into your own words." What are some other ways of getting feedback? What are some forms of indirect feedback that we can use to test or observe that inferences of others accurately reflect what you implied? Perhaps you can use any dissonance (disagreement) between what you felt was implied and what others inferred to help you learn more about the challenges, complexities, and wonders of group communication.

IMPOSSIBLE NUMBERS

Some numbers are impossible (they do not represent reality in the world). The name for this class of numbers is imaginary numbers. An example is one divided by zero. Is zero a number? There are other kinds of imaginary numbers. Try to compute the square root of a negative number. Find as many of them as you can. Do imaginary numbers have any usefulness (utility)?

Extensions

Imaginary words are nonsense words that make no sense. Aha! There are many nonsense words that have made their way into our language; for example; *Wow*! and *supercalifragilisticexpialidocious* (did I spell it correctly? Is there one correct spelling to an imaginary word?). List as many alternative spellings to this long word. What are some other examples of imaginary (nonsense) words that have become part of our language (thus making plenty of sense to many people)?

IMPOSSIBLE TIME

What day is it precisely at midnight? Is it today or is it tomorrow? When you are in the day labeled December 31, 1999, when it turns 12:00 midnight, what year, century, and millennium are you in? What argument could be made that the new millennium actually begins the moment after midnight of December 31, 2000? Hint: think in terms of the beginning of this millennium (which actually relates directly to the beginning of the first millennium of our Common Era). Was there a year zero? If not, how does this affect when the new millennium begins?

Precisely at midnight, could it be that you are neither in today nor tomorrow? Is there a point in time that is precisely midnight? If not, is there any other precise point in time? If so, then this point is in between time periods. Time is always described in periods that have some extension—duration (femtoseconds, picoseconds, nanoseconds, milliseconds, seconds, minutes, hours, days, weeks, years, centuries, millennium). What category of time is larger than a millennium? Hint: start with age, era, eon, and epoch.

Midnight stands out as maybe being outside of other time-related groupings. How can this be? Recall that zero is technically not a number marking neither time nor a distance. Twelve o'clock midnight is something like zero. Zero is not a number, but it is a concept upon which all numbers in our counting system depend. It is a prime reference point. Remember that all units of time have to do with duration of time. Is there a moment without duration? Is this a moment in time? Is there a moment out of time? Might there be an irreducible (can't be divided) fundamental unit that is itself timeless but which is the basic building block of what is known as time?

Ten o'clock A.M. is exactly ten hours after midnight. Ten o'clock A.M. signifies a specific span of time. We are dealing with a problem of the precise span between two points, each of which has no extension in space or time. (*See* "Dimensions—How Many?") When we are measuring something between two precise points that have no extension in space or time, these marker points become deeply problematical. Midnight (or any other marker in time) is a point without extension in space or duration in time, yet both space and time require these markers in order to make any sense of our physical world.

You could simply say that 12:00 midnight is exactly twenty-four hours after the last midnight and exactly twenty-four hours prior to the next midnight. This doesn't answer the question as to which day midnight falls in. Midnight is a prime reference. In most systems of any kind, there are prime reference points. These are like the core assumptions necessary in order for anything in the system to make sense. Learn to find the prime reference points in any system (including the way people act, think, and feel). There are many fascinating theories related to our most basic or prime assumptions. Every system of thought has its prime assumptions. How are they similar? In any system of thought or set of presumptions, there are irreducible basic or prime assumptions that can't be defined any further or defended. Is this actually true? How does this affect our capacity to communicate within groups composed of greatly divergent people with diverse prime assumptions? Do you believe we're capable of changing even our prime assumptions? How?

Back to midnight. Does an instant still involve duration of time? Is there a unit of time that is so small that it has no duration? Are there moments in between all the units of time? If someone thinks you're weird for wondering about such things, tell him or her that it directly relates to issues involving temporal anomalies issues. He or she will pretend to know exactly what you're talking about.

Extensions

If midnight is a concept, a point with no extension in time, then might it be the case that any other point in time is exactly the same thing—a useful concept? If so, what is time? Think about these related issues precisely at midnight.

IMPULSIVE ACTIONS

Impulsive behavior is related to not thinking about consequences. We just do them. There is an idea, feeling, suggestion, or set of circumstances, and we react. Identify the ways that you are impulsive sometimes. Is it when you're shopping, playing games, taking tests, being bored, angry, upset, or not thinking about what you're doing? See the patterns at play in your life. Once you become mindful of these patterns at play in your life, you start to gain wisdom about what forces energize you (negatively or positively). Seek this wisdom, and you will know yourself on a much deeper level. Most often, it is massively easier to see impulsivity in others rather than in our own selves. Why? Observe and take mental notes on the various kinds of impulsive acts you or others display.

Extensions

If we know that being impulsive is not usually good for us, why do we do these things? Is it ever good and productive to be impulsive? Recall the discussion on viewing an issue in discrete terms versus process terms. You get very different results depending upon your emphasis or creative use of both views. (*See* "Chicken and the Egg Question" and "First Human Being.") When you follow your passions and know your core energies, might it be good to sometimes drop the normal everyday things of your life and pursue something others think is slightly crazy or nuts? How do you know the difference between impulsive actions that are usually not productive or good for anybody and those occasional moments in which we have an opportunity to drop all the things that hold us back and pursue something that can really change us, or is just plain old playfulness without known negative consequences? When people reach these moments in their lives, others will usually judge them as being impulsive. Is it possible to be doing something without thinking about it? If you answer yes, might it be that you are concentrating on what you are doing in a nonconscious manner? Do we have different levels of awareness and different points of focus at the same time? We play with ideas and language a lot around our house. One of the humorous phrases we like to use with each other stems from the phrase, "Don't do what you're thinking." We invert it to say, "Don't think what you're doing!"

INCHES AND FEET

How long is a mile? How long is a foot? How long is an inch? We keep defining these units of measurement in terms of other units. Is there one inch, foot, or mile someplace against which all other inches, feet, and miles are measured? Hold a ruler in your hand and take a careful look at it. Then take another ruler and compare the two lengths. Are they exactly the same lengths? A machine in a factory made any given ruler. When the machine was set up to measure exactly one foot, did the workers use the other ruler in your other hand? Do these workers at these various factories have some magical one-foot ruler they use but never sell? Have a good time with your math and science teachers sometime and ask them how they really know that their yardstick measures up. If they think your getting smart with them, simply reply, "It's an issue related to analysis of presuppositions, and the concern about measurements is related to epistemological consistency!" Send them running for a dictionary. Hint: before you do this kind of thing, be sure you've looked up the words so you sound as though you really know what you're talking about. Somebody might actually say, "Tell me exactly in clear English what you are talking about!" It would really stun them if you could tell them in understandable straightforward English (or whatever is your chosen language)!

Extensions

Find out where we really do keep the big foot, yardstick, and clock of all clocks that keep us all on the mark and on time. (Could it be in the basement of your neighbor's house?) Do not read on if you do *not* want any direct hints.

In terms of physics research, there are three basic units for distance, time, and mass. In the Système International d'Unités (SI), these units are the meter, second, and kilogram.

- The meter is the SI unit for length. The meter is defined as being the length of space traveled by light in a vacuum during a period of 1/299,792,458 of a second. See if there is such a thing as a pure vacuum. The emptiness of outer space is filled with particles we never suspected before. Therefore, we can assume any vacuum we create will not be perfect. This means that maybe there is no perfect measurement of a meter. Is this why we continue to use yards as a basic length of measurement in the United States? Look up how a yard is precisely measured. If it is measured in the same way, maybe we should use the average length of everybody's index finger as our standard. Instead of the census, we could count and measure index fingers. Why not use the index finger as the standard if there are no more true vacuums anywhere?
- A second is the SI unit for time. A second is defined in terms of the period of radiation for the cesium-133 atom. Specifically, a second is the length of time equal to the duration of 9,192,631,770 periods of the radiation corresponding to the transition between two hyperfine levels of the ground state of the cesium-133 atom. The next time somebody asks you

what time is, make sure you quote this precise scientific definition. It will clear matters up quite quickly.

- The kilogram is the SI unit for weight. A kilogram is defined as being equivalent to the mass of a liter of water at the temperature of its maximum density, or approximately 2.2 pounds. This fundamental SI unit for weight is the only fundamental unit defined in terms of a physical thing held in a safe place. It is a platinum-iridium bar kept in the International Bureau of Weights and Measures at Sevres, France.

What are other SI units that measure for luminous intensity (light), electric current, temperature, and the amount of matter? How does the amount of mass differ from the amount of matter?

What are other standard units of measurement, and what are their standards for precise accuracy? For instance, the question about the foot-long ruler still stands. Where is the real one foot against which all the others are measured? As with the SI system, the actual definitions of what constitutes (makes up) the model against which all others are measured may not exist as an artifact. There may be no one, true, one-foot thing held in a safe place. The foot could be defined in other terms. Learn about the U.S. Customary System and the metric system, and then find out the basic ways they define their basic units. What are the basic units in the British Imperial System?

Find out what a furlong, league, rod, parsec, stone, gill, peck, hectare, grain, dram, mole, joule, and knot are. How do (or did) these systems guarantee that there is one definition of its basic units (mass, time, length)? For each of these units mentioned in the preceding systems, are there other associated measurements? When people used rods as a measurement of length, did this system have its own measurement of weight?

INDIAN NATIONS

Are the Native American tribes sovereign nations? If so, do they have diplomats and other rights and privileges of nationhood? What are some of the current issues related to sovereignty of Native American nations? What has been the history of the U.S. federal government relating to Native Americans and their rights signed in treaties?

Extensions

What are the basic requirements of being a nation? What are the smallest countries? Which are the countries with the smallest populations? When do you use the word *what* and the word *which* (as in the last two sentences)? Could there be a nation without land? What are other challenges related to the lives of Native Americans? Read about their history. What about the struggles of other aboriginal peoples (native residents of an area that was taken over by other groups) around the world? Who are they and what are their challenges?

INHERITED BEHAVIORS

As I was watching our first puppy mature, I noticed that he lifted one leg to urinate. No one taught him this behavior. The only conclusion I could draw was that this is an example of an inherited trait or behavior. What are other examples of inherited behaviors in any animal, including human beings?

Extensions

Make a list of possible candidates for behaviors that you think might be directly affected by or controlled by our genetic structure. Hint: this kind of list is growing longer, with a prolific (great) number of research publications related to human behavior and genetics. Can genetic structure really cause us to act in certain ways? Next time you go to a dance, a sports event, a concert, school, worship, or any other gathering of groups of people, ask yourself this question related to instinctual behaviors. Look around. What is the evidence? Keep in mind that one cutting-edge question is this: Why is it when the genetic code of a particular animal would indicate that it would be displaying certain traits, the individual animal often shows no such traits over the course of their entire lives?

INTELLIGENCES

Is there only one kind of intelligence? Who do you think of when you think of a very intelligent person? What is your own image of a very intelligent person? What kind of skills do they (you) have? Are there other forms of intelligence? Hint: intelligence might be a gift with many different kinds of manifestations. Could an auto mechanic be very intelligent in several ways? Could a bus driver be very intelligent in many ways? Could a dancer or basketball player be highly intelligent as evidenced in one's performance (physical or body realm)? Could someone be highly intelligent socially (social realm)? Could someone be highly intelligent with his or her feelings (affective realm)? Could someone be highly intelligent in math, physics, statistics, or other theoretical areas (the realm of abstract symbols)? Could someone be highly intelligent in the art and science of reasoning (the rational realm that may be related to an entirely practical process such as getting a fire started in a wet and cold situation)? Could someone be gifted in being aware of the mind's nuances and subtleties that are missed by most people? Could intelligence manifest itself through the inspiring and exceptional expression of language, stories, ideas, and concepts? Might there be forms of intelligence that reflect the unique combination of compassion, creativity, and faith in a context or being that is greater than the individual ego-defined self? Could there be forms of intelligence that enable persons to leap beyond all currently accepted definitions, names, and knowledge?

Maybe there are forms of intelligence that combine the rational/logical realm with the artistic/affective/intuitive realm. Are there forms of intelligence that are directly related to our senses? Someone might hear things and detect patterns that others fail to hear and comprehend (this may or may not have anything to do with hearing acuity—how well the physical sound waves are received). A professional cook may be able to detect taste patterns in foods that are being prepared and then apply this knowledge to alter the food preparation process. Could there be intelligences associated with the other senses? Try to list other possible realms of intelligence. After you list as many realms of intelligence as you can, try to define intelligence. Then record your observations of these various examples of intelligence at play. You may be surprised with your results.

Extensions

Might we all have different forms of intelligence for different situations? Might we all have forms of intelligence that are not apparent? If so, how do we find out about them? Try some of these possibilities:

- Participate in activities that are outside your usual engagements (like dancing if you've never danced).
- Talk to people who have different backgrounds from your usual circle of friends, acquaintances, or culture.
- Observe different people engaged in activities that you know very little about.
- Learn to discern your passions.
- Allow yourself to be curious about previously unexplored areas of human knowledge.
- Listen carefully to a wide range of people talking about greatly diverse topics.
- In the middle of the night when some flash of an idea, insight, or sense sweeps through your awareness with utter clarity, get up and record your experience.
- Carry with you a tiny voice recorder, and record the insights that occur to you in the middle of other tasks.
- Take time to do nothing. NOTHING! When you become fully relaxed, attentive, and alert, what occurs to you? What seems to attract your attention and curiosity?

You may be surprised at the kinds of gifts you have. Test yourself. Push yourself out of the comfort zones that you are so used to. Take some risks for the sake of learning and growth.

INTERSTATE HIGHWAYS

When was the legislation passed to develop a national artery of highways that would connect the entire nation and would come to be named the Interstate Highway System? What was one of its major purposes for the federal government? Hint: there was a distinct interest in the system of interstate highways on the part of one particular group within the federal government.

Extensions

When did the older U.S. Highway System come into being? What are the symbols for the U.S. highways, the interstate highways, state highways, and county highways? Is there one highway that connects Alaska to the southern part of South America? Is there a highway that extends all the way across Asia north to south and another one that connects Asia east to west? What is the longest continuous highway in North America? What is the longest continuous highway in the world?

ISTHMUS OF PANAMA AND THE ICE AGE

At one point in geological history, there was no isthmus connecting North and South America. When did the isthmus arise? What possible connection could you draw between its appearance and the onset (beginning) of the ice ages?

Think big. Think of ocean currents. Think of thermal energy (heat) being stored in these currents. Stop here and think about it before you go on and read about one possible answer.

What may have happened is that the warm equatorial waters (waters near the equator) may have been diverted (changed course) by the rising of the isthmus. These warm waters may have headed up the coast of North America and caused greater than normal precipitation amounts in the form of snow over eastern Canada. The increased amounts of snow would have reflected the energy of the sun back to outer space because white reflects solar energy. This may have had the impact of cooling off the Northern Hemisphere enough to have caused the onset of the ice age. It might be the case that an influx (input) of warm energy was a major contributing factor to the formation of glaciers across North America. (*See* "Glaciers.") Are there other geological formations that may have dramatically influenced weather systems?

Extensions

All dynamics in a system are related. If you change one element (even though it may appear to be something insignificant), it may alter the entire system dramatically and in unexpected and unpredictable manners. Even when one thing is changed in a far-off section of the system (like the isthmus in Central America), it may change something else in a distant place. What appears to be something that is entirely unrelated to something in the system under consideration might in fact be an element within the system being considered. There may be two different systems at play, but there might also be a larger, more encompassing system that is not observed or understood. Investigate the issues of including and excluding data, dynamics, factors, or elements. This is the issue of whether or not something is inside or outside the system under consideration. Look up Type One and Type Two errors in statistical analysis. Possessing some insight into these important issues can affect the way you look at many life issues. An entire system may change unpredictably. Look up a theory called dissipative structures. This has to do with systems that are sufficiently far from a state of equilibrium. In addition, look up something called bootstrap theory. This has to do with things occurring in one distant part of a system and simultaneously affecting other things in other parts of the system seemingly in such a manner that breaks the rule of nothing traveling faster than the speed of light.

ITCHING

Why does it feel so good to scratch an itch? Where did we ever get the weird-sounding word *itch*? What are other unusual-sounding words in our language?

Extensions

Have you ever tried to tell yourself to sit very quietly and concentrate on some image of, say, a flower or a flame? While you are concentrating on this image, tell yourself that you will not have any sensations of itching. What occurs? Why does this happen?

IT'S JUST IMPOSSIBLE, I TELL YOU!

For years, I would challenge people to spell an imaginary name for myself. It had odd sounds and letter combinations. According to me, there was only one correct spelling. It was such an odd-sounding name that most people could not repeat it back even after I had told them the name two to three times. Nobody got the spelling correct until one day I met a very bright young woman in a middle school who simply made up her mind that she would get the answer. She did. She listened very carefully and then recorded the phonetic spelling (what it sounded like to her). I taught her some basic methods of working with logical combinations. In this case, the combinations were the possible actual and phonetic spellings of the name. She went home and literally developed an extensive table of all the possible spelling possibilities. There were almost no trick spellings (letter combinations that would be unfamiliar to anybody else). She came up with the three most likely possibilities. One of them was correct. No one else even came close. The name was Porsnorfocus Schquieke Farquiere. Now, since you have seen this imaginary name in print, how would you pronounce it? Represent this pronunciation in phonetic spelling.

Extensions

How would you pronounce that name? Assign one consistent way of pronouncing the name. If you say it in normal tone and speed, see how many people can repeat it. If people can't repeat it, what is the challenge? Are they even hearing you? It is a very common pattern that if people decide that it takes too much work to hear or understand something, they shut down their listening process. The essence of this process is that some things appear to be too challenging. Something that is challenging can be complex, while something that is completely foreign can be quite simple. What are other reasons why something might appear to be overwhelmingly complex to somebody? What about past behavioral patterns? What about self-confidence? What about the person's history of being around others who either encouraged or discouraged the engagement with relatively complex material? What about the manner in which you ask the question and set the atmosphere or relationship with the listener? Try to discover other reasons why people often choose not to engage in things that appear to be complex. Remember that complexity is something relative to one's current understanding. Something terribly complex now may in fact be viewed as being incredibly simple or even simplistic in the future. Observe yourself and others very closely when you are faced with complexity. Do we sometimes try to convince ourselves that we are trying to comprehend the meaning, structure, and dynamics of something complex, when in fact we have already shut down and given up?

JUMPING PEOPLE

If all the people on the Earth were gathered together in one place and all at once they jumped up and down, would the Earth shake?

Extensions

If all the people were gathered in one spot and assuming that each person took one square yard, how much space would this be? How many pounds of food and water would they need to consume each year? Compare the weight of food and water available and used for those persons living in North America versus Asia. Compare the weight of the nutritional and caloric value of the food and the purity of the water consumed by the people in the upper three-fifths of income levels versus those in the bottom two-fifths of income brackets.

JUNK FOOD

Why does so much junk food taste so good? Is this true? Is junk and fast take-out food simply the lowest common denominator (lowest common kind of food that masses of people will consume and pay for)? When you taste excellent food that has taken time and care to concoct (make), what do you experience that is different from when you eat junk food? My family and I love to eat different ethnic foods. The first time I ate Middle Eastern food, I was amazed at the depth and complexity of the tastes. Then when I drank some tea, the tastes not only came back again but they were transformed! My most surprising incident while eating was in a Middle Eastern restaurant. At the end of the meal, the food server came up to each of us and sprinkled rose water on us all. We experienced yummy tastes and delicious smells of all kinds. We make one soup that has about eleven spices in it. It is not hot. It is simply delightful in complexity and depth.

The challenge with complexity and depth (character) is that everybody has her or his own tastes. When one goes through all the work to prepare such food, it is an act of love. Could there be a way of mass-producing such foods? One of my favorite foods is real strong lemon meringue pie. I have never tasted a single good slice of lemon meringue pie in any restaurant. Now I have given up trying to find wonderful lemon meringue pie in restaurants! My definition of greatness is obviously not the same definition as others. Thus, when people are cooking for large groups, simple tastes reign supreme. Try an experiment with strong-tasting cheeses. Get quite a variety of strong-tasting cheeses. See how many people like the samples. Next, put out bland-tasting cheeses. How many like these samples?

Extensions

Do our tastes for food change as we age? If so, why?

KEEPING THE GREAT QUESTIONS

When we keep something, we are holding or retaining it. The word *keep* also has the definition of being in harmony with something. For instance, "The painting is in perfect keeping with the room's decorations." When we are in keeping with our great questions, we are in harmony with a great creative power that can inspire us.

There are interesting times in which we encounter a question that is rich and intriguing. This kind of question continues to pop up in our minds even while we are focused on a completely different task. Once we have one extremely captivating question enticing us, it tends to lead us to other great questions. This process of intrigue and discovery opens doorways to human understanding that we would never have understood unless this passion to live in quest of dealing with the question had arisen. If we are in keeping with the question, surprising new insights will arise in our lives.

When I was younger, I was in a large building. I wandered around and found the basement. To my amazement, a little doorway led to a tunnel. The tunnel led to another large room. I felt like I was on an exploration of a lifetime. Something deep inside of me changed on that journey. For the rest of my life, I've been intrigued as to what is in the basements and subbasements of buildings. I love to find the interconnecting tunnels, hallways, doorways, caverns, and rooms. Some buildings are built right into natural caverns. Where the human-made structures end, nature's tunnelways begin. The big question for me is, where is the basement and might there be "secret" rooms or passageways?

Once I took my son and one of his friends into the subbasement of a large hotel. We got into a hallway that obviously led elsewhere. We needed to go see. (They needed just a little encouragement to become aware of their need.) As soon as the door shut behind us, I realized that this hallway had doors with locks that were completely different from any others that I had ever seen before. You had to have a key to get out of the hallway from the inside! Luckily, my wife was a few feet away. She had the common sense not to go into this hallway. She opened the door and out we walked—free people! I still wonder to this day where that hallway led.

There are so many startling and enigmatic questions that we can be thinking about! Don't just have one or two of them. Cultivate a whole garden full of interesting questions. What are your intriguing questions? They have a way of finding you if you develop your curiosity. Always be inquisitive and curious no matter what you are doing. Don't let others, don't allow circumstances, and don't permit the aging process to rob you of this most vital resource! Keep it a secret if you have to, but always be in keeping with intriguing questions!

Extensions

The most interesting questions can lead to startling and unexpected answers. Sometimes we get questions answered that we really didn't want answered. Sometimes it feels like the exploration into a question changes us. Occasionally, we run into a question that is so demanding that we give up the quest. Then there are those times in which finding answers can disturb the neatness of other assumptions we have in life.

When there are people around who have a great investment (interest) in keeping things the way they've been in the past, they often have a distinct interest in suppressing (preventing) significant questioning. Searching (challenging) questions lead to telling (revealing) responses. Certain persons in power who have some privileges that they feel are threatened by questions like to keep things quiet. At least in your own mind, encourage questions that challenge the way things are run. You may arrive at some interesting conclusions.

This kind of questioning can also lead to more efficient or effective ways to get work done. Be aware of the possibility of backlash (reactions) because you choose to raise central questions. Occasionally they are welcomed with open arms. Most of the time, they are treated as an interesting diversion from the real work of the group. Sometimes, there will be marked strongly negative responses not only to the question but also to you personally. Be careful but persistent (tenacious, never letting go) in your quest to learn how to be open to central life-altering questions. They can come popping into your life in the most unexpected moments and in the most unusual ways.

One of the biggest learning lessons of my entire life has been the simple insight that great questions lead to life material that necessarily changes your perspectives in ways that can in the short term cause more work for you. In the long term, you come out wiser for having entered the domain (territory) of the question. Questions that lead to the deep material of our values, hopes, dreams, assumptions, beliefs, and faiths can shake things up. Be careful to trust your feelings and share your explorations with other trusted and trustworthy people. The goal of all questions is to gain wisdom and insight for the sake of a fuller life. If your life is becoming richer and fuller because of these questions, you are on the right path. For instance, why is it that we eat desserts at the end of the meal when we all know that we are salivating (craving) to eat the dessert first thing? This is the perfect question to raise right when the mushy, pale-green, canned peas have been put on your plate to eat (because they are good for you).

Some questions are best left until we have gained more life experience. Some questions aren't ours to be impassioned about. It is not my passion to comprehend everything about the chemistry of soap suds. I'm glad that there are persons for whom this is an area of importance. It can be dangerous to pursue certain questions. I wonder what it would be like to walk on thin ice? I wonder what it would be like to jump out of an airplane without a parachute and then have somebody toss one to me on the way down? There are many questions whose answers I will never pursue.

Find your core passionate questions that give you a richer and fuller life. Once you start to find answers to your questions, don't be satisfied with safe havens. Keep pursuing great questions. In the presence of a person who is intrigued by great questions, there is a certain spark that is so apparent. It can be felt and seen. Seek out other people who have this spark blazing away. The core questions and pursuits of others may not be yours, but they will add greater dimensions to your life. Ever wonder why the sky is blue, so many leaves are green, and the stars keep on shining? Enjoy and play with your vital questions. If others aren't interested in them, keep them to yourself for a while. There will be others along your life course who will be impassioned and curious folks. Be patient. Try applying the way of living that is in keeping with a great question related to what is possible for your organization, company, family, school, or voluntary association. Unique and helpful ideas for goals, opportunities, or productivity will come to you. Teach others in your group to live in keeping with great questions. To be kept is to be beholden or dependent on something. If we're kept by creative, critical, and great questions, we resonate, identify, and associate with an unfolding productive novelty. If we are kept by nonproductive, uncreative, self-serving, and reactive concerns, our lives become a detriment to any group we are involved with. We need to be mindful and proactive in what we become absorbed, oriented, and kept in. There is a positive sense of being beholden to creative potential. There is also a negative sense of being beholden to reactive resistance to any change.

LAND AND OCEAN FORMATIONS

Look at some high-quality maps and find as many names for land formations as possible: isthmus, bay, point, sound, gulf, etc. Find and list one example of each formation. Look at maps and try to determine the difference between a lake, ocean, and sea.

Extensions

Land? I'm standing on land! Usually we assume that land stands for dry land. Would it be correct to call the bottom of the oceans "land?" Why or why not?

LATENT AND MANIFEST

What does it mean when we say that something is latent or that something is manifest?

Extensions

There are many aspects of life that are not on the surface, immediately observable, or directly detected, but they are important parts of life. Many persons have written about the unconscious mind. These are our thoughts, impressions, or memories that we are not directly aware of but which influence us greatly. Do you believe there is an unconscious part of us? What would be some evidence of this unconscious part of our lives?

LANGUAGES AND THEIR ROOTS

In the United States, our primary language is English. It is a member of what is known as the Indo-European languages. We derive our words from many other languages, but many of our words have their origins in Latin or Greek. Back in the days and places in which Latin and ancient Greek were spoken, what did these people look to as the origins of their own languages? See if you can find any information on this topic.

Extensions

Is there evidence that languages stem from one place? Some dictionaries can help you get started on this investigation.

LATITUDE AND LONGITUDE

We use degrees of latitude and longitude to figure out relative positions on the Earth. We need to know how to describe where we are relative to other positions on the Earth. On a family vacation when I was a child, my dad stopped the car and asked a person for directions. He pointed his hand in a general direction and said, "It's off yonder a fer-a-piece." My dad knew enough not to press for details. He drove on. We must have gotten there somehow. Most people, for most purposes, need directions that are more precise. That is why we have the system of latitude and longitude.

Lines of latitude run parallel to the equator. They never intersect. They are parallel concentric circles. As they approach the North or South Pole their radius, circumference, and diameter all decrease. Look up these important and basic terms if you don't already know them. Precisely at either pole, there is no radius, circumference, or diameter for any line of latitude. The poles are only a mathematical point. How far from a pole would you have to go in order to encounter a line of latitude? Draw a picture of a circle with a dot at the center. The dot could represent the North Pole. Draw a cross with its two intersecting lines at 90° to each other (perpendicular) running through the dot. Each one of these arms points due south. Now draw a second dot on the diagram close to the North Pole. Would there be a line of latitude running through this point? If so, would it be an ellipsis or a perfect circle? Make sure you ask, "Relative to what perspective?" Could it be measured in terms of degree, minutes, and seconds? If you were fifty meters from the North Pole, would there be an east and a west from this point? How long would it take to go around the world? If you were three feet from the pole, would there be an east and west from this point? How long would it take you to go around the world? (*See* "Signals—Beaming in One Direction.") Lines of latitude are called parallels.

Lines of longitude run north and south. They converge at either pole. Lines of longitude are called meridians. The prime meridian is 0°. It runs through Greenwich, England. Why? Is this a geographic necessity? (*See* "Maps and Grids, Old and New.") The meridian on the opposite side of the world is 180°. Is this 180° west or east? Boundaries are often interesting places. (*See* "Spiraling into Infinity" and "Impossible Numbers.") What is the relationship between the International Date Line and the meridian at 180°? Could the meridians be laid out like the parallels (in concentric circles parallel to each other)? Conversely (an opposite point of view), could the parallels be laid out like the meridians? If so, what would be the two new poles? Hint: they'd be at the equator. One would be somewhere southeast of India in the Indian Ocean, and the other one would be to the west of South America. What would we call these poles?

What kind of a grid system would this be? Would there be any advantages or disadvantages to it relative to the current system? Get out a tennis ball and draw this kind of coordinate system. Which would be the top and which would be the bottom? Couldn't they just as easily be called the A or B pole? Describe the coordinates of various places on the surface of the Earth using this system. When somebody asks you where you went on vacation, describe your answer in terms of this new system. See how people react.

A second coordinate system would use parallel concentric lines for both longitude and latitude. All points of intersection would be at 90° at the poles. There would be two sets of antipodal (opposite) poles. There would be no degrees, minutes, or seconds as units of measurement. There would be one hundred longitude and latitude lines, and the zero latitude line would be the South Pole and the one hundredth latitude line would be the North Pole. The zero longitude would pass through Africa at the equator near where human life probably emerged. The one hundredth longitude line would be in the Pacific Ocean. How would this system work?

Now for an entirely different third coordinate system. Imagine a perfect ball, a squished down bulging-at-the-center sphere, and an elongated sphere stretched at the poles. Do some research and find out which model fits the Earth's shape the best. Hint: find out what an oblated and prolated spheroid is. Another hint: the equatorial radius is greater than the polar radius. Whatever you decide is the best fit for our model, now imagine or draw this sphere as being encased (enclosed) within a 3-D box that is a little less than eight thousand miles across between any two faces. We have a three-coordinate system (height, width, and depth). All four poles (north-south and east-west) are the only places of the sphere that touch the cube. Because the Earth is an oblated spheroid (the equator has a greater diameter than the diameter between the poles), the length of the south-north axis will be slightly shorter.

Imagine there are three lines perpendicular to each other. The east-west line (E–W) begins at its easternmost point, which is the zero point located near the place where human life first evolved. This E–W line commences on the equator in Africa and has its one hundredth unit at the opposite end of the Earth just where the Earth touches this 3-D box. This would be in the Pacific Ocean (see if you can figure out where this point would be located). The south-north line (S–N) has its zero point at the South Pole, since this can be imagined to be the base of the world (if north is up) and has its one hundredth unit at the North Pole just where the Earth touches the 3-D box. The line for depth (D) is perpendicular (90°) relative to the E–W and the S–N lines (x, y, and z axes—plural for axis). The origin of this D line is at the equator in the middle of the rain forests of South America (a place of some of the richest, biodiverse plant and animal populations anywhere in the world). This makes the E–W line and the D line perpendicular to each other. The one hundredth unit of the D line would be at the opposite end of the world to the south of Asia. The easiest way to envision this system is to primarily be focused on the 3-D box, not the Earth itself.

Visualize the 3-D box from one of its faces. First, envision the E–W line. This line is inscribed (etched) on the surface of the cube. It begins on your right in Africa and ends in the Pacific Ocean. This is a horizontal line. The next line (S–N) is the vertical line commencing at the South Pole and ending at the North Pole. So far, this is simple. Now, the trick is this: keep the same perspective and you'll have to imagine the existence of a point that is at the intersection halfway across the E–W and S–N line. What you are observing is the beginning point from which a line extends precisely at 90° relative to the other two axes. If you envision looking at the 3-D box squarely, then you can only see two lines at once no matter which face you are observing. As soon as you face the cube from any other angle, you can see all the coordinate lines (E–W, S–N, D). If you are squarely facing the cube's face containing the commencement point of the D line, then you are looking directly at the Amazonian rain forests.

In this system, there are no degrees of arc, minutes, or seconds. Rather, we use decimal places to whatever place we need in order to locate something within the system with any degree of accuracy desired. You locate anything down to nanometer, picometer, or femtometer.

Thus, some imagined coordinate could be 50EW, 50SN, 50D. This would be the precise center of the Earth. Remember, it is easiest to envision this coordinate system if you remain focused on the 3-D box and its x, y, z, coordinate system initially and secondarily on the Earth itself. Where would 100EW,100SN, 100D be located? Hint: you wouldn't want to be there in your summer swimsuit, goggles, and snorkel only. This would be a nasty and lonely corner to be stuck in. You would be in an extreme corner of the 3-D box in outer space. If we say that numbers greater than one hundred and less than zero could be used, then we could easily compute locations for any position beyond this eight thousand–mile artificial limit. Any point of any Earth orbit could be precisely plotted. A point defined by the coordinates 50, –10, 50 would be 10 units south of the South Pole. In this coordinate system, you can go south of the South Pole, north of the North Pole, east of the East Pole, and west of the West Pole because we are viewing the system imposed on the 3-D box within which the Earth exists.

Every place has a coordinate. The limit is if we wish to locate the precise location of a mathematical point. How many decimal places would this require? You could use any number of decimal points, depending on the necessary degree of precision. All we need to know is the exact number of units between zero and one hundred for every axis. In real life, more decimal places require more sensitive and accurate measuring devices. These units could be converted to units of feet or meters. Remember that the conversion factor for the E–W and D axes would be identical because of the identical equatorial diameter for both lines, and the conversion factor for the S–N line would be different because the S–N diameter is approximately twenty-six miles shorter than the equatorial factor.

The position of any satellite, any sunken boat or ship, any point on the surface of the Earth (in the deepest valleys to the highest mountains), any grain of sand or molecule and any point in the interior of the Earth could be plotted and described with extreme accuracy. In such a system, where would the new day begin?

Extensions

Play with different coordinates for different well-known places. How many decimal places would be needed to delineate the distance between a friend's front door and yours?

Three alternatives have been presented. The assumptions are: uniform mass of the Earth, no ongoing deformation of the shape of the Earth, and a stationary globe. As soon as we begin to spin the Earth, the system becomes dynamic. We are now dealing with an ellipsoid with a mathematically generated universal reference system as the surface. Since the Earth doesn't possess uniformly distributed mass, and since its surfaces deform in many dynamic ways, we need a uniform world geodetic system that includes a fourth dimension of time. This system is massively more complex. Learn what you can about these established systems.

LEAP YEARS

In a leap year, we get an extra day. Does this lengthen life? Why do we have leap years? If you can figure out why we have leap years, you'll be able to know how we got the length of time we call a year. Look up sidereal time relative to this issue of the length of one day. What is true of other scales used to measure many different things is that there is a primary unit determined by some precise means from which all other measuring units are derived. In the case of a year, the prime measurement is in terms of a single sidereal day. Find other systems of measurement and discover the prime measuring units and how they are derived.

Extensions

What are the rules for how often leap years occur? Be sure to look up the exceptions and whether or not the turn of a century or millennium has anything to do with it.

LEAVES AND THE WEIGHT OF THE EARTH

If all the leaves on the Earth were to fall to Earth at once, while they were falling, would the Earth weigh less?

Extensions

Once the leaves fall off a branch, at the point where they were connected, is there another bud ready for the next year? Beneath this place, is there some kind of material that will become the bud for two years down the line?

LEGOS

How many individual Lego pieces has the company manufactured? How many different kinds of pieces has the company manufactured?

Extensions

Find out how the Lego Company (or any other toy company) designs its toys. How are they manufactured? Is it environmentally safe? What does the company do with its leftover solvents, paints, and other chemicals? Where are they manufactured? Does the company treat its workers decently?

LEVELING OTHERS

There are persons who have a tendency to try to knock down (be against) anyone in a leadership role. Have you ever heard people being put down because the other person excels in some manner (sports, arts, academics, organizational roles)? Why would people try to level or pull down those who take stands on issues or excel in some manner? If you were a leader of some group, would it be safer for you if you led without taking any significant stands on issues? Would you be safer if you tried to make everybody happy all the time? Would you be providing significant leadership?

Extensions

Think of different groups you are related to or involved in right now. How willing are you to express your real feelings and ideas? What is it that can hold us back from such expression? What does it feel like not to express what you vitally and passionately feel and value? What are the consequences when you do? What are some lessons you are learning in terms of expressing yourself while also being mindful and responsive to (but not controlled by) the sentiments of others? Are there some leadership positions that make the leader too vulnerable and thus should be avoided? How can we know in advance? Does the interview process reveal the real issues in the life of the organization or group? Because the finalist is presumably the top candidate for the position, there often occurs between the selection committee and the candidate something like a romance wherein people tend to see what is best, and critical judgment is suspended in the worst scenario or affected in most cases.

LIES BECOMING TRUTH

I listen carefully to people talk, and the same kind of thing goes on all the time. The most common form of not being entirely truthful is stretching something that is true. (*See* "Confabulated, Conflated, Inflated, and Genuine Stories.") Listen to people talk, and there will be many claims of knowing something to be true when in fact they are expressing something valid in a contorted fashion. I sense that part of this is psychologically related to our development as human beings. At some stages in our growth, we simply do not know that we are taking one thing from our information sources and converting it into something that we want to believe about our world. Some adults do this consistently all through their lives. Also, as I listen very closely to conversations, certain kinds of information are seen as giving the spokesperson power. Observe a group of adolescents and listen for the ones who have just seen the hottest movie that is driving parents nuts. The person who is telling the story of the movie accrues (gets) tremendous power.

It is one thing to imagine some things about yourself or the extent of your knowledge. It is another thing to tell others stories that are not true. As a child, I experimented with this art of not being truthful. I quickly realized that one lie led to another. Soon life got excessively complicated. I had to work hard to try to remember what had been said to one person and what was said to another. The clear and swift conclusion was that life is much easier if I simply tell the truth. Life is not only simpler but it is massively more enjoyable when we live with an innocence and sincerity that allows us to be transparent to others (what you see is what you get). I still love the gift of using my imagination to see the world in many different ways. Imagination is not the problem. How is it that some people who lie on a consistent basis come to believe the lies are truth?

You can learn to be truthful to all persons and reserve how open you are to certain persons and groups relative to your trust in their capacities to relate to others in a trustworthy, compassionate, gentle, and nonviolent fashion. To thrive in life, we need to learn this art very well without becoming twisted by the machinations (internal twisted deceptions) of others. If we keep making adjustments in the way we relate, act, feel, and think, we can find that we have compromised our essential selves. It is important to know in real time (while you are going through a process) that you are adjusting yourself to the presence of controlling, untrustworthy, unloving, harsh, or violent people or situations. As soon as we find out that this is occurring, we need to get back to our center of true values and life-offering behaviors.

We need to make decisions about taking risks related to changing the quality of our relationships. We need to act in accord with what is essential and true for us. We may choose to take risks to keep these relationships. In doing so, we need to be clear in our own minds and with others that certain core personal or systemic (group) issues be addressed and changed. If they are not addressed and changed, we may need to withdraw from this individual or network of relationships. If we do not address these issues, we can maintain our desire to keep the relationships intact, but we can become embedded (trapped) within a series of compromising and disastrous consequences:

- We can put more and more energy into making these relationships work while we become unconscious of the basic fact that the basic relationships are not going to change.
- We become consumed in attempting to keep something going that is not good for us nor is consistent with our core values, energies, sentiments, feelings, ideas, and behaviors.
- We can place ourselves at extreme risk by attempting to make the unworkable workable.
- In the act of trying to balance things, we lose our self-awareness of what makes us vitally alive.
- We can lose sight of the fact that we are living constantly in an off-balance way because we're trying to balance too many things that can't be balanced.
- We can exhaust ourselves by trying to juggle too many things that are in fact detrimental (bad) for our well-being.

There are three fundamental choices concerning your well-being:

- change yourself and act in a conscious manner that reflects your core values, feelings, and behaviors while not confronting anything or anybody in the system, or
- change yourself and act in a conscious manner that reflects your core values, feelings, and behaviors while effectively advocating for changes while addressing the core unhealthful dynamics, or
- make the decision and start to actively plan your exit out of a debilitating relationship or network of relationships.

Gather a group of friends who will bring to you wisdom, courage, strength, compassion, and the sense of valuing acting with integrity. In every lived moment, we carry with us a few totally essential qualities. One of them is integrity. That means that nobody can take this gift away from you. You can give it away or lose it in your desperate attempts to hold onto a relationship or network of relationships that are not healthful for you. This is the metaphor of losing your soul. It is also the metaphor of the Faustian bargain. Look this one up. What are other qualities that are totally essential in every lived moment?

From what life has taught me, what abides with us (stays with us and defines who we essentially are) are the gifts of sanity, integrity, creativity, vision, compassion, conscience, and involvement. These are our treasures that nobody, no group, or no force in the world can take from us. These are our great gifts that we bear with us in every lived moment. As we manifest and share them, the lasting influences we leave behind that truly make a difference stem from these qualities. These are the most vital qualities of a life that is dedicated to the pathway of growth and honoring life. These qualities serve as something like a compass. We can know that something is not right in our life when any of these qualities are being compromised. If we sense that any of them are being compromised, we need to understand what is happening and then act before we get too deeply into something that robs us of our vitality.

Extensions

What would your life be like if you convinced yourself that lies were critical to surviving? Under what kind of circumstances would this kind of dependence upon lies and deception emerge? What are the biggest possible lies? Hint: it may have something to do with deceiving ourselves as to what is essential to living and what compromises are necessary.

LIFE—WHAT MAKES THE DIFFERENCE?

I'm alive. We take this for granted. What is the difference between something that is alive versus something that is not alive (inanimate)?

Here are some basic qualities that we use to describe things that are alive: they grow, reproduce, move, utilize (use) energy, and respond to their environment in some fashion. In the simplest forms of life, this response to the environment is a mere chemical interchange with certain patterns determined by the organism's genetic code. In the most complex forms of life, this response to the environment includes intellect, intention, imagination, and feelings. What are some other qualities that define living things? Develop a list of qualities that are necessary in order for us to say that something is alive. This will help you define the difference between living and inanimate things.

Develop your list on your own. Talk to your friends who are curious and inquisitive. Then go to books or the World Wide Web and ask your parents and teachers. In school, you could have various groups working on the same task (as independently of each other as possible). Compare the results of the process. When you are setting up independent groups, make sure that you learn all you can about how not to predispose the groups toward certain outcomes by giving them too many specifics on methods in advance. Be as general as possible. This gives them the most options for diverse methods and answers.

Once you have this list of qualities that distinguish living from nonliving things, explore the realm of things that might be alive and might not be. There are organisms that are dormant yet alive in some sense. They require some changes internally (genetic codes) or externally (the environment). Explore and learn about the simplest forms of life.

Extensions

Is there anything that may have one of the qualities that you've listed above and not be alive? Play with the various combinations of qualities of life and see if there are exceptions. The anomalies (exceptions) point in the direction of possible new patterns that have not been known before.

LIFE WITHOUT . . .

Would there be any life on Earth if there were no water? Hint: most life-forms are either in the animal or plant kingdom. Some very small forms of life are neither plant nor animal and appear to be like animals in some respects; in other ways, they appear to act like plants. Are there any forms of life you can find that do not depend on water?

Extensions

If everything were frozen at absolute zero, do you think life could exist? This is a tricky question. We have found seeds and other simple forms of life that are solidly frozen. If they are warmed up under the right conditions, they come back to life. Therefore, while they are frozen solid, are they alive? Are they dead while they are frozen? If they are dead, can the dead be brought back to life? If you're frozen, are you dead or alive? If you decide that you are neither dead nor alive, is there another state of existence other than life and death?

LIGHT'S PATH

When light is emitted from its source, it expands equally in all directions. How can we talk about light traveling in straight lines (in the absence of mass)?

Extensions

How do we get lasers to travel in such precisely straight lines?

LIGHT, HEAT, AND ELECTRONS

It seems like a simple enough procedure. You flick your finger and the light switch changes from its "off" to its "on" position. What is taking place?

When the switch is on, it completes a circuit. Electricity then flows to the lightbulb. What in the wire is actually flowing? The wire itself is not flowing. A river has water flowing in it. The stuff is moving. It can be felt and seen. Are the electrons flowing in the wire? What about the electric field around the wire? What are electrons? Are they matter? If something is flowing, doesn't some physical thing have to be moving? If it is energy that is flowing (or moving), what is energy? If you investigate what is actually moving (exchanged, communicated, or transmitted), you will be led to some of the most profound mysteries in the universe.

Once the electricity gets to the lightbulb, how and why does it light up? What creates the light? Why is so much heat produced?

Extensions

Different processes like an automobile engine, an electric motor, our human bodies, and many chemical reactions give off heat. The more heat dissipated (lost) means that the process is more inefficient (wasteful). Scientists and engineers are able to figure out how efficient the process is (how effectively a process uses energy relative to its purpose). They are able to assign percentage figures, such as a home water heater or home furnace could be 85 percent or 90 percent efficient. Investigate how these numbers are assigned (derived or figured out).

Now that you know how the numbers are assigned, try to figure out how efficient the human body is. This is a complex issue. Remember all the tips you've been learning about investigating your world. Compare the process of the body to other processes that you already know. When things get very complex, create a model that will help you see (visualize) the process. In this manner, you can break down the major parts (components) into chunks that you can understand while at the same time you can get and keep (retain) the big picture.

For any complex or challenging tasks, try to see and understand the few most important (critical) factors (dynamics). Keep these few most critical facts clearly in mind so you do not get lost in the maze of the problem or challenge. Keep referring back to the basic facts. Then you must be open to the possibility that the basic facts need to be reappraised (seen in a new light).

Another way of visualizing how to approach a complex task is to view the task in terms of a map. We all need maps to get through complex tasks. Try to get and retain the picture of the big outline of what you are attempting to do. Keep this outline or overview clearly in mind as you begin dealing with the pieces of the puzzle. Keep in mind also that things you discover may in fact cause you to alter the big picture. You may have started out looking for one thing but in midcourse discover that something else is much more interesting and important. If this occurs, then change your big picture or map. Don't get lost in details. This is a metaphor related to the necessity of understanding the details. All the detailed analysis in the world will not help us if we do not have a clear picture of what we are searching for in the first place. Be mindful of details but keep the big picture always in sharp focus. At the same time you need to have a crystal-clear picture of what you're looking for, it is very helpful to be receptive to anomalies that can't be explained by your current understanding. Some of the anomalies may prove to be vastly more important than the original thing you are looking for.

The process of discovery is an art form, and it requires a high level of curiosity. Continue to be curious and let your intelligence loose. Play with the issues. Invent paths to the answer. Discover new ways to look at the issues. The first issue you begin to investigate may turn out to be only a minor issue, and you may uncover something much larger and so vast (big) that an entire new universe of understanding opens for you.

Let your genius out and see where it leads you. Listen to that still inner voice that guides you as to what is most important in the present moment. Enjoy! Play! Discover! Don't forget to always be thinking in terms of the resources available to you that can assist you in your task. Always be resource rich. Remember that the greatest resource in the world is inside of you.

LIGHT—ITS SPEED

Who says that the speed of light is the fastest moving thing in the universe? Who says that light cannot travel faster than 186,000 miles per second? The answer, of course, is almost everybody. Just because everybody who subscribes to the accepted laws of physics believes that nothing can travel faster than light, why couldn't anything travel faster than light? We would have to alter our basic perceptions of our space-time continuum if we were to allow for something to move faster than the speed of light. Why? What might some of the changes be? For one imaginary venture into this realm, find a reference to the term *tesser,* or *tesseract*. Hint: it's in a well-known children's fiction book. You do not have to go to the realm of fiction in order to find theoretical constructs (ideas) that would posit (support the idea) that there could be things that travel faster than the speed of light. Incidentally, scientists at Princeton University recently claimed to have shot light through a sealed chamber filled with cesium gas. If their calculations are correct, the light exceeded the maximum speed of light thought possible. Keep your eyes out for the further research released on this topic. Some scientists argue that these results are of no significance.

Extensions

If light were traveling with no reference points, could we imagine that it would be simultaneously moving at an unknown rate of speed and standing still? If it were standing still with no outside reference points, how fast would you be moving while observing the light? Would you become the reference point? Do the laws of physics need an observer in order to be valid (if you weren't observing, who is to say that the speed of light can't exceed its assumed limits)? What would light look like if it were standing still? Could there be light with no motion? There have been some recent experiments that projected laser beams through Bose-Einstein condensate. The results are stunning. They have slowed the speed of light down to thirty-eight miles per hour. That's slower than some people drive past your house! This is twenty million times slower than the speed of light in a vacuum. The same scientists are now working on slowing this obtained speed another one thousand times slower. Find out what theoretical and very practical effects this will have on us. Imagine light actually standing still! Find out whatever is available on this topic.

Back to the maximum speed of light. Recall the little humble-looking formula $E = mc^2$. Contained in this little eloquent and phenomenal phrase is the answer to why supposedly nothing can travel faster than the speed of light. It states that energy and mass are equivalents. If they are equivalents, the units needed to measure one need to be converted into the units used to measure the other. The means of converting these units into the other is to use the speed of light as the conversion factor. This is one kind of explanation. Other explanations have to do with inertial frames of reference. Another explanation has to do with the fact that it is not only the speed of light that can't be exceeded, but there are other particles that travel at this particular speed. Still the question stands, "Why can't something, anything, exceed the limit of the speed of light?" When we get to prime assumptions upon which entire systems of thought rest, it is very difficult to get answers as to why these core postulate or axioms (foundational assumptions) can't be seen in a new light. One of the reasons is that, in order to change a prime assumption, the entire system of thought would have to be altered in a major way. There is an accumulated mass of evidence and cultural momentum of energy supporting the current knowledge base. To move something with such tremendous mass requires stupendous energy. It also requires risks that few people are willing to take because it would entail altering the entire edifice of presumptions and the mass of intellectual insights rooted in these presumptions.

LIMITS

Things within systems have limits. Trees only grow so tall, human beings only grow so tall, people build homes only so large, people can only walk so far at certain temperatures without drinking more water or having more food, or insects and rabbits can only multiply so fast. Identify many things and processes with limits, and then try to name the factors that set these limits. For instance, there are limits to how long somebody can survive in cold water. What are the factors involved? These are all maximum (largest) limits. What are some examples of minimum (smallest) limits?

Extensions

For the things you've identified, how can the factors you've named be altered so that the limits can be changed? For instance, when people swim across the English Channel, they grease up their bodies and wear wet suits. If they were to try to swim the same waters without a wet suit and without greasing up, the maximum limits would be much lower. Some factors have been altered. Limits are dynamic and change. A man crawled up into the wheel housing of a 747 jet right before it left Asia. It landed in the United States and the man was discovered. He was almost dead. His core body temperature had plummeted down into the 70°F range. One doctor reported that there is nothing in the medical records reporting anyone with such low body temperature who survived the hypothermia. Was he superhuman? Had he exceeded all known limits and yet survived? He has survived something like –50°F with massive wind-chill factor. (Look up in a wind-chill table the effect of winds of several hundred miles per hour at –50°F!) The one factor that was interesting was that he was completely covered with brake fluid and oil. Here is one major factor that had been altered.

LIQUIDS

Nearly all substances at a certain temperature turn into a liquid state. Which substances do not turn into liquid at any temperature?

Extensions

If anything is in a liquid state, how do the atoms and molecules interact with each other? If something is in a solid or gaseous state, how do the atoms and molecules interact with each other?

LIQUIDS—WHAT IS THIS STUFF?

I was quite surprised to find out from my supplier of ink for my computer printer that the ink is not a liquid. It comes in a tube, and if it gets out of the tube, it runs all over everything. I was told that this stuff is not a liquid; rather, it is finely compressed powder that acts like a liquid. How does it mimic (copy) the behaviors of a liquid? (*See* "Forms of Matter.")

Extensions

Find other examples of this kind of stuff (powders that act and look like liquids).

LIVING THINGS

What is the biggest living thing? What is the oldest currently living thing? Of all things that have ever lived, which one had the longest life span for an individual organism? What is the smallest living thing? Try to find which species of living things are the oldest. Do not read any farther if you do not want any hints.

Hints: for a while it was thought one of the whales was the largest living thing. Which whale? Then a large fungus was discovered in Michigan that was thought to be the world's largest living thing. It is one huge group of fungi completely interconnected so it lives as a single organism. Now researchers believe that the largest living thing is a tree. This last sentence is tricky. It is not a trick question. Once you know the answer, you will see why it is not a trick question, but it is very misleading. Be careful about what you assume "a tree" is. The answer is not as easy as looking up the world's largest trees. As with the fungi, some trees grow from a single source and manifest as what appears to be an entire grove of separate trees but they are actually one completely interconnected organism. How could this occur? The question related to the world's oldest living thing is also tricky because of the definition you choose to use for life. (*See* "Life—What Makes the Difference?") The question pertaining to the longest living single organism is not simple, because there are organisms that keep producing new parts of itself. This occurs in different ways. Of course, the questions related to cloning greatly complicate the issue of longevity. Is a clone a piece of the former organism that continues forward? If so, what is death relative to cloned populations of living organisms?

Extensions

Do all living things have feelings? How could we know? Start with your pets—do they have feelings? Some studies have shown that plants have feelings. Is that a valid proposition (proposal)? How could this be?

LOGIC—BE CAREFUL

If statements are made about anything, it is helpful to know if these statements are both valid and sound. Look up the difference between a line of reasoning being valid versus being sound. Can a series of statements be valid but not sound? Can a series of statements be sound but not valid?

Extensions

There is a big difference between "and" and "or." If I say that "I'll clean the house, mow the grass, and trim the hedges," is this statement different from "I'll clean the house, mow the grass, or trim the hedges?" Is this statement different:

"I'll clean the house and mow the grass or trim the hedges." This is from an area of study called symbolic logic. It is quite interesting. Look for statements containing the words "if . . . then," "if and only if," "and," and "or."

LONGEST STREET

Where do you think the longest street is located? Would it necessarily be in a city with the greatest population? Would it necessarily be straight?

Extensions

Which would be the widest street? What are some very famous very short streets?

LONG ISLAND

Where is the longest island in North America? Be careful with the name of this section. It is meant to be ambiguous, because many people do in fact jump to conclusions because of the names used and the form of the question asked. (*See* "Life—What Makes the Difference?" and "Home, Sweet Home.")

Extensions

Where is the longest continuous sand beach in North America?

LOST TREASURE

Have you ever felt that you've lost something that can never be recovered? A best friend moves, you get permanently injured, a life companion dies, a divorce occurs, a job or career is lost, you're having to move and leave behind all your family and friends—these are big significant losses. When we've lost something, we are affected by this a sense of loss. Something arises within us that gets us back into life. Have you had this experience? It is something that rises deep inside of us. It is not something that is necessarily dependent upon outer circumstances getting better. It is a change within us that allows us to experience ourselves differently. In order to experience it, we need some kind of commitment to openness, risk, work, discipline, faith, and courage.

Extensions

When other persons are suffering some kind of significant loss, will you extend yourself to that person? It takes openness, risk, work, discipline, faith, and courage to enter the other person's experience. Sometimes all we can do is listen with care.

LOVE'S SWEET MYSTERY

There is simply no one simple explanation for the depth and breadth of the number and kinds of love. Describe to yourself the different kinds of love in your life. What are the feelings associated with each of these kinds of love? Try to describe to yourself different explanations of each kind of love. Then try to find something in that kind of love that can't be explained. For instance, why is it so enjoyable to touch those whom we love? Why is it so liberating to let down all our defenses with those whom we love? Why are we set free to truly love when we reveal to the ones we love who we really are? Why does deep love cast out fear? How and why is it that we can tangle with those whom we love in ways that we don't tangle with others who are mere acquaintances? How can the deepest loves be more than feelings? How is it that love finds a way of presenting itself to us even when we've felt that love has died for us? Are there instances of love emerging in our life, where we've rejected it and held it off? Is love always personal with the expectation of getting something back? How is compassion for the sake of all others related to our assumptions, experience, and behaviors related to personal love? Is there, in any sense, a self-centered quality involved in the ways we love? How can compassion for all others become a real part of our lives? How can personal love and compassion for all others be balanced?

Extensions

If love is the fulfillment of being human, and if hatred is the collapse of the human spirit, then what is the opposite of love? Could the opposite of love be fear that holds us back from fully experiencing the beauty and wonder of others and ourselves? Might fear hold us back from accepting our own foibles (shortcomings)? Could it be that the stuff of life that we reject for ourselves gets projected outward onto others? Could it be that the scorn (bad feelings) and harsh judgments that some of us hold against others are rooted in material that we've rejected about ourselves? Might we be making others into objects that are easy to uphold as something negative so that we do not have to face certain things about ourselves? Keep track of the number and kinds of fear that you have. Carefully sense what this fear does to you. You will be a wiser person. To be aware of the different kinds of fear leads us to wisdom. To be focused on our fears leads us into reactive energies, delusions, and severe unhappiness that become projected outward, causing suffering within us and in others.

MAGIC WAND—WHAT IF?

What would it be like if you had a magic wand? Would you really want to have one? Create a list of all the things you'd like to do with a magic wand. Keep adding to the list when anything comes to your mind. What patterns or kinds of things are obvious on your list? Would it be a good idea for us to really have a magic wand? If you could have one wish, what would it be? Now if you had three wishes, what would they be?

Extensions

What is it that would fulfill your desires? Do you have some desires in life that contradict each other? Would the pursuit of some desires cause us to be diminished or hurt other people? What does it mean to be happy or contented? To be contented with who you are in life and to be contented with your life circumstances, does this require that all your desires become fulfilled? Might it help create a strong and compassionate character if we didn't have all our desires fulfilled? Might we be more mindful of the needs of others if we didn't have all our desires met? Is there a difference between having our desires met and our real needs met?

MAGNETISM

The Chinese discovered that if you take iron and heat it red-hot, then allow it to cool and align it north-south, it will become magnetic. How does this happen?

Extensions

What are some other examples of major discoveries that result from doing common operations in a slightly different manner? Sometimes these discoveries take place because someone had special sensitivities and could spot unusual patterns emerging.

MAGNIFYING GLASSES AND THE UNLUCKY INSECT

Why do some kids go out of their way to use a magnifying glass to fry an insect? Why do some go out of their way to step on insects that are not hurting anything related to the human species?

Extensions

What are other forms of intentional meanness? Why do people do such things? Can we know the mind of another person who has behaviors and values very different from our own? Are we really so different, or do we like to make ourselves believe that we are? Under what conditions have you ever been mean to somebody (if ever)?

MANUFACTURED GOODS

Look up the definition of planned obsolescence. For instance, Mercedes Benz and Rolls Royce engines are designed for long-term use. Most of the engines by the mass production automobile companies don't last nearly as long as those by Mercedes Benz and Rolls Royce. Why? If the technology were there to build better engines, why wouldn't they do it? What are other examples of manufactured items not lasting as long as they could? Why do so many people accept and conform to a culture of planned obsolescence for things and people?

Extensions

What could be done differently to build engines that would last longer? You might begin by looking up something called tolerances. List as many factors as you can think of that would affect the longevity of an engine. Look up the topic of tolerances, quality control, quality of materials, and mass production. While you are researching engines, learn about the new kinds of engines that are projected to be put into mass production in the future. Start with something called a hybrid engine. Look up anything on fuel cells supplying energy for engines.

MAPS AND GRIDS, OLD AND NEW

Once when I was visiting a family member, I looked at the old map framed and hanging on the wall. It was a map showing the area where his ancestors had lived. It happened to be in Eastern Europe. I noticed that the longitude and latitude numbers did not correspond (match) to the present-day numbers. I asked about this odd set of numbers, and I was told that the lines of longitude were not measured from Greenwich, England, as the prime meridian. On the bottom of the map were the mysterious words "Oestlich v. Ferrow." It took some concerted research to figure out that those words indicated the prime reference point. If you want to research this question, a hint is that this prime reference dates all the way back to the times of Ptolemy. This was a map from the old Ottoman Empire. Have some fun, investigate old maps, and look at how they locate the portion of the world relative to the rest of the world in terms of some grid. When did people start to make maps with reference to the entire world? This is a tricky question. In order to answer it, you might assume the view of the mapmaker and the culture of the times. There are different ways to answer this question.

Extensions

You may want to look up how and why von Farrow was used as a guide, zero, or prime reference point. At that time, how many countries claimed to have their own prime meridian? Why was this so important an issue? What are the various ways in which different cultures like to think of themselves as being the true measure of what is real, best, highest, sophisticated, cultured, or advanced?

MASK OF A SIMPLE QUESTION

There are certain questions that have a façade (face) of being so simple but once they are asked, they tend to incite or excite (cause) a complex of challenging issues. Some examples of searching and startling questions may be:

- Who are you?
- Why are you here?
- What is most important in your life?
- Do you know what really makes you tick? (What gives you the sense of being fully alive?)
- What do you really trust in the deepest place of your heart?
- What or whom do you truly love?
- What is the prime intention or sense of purpose for your life? (What are you up to in life?)
- What is your core passion in life?
- What scares you?
- What inspires you?
- What do you hope in?
- Do your outward commitments reflect your true self?
- Are your deepest inner commitments reflected in your outward actions?
- Are you able to apologize for mistakes?
- What is the most difficult thing that you are facing right now in your life?
- Does death scare you?
- Does life frighten you?
- What makes you feel secure?
- What makes you feel contented?
- What makes you feel smart?
- What makes you feel untalented?
- Do you find yourself a good and beautiful human being?
- What is the most important characteristic (habit) that you really need to be working on?
- What do other people like about you?
- What do other people dislike about you?
- Are you truthful in all things with yourself and with others?
- What is the greatest moment of moral integrity in your life (when you were really challenged)?
- What are the things in life that really grab you and make you react quickly?

- Is it true that outside things really force you to be reactive?
- In what circumstances were you challenged and you did or did not rise with courage, strength, and conviction?

Next time you are at some social gathering and the talk seems a little trite (stale or boring), try some of these questions with somebody. Whenever we start to delve into (go into) the deeper substance of our lives, we find points we share in common with others. Life is much less lonely when we learn to share the deeper real stuff that we all hold inside of ourselves. It is amazing what can occur when we reveal something of ourselves to somebody who is trustworthy. How can you tell if somebody is trustworthy?

Extensions

Next time you're in a social gathering, be genuine (real), direct, and caring while being curious about other people. Really care to know about the person. Be discreet (showing good judgment) and direct. See what happens. Every person is like a walking encyclopedia of human wisdom and experience. Most often, we just pass by each other with phrases like "How are you?" Next time, mean what you say, stay and look the person in the eye, and really care to know how they are.

Who are people in groups who are always or almost always alone? Some persons react to the presence of others in a manner that makes it difficult for people to relate to them. What are some of these qualities? How do groups exclude those who don't match certain social criteria (standards)? What are some of these criteria? I recall in grade school watching two young girls being pushed into snowbanks because they had plastic bags tied around their feet (their families could not afford snow boots). Have you ever seen people standing around laughing while others are being hurt in some way? Why does anybody stand around when others are getting hurt intentionally and unnecessarily?

MASS—WHAT IS IT?

Mass is a property of matter. If mass is said to be the amount of matter contained in a given object, we have only shifted the question to "What is matter?" We haven't answered the question. Can mass be defined?

What are mass and matter? How are they related to each other? Does mass have to do with a property of certain particles in the universe that react to gravity? If these particles do not react to gravity, can we say they have no mass? Exactly what is this force called gravity? Would it be accurate to say that a collection of particles with mass will alter the space-time continuum? Why does gravity act on certain particles and not on others? What does inertia (the tendency of a body to remain at rest or in the same path unless other forces act upon it) have to do with mass?

Extensions

What would it mean to have infinite mass? Under what conditions could this occur? What would it mean to have no mass? Under what conditions could this occur?

MEANS AND ENDS

Is it possible to have good ends (goals, objectives, and intentions) and use bad means (the way you choose to get to your goal)? Here are some possible examples of issues related to means and ends.

- I want peace in the world, so I have to destroy my enemies.
- I love the Earth and want to help clean up its ecology. In order to help clean up the Earth, I want to work on recycling and picking up trash. In order to have time to do these things, should my family be using chemicals to kill the weeds in our yard so I don't have to spend so much time picking weeds?

Name as many issues as you can that raise questions related to the consistency of means and ends.

Extensions

Is it possible to have good means and bad ends? Play with the metaphors and see what you conclude.

MEASURING PROGRESS

Some things are easy to measure—like progress in the number of assignments we've completed. Others things are much more difficult to measure. How do we measure our progress in moving toward our personal goals in life? Very frequently, we measure ourselves against others. This is awkward, imprecise, most often highly inaccurate, and usually unfair to ourselves and to others. How do we measure where we are in life compared to our life goals? How do we gauge, measure, or estimate progress when we haven't determined for ourselves what it is we want out of life? What do you want out of life? You can be very specific or you can be very general. Some of these things will change over the course of time. Some of the things we want out of life may not change so much as they become more refined (like the desire for love and the desire to be able to love).

Extensions

How much energy does it waste to be measuring yourself against others? What are positive and useful ways that we can be measuring some areas of performance? How can this metaphor of measuring be changed? Can we help each other define for ourselves what it is we are searching for and desiring out of life?

MEASURING THE YEARS

What year is it right now? Do all people in the world have the same year on their calendars? What are some alternative numbering systems for calendars that people are using in the present time?

Extensions

What are some alternative numbering systems for calendars that people have used in the past? Invent another kind of calendar. What are its various advantages and disadvantages? Who says there have to be seven days in a week? Couldn't there be ten months instead of twelve? Does one year need to be related to the time it takes for the Earth to spin around the sun? Why are there twenty-four hours in a day? Is this necessary? Change some basic assumptions about calendars and time. See what you come up with.

MEETING PLACES

Drive through some small towns and you will see a common area of green grass at the center of the town. It was the center of the life in the community. The community had a geographic and social center point. Often there is a town hall located on the commons area. This is where people met to discuss and work through their shared vital issues. It's where people held major celebrations. In what sense is there a center to your community? Where do people congregate? Under what conditions do people congregate? How has television affected our patterns of gathering together as groups? What else has affected these patterns of gathering? Are there places in which people gather to discuss vital shared issues?

Extensions

One place people meet is while driving on the highways. We drive from our little pockets of neighborhoods and frequently, in order to connect to others, we need to drive on the highways. They are public gathering places. What kind of behaviors do you see on the highways? What does this suggest about how we relate to each other?

One recent study suggested that the biggest and most expensive of the highway construction and repair projects will decrease driving times on average about thirty seconds. When this time saving is compared to the huge number of lengthy delays caused by the construction, it is figured that it would take years of constant driving to make up for the time lost during construction.

Where there is high-volume traffic and where there are both construction delays and varied kinds of vehicles driving at varied speeds, certain persons will drive very dangerously in order to pass several vehicles at once. What does this say about our values and us when so many lives are risked for one person to save a few seconds of driving time (that results in others being slowed down)? Maybe this person was not trying to save time; instead, perhaps the person was simply trying to be in front of somebody else. What are some alternatives? How is the car valued in our culture? What does it represent to us? Would it be possible to reemphasize train travel again? If trains and safe dependable personal rapid transit in the metro areas were available, would this make a difference in our patterns of how to travel?

MEMORIES

What are your earliest memories? Keep track of them. These memories can teach you some important things about yourself. When we are recalling things at the edges of our awareness and memory, some very interesting things occur. One of them is that we can become confused as to what actually occurred and what has been suggested to us by various cues related to memory. An example is about me remembering sitting on my grandmother's lap as a three-year-old. When I thought about this memory, I realized that my image of that experience was almost identical to a picture I had seen of me sitting on her lap at that age. At the edges of our awareness and memory, what are some other interesting phenomena that have occurred for you? Some of these experiences may not just be interesting, but they may also be extremely important to understand.

Extensions

Try keeping a journal of your interesting memories and dreams. Teach yourself to be aware of when certain senses can trigger memories (smell, sight, touch, taste, and hearing). For instance, when I hear the sound of the mourning dove, I remember sleeping overnight at my aunt and grandfather's home as a child. Certain kinds of wonderful feelings come to me when I hear the mourning dove cooing. These powerful associations bring back vivid memories. At the edges of our awareness are vast resources we can use to help us face and resolve many issues. Train yourself to be attentive in a way that is not narrowly concentrated and confining. Our natural awareness is expansive and inclusive, but many of us become dependent upon a fragmenting smallness that excludes vast resources that otherwise could yield to us a creative fullness that is astonishing.

MEN AND WOMEN

Do you sense that men and women communicate differently in some significant ways? What are these differences?

Extensions

What are the manners of communicating and relating that women and men share in common? What are the exceptions to your observations and experiences? Are these patterns a result of our genetics, given to us because of our gender? To what degree do you believe that these patterns of communication and relationships are culturally based and reinforced? If they are reinforced by culture, in what manners are we free to change any of them?

METALS AND MAGNETS

In order for something to be attracted or repelled by a magnet, it must be metallic. Is this right?

Extensions

Are all metals affected by magnetism?

METEORITE, ASTEROID, COMET, METEOR

What are the differences among an asteroid, meteoroid, meteorite, meteor, and a comet? What are their origins?

Extensions

A chunk of the planet Mars was discovered on the Earth. How could it have gotten here? Has it been proven to be from Mars? Some scientists are claiming that it contains fragments of materials that are related to life. Look up some information on this topic. Has there been life on Mars? How could anything living survive the high-temperature crash into our Earth's atmosphere? How could anything living survive the barrage (bombardment, pummeling, or blasts) of different kinds of high-energy electromagnetic waves racing around all regions of space?

MIGRATING

If human beings can get lost a few blocks from home, how can animals and butterflies migrate so successfully and precisely? Who has the brains around here anyway?

Extensions

Do other life-forms have talents, skills, and capacities that we human beings don't have? Can we learn anything from these other life-forms? Might we have more talents than we realize? Might we be masking over some interesting talents that other animals possess and use? What might be some examples?

MIGRATING ANIMALS

Other than birds that fly south every fall, what group of animals has the greatest north-south trek (trip) in the fall and then south-north mass migration every spring? The word *great* is defined in terms of the amount of stuff they manage to carry with them. Hints: it may not be an animal you'd think of as being migratory. These animals congregate in Florida, Texas, and Arizona mainly. They're nicknamed by other nonmigrating animals of the same species "snowbirds." These animals are not geese but they do honk a lot (no more than other members of the same species who do not migrate).

Extensions

Do all animals migrate from the north to the south in the fall? Think of the Northern and Southern Hemispheres. Find out about migration patterns for animals in both the Northern and Southern Hemisphere. What are the main forces in nature that cause animals to migrate? Are there examples of migrating animals near the equator? Are all migrations mainly north or south in orientation? What are some other migration patterns that are not mainly north or south in orientation? Hint: think of animals that live at different altitudes at different times of the year. How do they migrate? What about animals that live in the oceans? What are various migration patterns at play? What about certain animals that migrate in both oceans and rivers? Are there any animals that migrate both on land and in the seas? How has human development affected migration patterns (routes and timing of migration)? Has global warming affected migration patterns? What are the most interesting examples of human migration?

MILLIPEDES DANCING

Yup, they really do dance. It has to be live music played by musicians who are not much bigger than the millipedes, under the red shifted light of a blue moon right at moonrise, and then only when there is plenty of earthshine. (*See* "Earthshine" and "Blue Moon.") Seriously, can you imagine a millipede or a centipede dancing? Whenever these cute little critters scramble anywhere, it is like they are dancing. How do they keep all those legs moving in synchrony (in a uniform step)? Imagine the size of their brains. Do insects have brains? What are the largest living things without brains? What are the smallest living things with brains? If you want a really simple little bedtime issue to think about right before you fall asleep, try to figure out the relationship between what we mean by mind and brain.

Extensions

Have you ever had the experience of learning some rather complex physical motion, and then once you've really learned it, you can do it without thinking about every step of the process? You get the feeling for it. You see the entire complex process as one integrated whole. Then, something happens and you get very self-conscious. Suddenly, it's as though you are a beginner all over again. A few seconds later, you recover your self-confidence, and it's like you're back in some kind of groove or rhythm. This can occur for physical, social, intellectual, and emotional experiences of all different kinds. Under what conditions has this ever occurred to you?

MINIMUM, OPTIMUM, MAXIMUM

In real life, there are always multiple things happening. We have diverse desires. At different times, we like to have more of something, less of something, and just the right mixture of things. This is like an ongoing balancing act. Learn what it means to maximize, minimize, and optimize something. For instance, if you go on a vacation, what are the things you'd like to minimize, maximize, and optimize? If you don't know the meaning of the term *optimum*, look it up.

Extensions

Might it be that if we maximize something (like having all the candy we want all the time), there will be consequences we do not intend? If we minimize everything we want to reduce or eliminate (like food we don't like or challenging people), might there be negative consequences? Can we ever perfectly optimize our lives relative to our needs and wants? In many ways, we carry within us contradictory needs, desires, attachments, and aversions. This adds considerable complexity to our lives (and to the lives of those around us).

MIRACLES?

What is a miracle to you? Given your definition of miracles, have you ever experienced one? Remember that the basic way we look at something determines the outcome (our assessment, judgment, opinion, and bias). There is a great difference between viewing life issues in terms of outcomes in discrete terms instead of process terms. (*See* "First Human Being" and "Chicken and the Egg Question.")

Extensions

What are some other definitions of miracles? Can miracles be defined? Might there be a sense or experience of the miraculous nature of existence without being able to define it precisely? What are other examples of important things that you can't define exactly? Ironically, some things that are greatly difficult, complex, and demanding can be defined in a simple yet profound way.

MISSING AIR

If air pressure is 14.2 pounds per square inch, why don't we implode? If your answer is that there is air inside of us with equal pressure, where is this air (other than our lungs and heads at certain times)?

Extensions

All life-forms are suited or adjusted to the demands of the environment in which they live. What are some peculiar behaviors and some peculiar (from our perspective) adaptations in terms of body types that allow certain organisms to survive in their environments? Be sure to consider those life-forms that are under the water. Don't forget the microscopic life-forms. Look at our human bodies, the social contexts we create, the physical settings we generate, and how we affect the Earth's ecology. Are all of our adaptive mechanisms and behaviors ecologically sound? If not, in what sense are the behaviors and mechanisms we employ adaptive? Adaptive to what?

MITOCHONDRIA—THEY'RE EVERYWHERE (ALMOST)

Mitochondria are organelles within the cells of our bodies. Their job is to help us metabolize energy. Study these vital little things. During our evolutionary process, might it be possible that these mitochondria were once independent organisms that became associated with the cells of animals? Are there any other parts of our bodies that may have once been independent living organisms? Are there living organisms within our bodies that help us maintain life? Look up *symbiosis*.

Extensions

Mitochondria are examples of eukaryote cells. What is a eukaryote cell? What kinds of life-forms have eukaryote cells? What are non-eukaryote cells? What kinds of life-forms have non-eukaryote cells?

MOMENTS OF JOY

Do you recall having moments in which you feel joyful and peaceful, when everything seems right? What words would you use for such moments? Do you think there is anything you can do to have more of these moments? Are these moments mostly due to circumstances and the environment (things happen to go your way for a moment or period of your life), or are these moments mostly because of something internal within yourself? Can you cultivate a way of living in which these moments are encouraged, recognized, and honored?

Extensions

When you've felt sad, mad, off-balance, scattered in your thoughts, a lack of self-confidence, the world's against you, and not very creative, are there any patterns in your life that give clues as to why such moments or periods of your life occur?

MOON CYCLES

What are the most famous regularly occurring holy days from any religion that are based on cycles of the moon?

Extensions

How are the dates of these holy days calculated? Hint: for the Christian holy day of Easter, look up the formula sometime. There are others.

MOON—MYSTERIOUS PRESENCE

How did our moon get there? Was it a captured asteroid, a burped-up hunk from the Earth while it was molten, or a body formed at the same time as the Earth that evolved into a binary planet system? (Some people do consider the Earth-moon system as a dual planetary system since the size of the moon relative to the size of the Earth is substantial.) What are some other possibilities?

Extensions

Could the sun have any moons? Could a moon have a moon?

MOONSTRUCK

How are the terms *moonstruck*, *hysterical*, and *hysteria* related?

Extensions

What are some ways that some people claim the moon is related to various forms of human behaviors? We've heard of behaviors related to the full moon. Is there any cultural lore related to the waxing, waning, or new moon? Where do we get the words *waxing* and *waning*? What else, other than the moon, waxes and wanes? (*See* "Earthshine.")

MORALITY AND RESEARCH

During World War II, the Germans conducted biological research on Jewish and other hostages. They did terrible things to these victims in order to obtain (get) information related to the human body. It is obvious that this was wrong and immoral. Why did medically trained personnel do this research? Are there German documents that reflect that some people did protest this form of greatly inhumane behavior? During World War II, while the Japanese occupied major portions of China, they conducted biological research on the Chinese. When such atrocities occur, where are the people of conscience? How does society neutralize the persons of conscience when that society wishes to violate life in such systematic and intentional ways? Do most people in the society know what is happening? Who is responsible? Are there state secrets that our own country holds that cover up unethical behaviors? If so, what does this do to the moral fiber of the entire society? Are there practices within our own society that are openly practiced and rarely talked about that are highly detrimental to human beings and other life-forms? What are the social and cultural mechanisms at play that prevent us from confronting such behaviors?

Extensions

The Nazis gathered large amounts of information and stored it in databanks that are still in existence. If some of this information could help people today, is it morally acceptable to use the information in these databanks? List as many ethical requirements that you can think of that would justify certain research and justify using the information derived from that research. List things that ought never be done. What are forms of research conducted today that are questionable in terms of morality? One example could be whether fetal brain tissue from aborted fetuses ought to be used in studying brain degenerative conditions that affect many adults. What are possible forms of research that might be conducted in the future that you would definitely find immoral and unethical? What are some forms of research that you find questionable in terms of ethics but necessary for some reason? Find out all you can on the greatly complex issues related to stem cell research.

MORPHING

Many movies have used the technique called morphing: dragons turning into monkeys, flowers turning into trees, or people turning into stones. When we see one form turn into another form right in front of our eyes, we see directly what our minds say can't happen. The term *morphing* comes from a Greek word *morphe*, which means "having one form." If we are human beings, we're not birds. If we are fish, we are not spiders. We organize our world by using categories by which we can distinguish many diverse things in life. Our minds do not easily adjust when one form either instantly or gradually but steadily turns into another form.

People have challenges in adjusting between the forms of being a child, an adolescent, a young adult, a middle-aged person, a young-old person, and a very old person. We look at ourselves in the mirror and see our bodies changing. The way we process our feelings and thoughts changes. The way people value us and the manner in which we value others change. In a way, this aging process can look as though we are being morphed. Look up how much money is spent annually by people on goods that supposedly make them look younger. This huge industry is based on our difficulty in making transitions and aging. What other industries make huge profits from the same human tendency of not being able to accept change and transitions?

One kind of morphing is a process produced by computers. Another kind of morphing occurs when there are significant transitions in our lives. To morph is to change form. This can refer to outer form or inner substance. Some kinds of morphing blur the edges of what we believe possible and what we believe to be impossible. The lines between fantasy and reality become less clear. If it looks real, are the images we are seeing real? Look up how much money is spent every year by people surgically altering their bodies. What is real and what is fantasy?

Extensions

There is a branch of biological sciences called morphology. This discipline studies the similarities and differences between the various forms of life. One day I was studying some photomicrographs (photographs of extremely small objects taken through microscopes). The pictures were all of dust mites. When I examined these photomicrographs, I was amazed at how similar the dust mites were to some insects. The morphology (outward form) was similar.

I began to wonder whether very small things like the dust mites could be enlarged. Would we call it an insect? Are there other small things that you can imagine being large in real life? Are there large living things that you can imagine to be extremely small (like a bully, a pest, a teacher who consistently assigns too much homework, or a supervisor who always demands the impossible from you)? Try to imagine large animals being exactly as they are but in much smaller renditions (versions). Remember this is not just fantasy, because there once were giant-sized beavers on the face of this Earth. There are examples of animals that were once large that evolved into smaller animals. The last surviving mastodons lived in an isolated area in which the environment would not allow for the survival of giant-sized mastodons, so they evolved into mastodons that were much smaller. Imagine a mastodon being the size of your dog, and imagine a horse being the size of your cat. Could you imagine a virus being large in real life? What would the environment have to be like in order to allow viruses or bacteria to be much larger (like the size of a dog)? In such an environment, would humans survive? Would we ever get sick from them again? How would a dog react to a barking virus?

MOUNTAIN PEAKS

What is the highest mountain in the world? Be careful not to give the most obvious answer. Hint: highest can mean different things. One sense of highest means the point of a mountain that is farthest from the center of the Earth. Another way of looking at the question is to measure the mountain from its base to its peak. If you do this, there is a very unexpected answer. Hint: the mountain may be next to an ocean and adjacent to a deep ocean trench; then again, maybe not!

Extensions

The manner in which any question is asked is not necessarily the way in which you must answer it. Change the way you look at the question. Get a picture of the question in your mind, then alter the picture. Very complex problems can be pictured or imaged. The image contains vast information. Each piece and the picture as a whole contain information. Try it out. Especially with such creative kinds of tests as multiple choice or true-false tests, any teacher will especially enjoy your efforts to rephrase the questions.

MOUNTAINS AND THE PLAINS

If you were to drive through the mountains with exactly the same number of ascents and descents of the same altitude differentials (differences), would your gas mileage (number of gallons consumed per mile) equal that of driving the same distance on a flat plain? Assume all the other factors are the same: wind resistance, car, tires, speed, acceleration, and cargo weights.

Extensions

Talk to a pilot and see how fuel consumption varies because of different factors (tail wind, frontal wind, air temperature, air density, load, types of fuel, uplifts, downdrafts, and humidity). Before talking to the pilot, list as many factors as you can think of that might affect fuel consumption. If a jet were to suddenly fly into a huge pocket of low-density air, could the jet fall out of the sky? Would it require more engine power to maintain the same altitude and speed? What would happen if the jet ran into a sudden and unexpected area of high pressure?

MOVIE STARS

If you were to see a movie or musical star, your very favorite one in the whole world, how would you react to her or him? Would you treat the person as an object that you've adored or identified with because of the movies or because of her or his music? For instance, he or she might be the symbol of power, fame, riches, beauty, wisdom, compassion, or ruggedness for you. Might you be able to talk to your favorite movie star as you would to another human being? Are these performing artists more than regular human beings? If so, why and how?

Extensions

How do we treat other people as objects?

MOVING WHILE STILL IN HOW MANY WAYS?

If you are holding your breath, lying flat on your back, not moving a muscle and perfectly relaxed, in how many different directions at once is your body moving?

Think about your body being affected by many different forces of the universe. The same forces that govern the motion of planets and stars affect your body.

You are lying still. If you live in eastern Canada or Scandinavia, the surface of the Earth is rising—springing up due to the melting of the last ice age's glaciers. However, your tectonic plate is moving ever so slowly. The Earth is rotating on its own axis. While the Earth rotates it has a slight wobble. There are ocean tides related to gravitational influences of other celestial bodies, and there are Earth tides related to the same forces of nature. The Earth's surface rises and falls (deforms) due to external gravitational influences! While the Earth is rotating relative to its own axis, there is such a thing called the precession of the equinoxes. The Earth's axis is an imaginary line. If you extend this line straight out and north, you will get to the planet Polaris, which is otherwise known as the North Star. (While you are looking up any information on precession of the equinoxes, you might as well also look up information on something called obliquity of the elliptic. You'll be glad you learned about the obliquity of the elliptic the next time you play Scrabble.) Back to the precession of the equinoxes. Thousands of years from now, Earth's axis will be pointing at the planet Vegas. This is a shift of twenty-six degrees in the angle of the Earth's rotation around its own axis. Thus, the Earth is shifting toward the direction of Vegas from Polaris. The Earth is rotating around the sun. There is such a thing as the precession of elliptical orbits. The orbits of the planets rotating around the sun are moving relative to each other. In other words, the path we travel around the sun is changing all the time. Our planet is part of the galaxy named the Milky Way. The galaxy is rotating around its center. Therefore, we are spinning around the center of the galaxy. All galaxies appear to be moving away from each other. If the space-time continuum is warped by the concentration of matter, we might also be moving in relation to the warping of the time-space continuum. Try this one—if the universe (space-time continuum) is expanding from every point, since your body is part of the universe, then your body is expanding away from its center point. Check out this possibility with an astrophysicist and maybe your doctor. Ask if there is any medicine to help prevent body-based space-time continuum expansion. I'm sure your doctor will know exactly what you're talking about, but you may be referred to somebody else. Actually, this is an issue of space dilation (expansion), but it doesn't affect things like our bodies. (*See* "Dimensions—How Many?")

Can you name any more ways in which your still and supposedly motionless body is moving all at once? Next time anybody wants you to be still and just be quiet, ask him or her this question about the different kinds of motion. Make sure you ask when he or she is not feeling pulled in too many directions at once due to a busy schedule. Be careful not to be oblique (indirect) or elliptical (obscure or unclear) in your manner of describing the problem with sitting still. This kind of question at the wrong time might set off some strong reactions and he or she might do something crazy—like wanting you to order out supper from a junk-food palace.

Extensions

Look up the definition of a paradox and another fancy word—conundrum. Some things the mind has a difficult time figuring out. Some things are impossible to figure out. For instance, can anything be moving in more than one direction at the same time and retain its integrity and shape? The answer is yes, but how can this be? This is a riddle that can only be answered in a larger and more encompassing context.

MUSCLES THAT KEEP GOING AND GOING AND GOING . . .

Try lifting some relatively light object a few times with your arm. Nothing to it! You're a real muscle-bound creature! Now take a slightly lighter weight and keep doing the exact lifting action for eighty years (give or take a few moments).

Did you get to even one year? If you did this for one year, you really need to get a life! If you did this experiment for even a few hours, you're going to regret it tomorrow. Did you notice how tired your muscles got? If you kept going after the muscles were tired, they began to ache. If you kept going, you may have noticed that you actually can exercise mind control over your pain sensations. Even if you can do this mind control stuff, eventually it all stops working. The muscles need rest. You would severely injure yourself if you kept on going through the various levels of pain and exhaustion. These are all signals from your body that it needs to rest. How often do you listen carefully to the needs of your body? Can the body yield (reveal) wisdom to us that the rational mind is unaware of? Are there certain soma (body) communications that are part of our deep consciousness (prior to conscious awareness)?

Now stop to think about the fact that your heart is a muscle. It keeps on going and going over the course of your whole life. Ever had heartache? This kind of aching can be from food being digested in a weird way. One's heart can hurt from different kinds of heart attacks or love lost, but let's not talk about those related phenomena now. Assume that your heart itself isn't hurting. Why don't the muscles of the heart become tired and exhausted?

Extensions

How many different kinds of muscle tissue do we have in our bodies?

MUTUAL PACTS OF CIVILITY

There are explicit (outward, visible, direct) agreements and there are implicit (inward, not always obvious, indirect, tacit) agreements upon which we all depend. We trust that when there is a green light at an intersection we can proceed without someone racing through a red light from a side street. We trust that people will not drive drunk. We trust that people will safeguard the rights of all persons. These are all implicit agreements. Explicit agreements are those pacts (agreements) that are formal in nature. I agree to buy a car. This also entails (involves) being responsible to pay for it. This is a formal written agreement. It is the implicit (not directly spoken) agreements that keep us civilized. What does it mean to act in a civilized fashion? What are other forms of implicit agreements that make us better, safer, and more enjoyable?

Extensions

Many civilizations have produced groups that have done horrible things in the name of their civilization. One example is what people did and are doing to native peoples all over the world. Another example is what has been done to women over the course of history in the name of civilization. Delve into (examine) the history of how adults have treated children in the name of being civilized. What are the other forms of implicit agreements that have disastrous influences on both the victimizer and the victims? How are these implicit agreements communicated? What are the various reasons people agree to act in accord with these implicit agreements? How are they reinforced?

MYSTERIOUS BAR CODES

How do bar codes work? When you go to the grocery or large general merchandise stores, the checkout people use scanners to electronically scan for bar codes. How can these bar codes contain so much information embedded in a series of lines?

Extensions

Who designed this system? How long has it been in use? How do the bar codes work that we can print onto our own envelopes at home with the use of our computer?

MYSTERY TIME

Do you have anything in your life that is a real mystery? Once when I was young, I camped deep in the woods with my family. We were in the huge wilderness area of a national park. I awakened in the middle of the night to hear a sound that was like a big rope being pulled back and forth over a branch. The loons and the wolves started to make their sounds. It sounded like the rope was being tugged back and forth over a branch with increased speed and energy. Then the ropelike sound ceased and the loons and wolves became silent. I was left to wonder, what had happened?

When I look at an eye or think of the heart or brain, I am left to wonder about how life could have evolved from hydrogen (from the big bang). How could we have gotten hydrogen from the original stuff of the big bang? What are some real mysteries for you? They could be related to relationships, nature's patterns, who did what to whom, do certain things really exist, or do some things exist in reality in a vastly different way than we suppose they exist, period. If we think about it, life is filled with interesting and some inspiring mysteries.

Extensions

Because something is unexplained or because there is a gap in our understanding, does this mean that the unexplained phenomenon or mystery is supernatural, extraterrestrial, or unnatural in some sense? Could there be an order to the universe that is not explained by our present-day knowledge? Is it possible that there is a much larger and more encompassing reality than we even imagine? Could it be that what we see as the universe is like an atom inside another universe? Might it be that what we refer to as atoms might contain entire universes? Could everything be infinitely divisible (existing in smaller and smaller units relative to our perspective)? Could everything be extended into very small or very large scales that are so different from our ordinary reality that we fail to be able to detect their presence? What would be a reality so large that we would not be able to detect or sense its presence? How about certain rhythms and cycles that occur so infrequently that we are not able to detect their cycle or rhythm? What are some other possible phenomena that we actually do see but we do not notice?

NAMERS AND ECHTHROI

In a wonderful book entitled *A Wind in the Door* by Madeleine L'Engle, there are powers in the universe who care about all others. They are the Namers. They help you become what you potentially might be. They are friendly and nice to have around. Then there are the Echthroi. "War and hate are their business, and one of their chief weapons is un-naming—making people forget who they are. If someone knows who she or he is, really knows, then this person doesn't need to hate. That's why we still need Namers, because there are places throughout the universe like your planet Earth. When everyone is really and truly Named, then the Echthroi will be vanquished."

Imagine the power of names. Think back to all the encounters in school, playgrounds, work sites, and in our homes in which names have been used. Sometimes names given to us by others are meant to hurt us, limit us, put us in a place of being without power, or make us feel bad about ourselves. Then there are those people who have a talent for making other people feel good about themselves and feel empowered and secure enough to venture into new life territory. The names these people use for others are names that help us feel a kind of power that builds up relationships, self-esteem, compassion, and a sense of justice. This is the true gift of naming.

Once we begin to accept the names others have given to us, we start to believe them. You have your legal name and nicknames. Over the course of time, we listen to the other names that other people use for us, we take them into our lives, and they become names that we begin to use to identify who we are. Then something like an inner voice comes up that starts to convince us that we are this name. Names are words we use to describe ourselves or words others have used about us that we have believed in some manner. Think about all the names you have assumed are true about you and names you have used (or thought of) for others.

Extensions

What is the impact of these names? Labels that hurt include: stupid, bad, dork, clumsy, dumb, mean, I'm not very good at . . . , I'm not very good looking, I'm not too popular. Labels that build us up include: talented, good, enjoyable, fun, imaginative, bright, loving, caring, gentle.

Create your own list of both kinds of names and labels. Who have you heard these names from? Which ones do you believe, and why do you believe them?

NANOCARBON TUBES

Imagine millions of little tubes that are too small to be seen even with our optical microscopes. Materials made out of these tubes could be up to one hundred times stronger than steel and weigh as little as one-sixth the weight of steel. These little tubes are approximately a billionth of a meter in diameter (across). They are very strong, conduct electricity very well, and they conduct thermal energy (heat) better than most known materials. Put your mind to work on as many possible applications for this stuff as possible. See if they sell this stuff by the pound at your local hardware store. A recent experiment successfully used these nanocarbon tubes to create a working carbon-based microchip. It is a very simple machine but its importance is that it is not silicon-based. Might this be the material of the future for computers?

Extensions

Try to imagine the applications of a material that is superstretchable. Imagine a balloon that could be stretched for fifteen miles without losing strength. What could this material possibly be made of?

NAUGHTY!

Naughty is a funny word because it has different meanings. In one sense, naughty means that some behavior is outright bad. In another sense, being naughty is something that is a natural part of growing up when it has to do with differentiating yourself from the authority figures in your life. People bend the rules that have been handed to them by persons in power. We can't discover our own power and reality until we know certain truths for ourselves on our own terms.

We need to learn how to apply the great wisdom of the ages. Others can't do this work for us. Some of this exploration and growth can be called naughty. Listen to young children talk on the playgrounds. Some of it is naughty talk. They think they are out of earshot (listening distance) from any authority figure who has power over them. This behavior starts early in life. There are benign forms of this naughty behavior, such as sneaking a piece of candy from your parents' stash of chocolate goodies. There are also detrimental (damaging) forms of naughty behaviors. What are the various benign and detrimental forms of naughty behaviors that you've participated in and have observed? What kinds of persons have we observed who are not able to distinguish for themselves the line between benign and detrimental behaviors?

One of the challenges in this area of behavior is that real lasting damage can be done to others and ourselves. An associated challenge is that power and authority are often abused in such a manner that youngsters grow up in a very reactive manner; thus they are more likely to cross the line from the benign side to the detrimental side. This is a sorry state of affairs, because the testing of these lines is exactly what is needed in order to become your own unique self. Naughty behavior is not necessarily "bad" behavior. It is experimental behavior done at the edges of our understanding and wisdom. It is reality testing. This is why the benign and wise presence of others is so critical to our development. This is why it is ever so important whom we choose as our role models. If there are no positive ones, there certainly will be a host (a lot) of negative ones available (then it will be very difficult to distinguish between harmless and destructive behaviors and values). Ultimately, something inside of us tells us what is right and wrong, where the lines are, what is life giving and what is life diminishing (robbing). The development of this inner voice is a most crucial gift in life. This is why it is so critically important that we are in relationships that honor the development of our own inner voice of conscience and wisdom.

Extensions

Have you ever done something that is bad for you or others? You knew it in advance. You went ahead and did it anyway. Why? Were you reacting to something? Were you trying to get one thing but got another?

NECESSARY AND SUFFICIENT

In the art of thinking and investigation, what is the difference between something that is necessary and something that is sufficient? Clue: it has to do with logic.

It is Friday afternoon and you've agreed with a parent that a certain set of five jobs must be done around the house before you go out to play with friends. It is necessary that all five jobs be finished before departure. One of the jobs is cleaning your room. Is it necessary to do this job? Is it sufficient to do this one job? Is it necessary to do all the jobs?

Extensions

Can you come up with other examples of things that illustrate the relationship and the distinctions between things that are necessary and things that are sufficient?

NEIGHBORHOODS OF POVERTY

Drive through many of our major metropolitan areas in our country and we begin to notice that the poorest neighborhoods are often concentrated in certain confined areas. Why are they confined? Who or what causes the poorest of the poor to be located in confined areas? Is this good for the persons living in poverty? Does having the poor concentrated in certain areas benefit others who are not poor? Is this concentration of poverty intentional or accidental? There are some facets of our lives that are not consciously instituted (caused) and yet are part of the cultural design of how we choose to share life. These are systemic flaws in the basic fabric of our culture that cause massive suffering on large scales over protracted periods of time. If these pockets of concentrated poverty are causing massive human suffering, what things can the human community be doing to prevent this concentration of poverty? Is it the moral responsibility of those in poverty to do something for themselves? Is it the moral responsibility of the entire society to help the poor make it in life? How do we all become aware of the flaws in our cultural fabric of life that cause unnecessary suffering? How do we gain the courage and moral conviction to do something about what we are aware is damaging and detrimental? How do we learn to act together to face these challenges?

Extensions

Do most nonpoor neighborhoods welcome poor people to live in the same area? Why or why not? How do we practice segregation based on economic status? What are the other forms of segregation that we practice?

NEWTON'S OTHER LAWS

Isaac Newton was a famous scientist. Among his accomplishments are the laws of motion. The third one states that the actions of two bodies on each other are equal and opposite (any action will have its equal opposite reaction). What are the first and the second laws of motion defined by Newton?

Extensions

Do you think that if a body were moving at a constant rate in a straight lines, it would keep moving in that direction with the same speed forever if nothing interfered with it? Wouldn't it run out of oomph (energy)? What is a unit of measurement for oomph?

NICE GAS!

This is something nice people don't talk about—at least, nice people can't talk about it in a polite manner. However, President Reagan once said that trees pollute the Earth more than cars. So let's ask which one of the following gives off more gas each year:

1. cars
2. trucks
3. dogs
4. cows
5. cats
6. trees
7. human beings
8. the Old Faithful geyser in Yellowstone National Park
9. politicians
10. magma rising to the surface of the Earth
11. food you can't stand to smell
12. northern tundra (that covers about one-fifth of the Earth's surface)

Extensions

What are other sources of gases?

NORMAL AND NECESSARY

When we look back at a set of circumstances, it can seem as though everything is right and things "were meant to be." Some examples might be:

- who we married
- the number of children in the family
- where we live
- the course of our lives
- that a certain race is the dominant race in a society
- that a certain religion is the dominant religion in a culture
- the language we speak
- the way we've evolved
- the very fact that we human beings ever evolved at all
- the Earth with its atmosphere and forms of life
- what we see as the universe

We can easily forget that things might have been very different if any one thing would have been different. Everything in our lives, anything we call reality, could have been very different with the slightest difference in the course of events. Name twenty things that easily could have been different in your life. In the evolution of the universe, billions upon billions of things could have been different. Imagine if people would have risen up against racism long before the civil rights campaigns.

Extensions

Some persons believe that, because things are a certain way, it is by design and purpose. This is the way things are supposed to be. Did the universe come into existence to support human life? This is called the anthropic principle. There are "weak" and "strong" forms of this principle. Learn some things about the anthropic principle.

NORTH STAR—AN ANTIPODES?

The North Star is that star toward which the axis of the Earth points. Is there a South Star? Find resources to deal with this issue. The only clue I've found is one single reference to a constellation named Octans that contains what is called the southern celestial pole.

Extensions

What are antipodes? Would the Northern and Southern Pole stars be antipodes? After Polaris is replaced by Vegas as the Northern Pole star, what will be the Southern Pole star?

NUMBER THIRTEEN

The number thirteen is considered an unlucky number in our culture. Many hotels do not have thirteenth floors (or at least, do not have floors that are labeled "thirteen"). How did this custom come about? What are other examples of myth, lore, fear, or misperception that cause entire groups to react in ways that reflect persistent and continuing belief in irrational (or magical) beliefs? How do these inclinations and tendencies affect peoples' willingness to take risks that could affect their careers?

Extensions

In some cultures, a certain number is seen as a symbol for transformation and growth. Which number is it? What are other numbers with special cultural significance? Look up how they became significant.

NUMBERS—LARGE AND SMALL

Very small numbers and very large numbers have names to them. These numbers are grouped for our convenience so that we can understand them better. For instance, one grouping is composed of the numbers less than one hundred. These are called the tens (ten, twenty, etc.).

An aside: Find out what *etc.* stands for—what language does it come from? While you're at it, look up what *i.e.* and *e.g.* stand for. These three terms (*etc.*, *i.e.*, and *e.g.*) will help you write and record ideas.

If we move from the tens, the hundreds are next in order, then the thousands, then the millions, billions, trillions, etc. What comes next? Look up the word *numbers* in an unabridged dictionary. What language do the names for numbers come from? Can you memorize several of these numbers? It is quite easy. Now that you have discovered quintillion and octillion, learn about the names of small numbers.

To describe brief moments of time, we need names of numbers. Try to find the names of portions of a second. A thousandth of a second is called a millisecond. A millionth of a second is called a microsecond. See if you can find out what femtoseconds, picoseconds, and nanoseconds are. Are there names for portions of a second smaller than any of these mentioned names? What kind of resources would talk about this kind of information? What kinds of processes in nature do these numbers describe?

Computer floppy disks are often measured in terms of how much information they can store. One measure is in terms of kilobytes (one thousand bytes of electronic information). Another larger measure that has become much more common is megabytes (one million bytes of electronic information). Now the largest hard-disk drives measure their capacity in terms of gigabytes (billions of bytes). Computers are starting to be manufactured that measure size of storage in terms of terabytes (trillions of bytes). Computers of the future may be so powerful that we have to measure information storage in even larger terms like petabytes and exabytes. Decide on a certain kind of database like the Bible, the *Encyclopedia Britannica*, the entire works of Shakespeare, all the books in the Library of Congress, or all the recorded music in the world. Select some database that is well known so that you can consult with a computer expert and find out how much computer memory space these databases would require. Then go back and compare computer memory limits. Would your selected database require kilo-, mega-, giga-, tera-, peta-, or exabytes of memory? This will help you define how big some of these numbers are. Can the information contained in the brain be estimated in terms of the amount of data? Is it stored in the brain in digital form? If there is memory, then how does it relate to memory in a computer?

There have been estimates made about how much computer memory would be needed to store all human knowledge. What is the largest database you can think of (don't forget that everything that exists can be interpreted in terms of information or data)? A tree, a human being, a planet, a solar system, a star, and an entire universe can all be interpreted in terms of information. Could any computer, in any age or time, given any technology, contain all the information in all systems? Look up the term *epistemology*. Can we know everything? Can we know everything in real time (the current moment)? Can human beings only be conscious of so much at once?

Can computers hold in their databanks wisdom and the means to continually grow, evolve, and learn? If not, then they can never hold all the information there is in life. If they can grow, evolve, and learn, then there is a problem because the very process of growth, evolution, and learning is information. To grow, evolve, and learn is not a simple matter of changing something for another. It is a fundamental transformation of what is real, valued, experienced, and imagined. Growth, evolution, and learning are not simple pieces of information that can be digitally stored. One form of genius is the capacity to leap beyond all prime presumptions and prior tendencies and to manifest an entirely different (maybe original) basis for living or solving an issue. Computers might be intelligent (A.I.) but can they ever be ingenious? Could they ever be self-conscious?

True growth, evolution, and learning are requirements of self-consciousness. Self-consciousness is not some datum that can be written into a computer program. What would have to happen is that the computer software designer would have to comprehend self-consciousness and then ingeniously transfer the quality to computers. It is not the case that we know that there never could be artificial intelligence rooted in its own variety self-consciousness. (*See* "Dimensions—How Many?") The very capacity for growth, evolution, and learning is rooted in the fact that our consciousness is riddled with mystery. We can't know the future and can't know every aspect of our potential in the current movement.

The existence of the holes in understanding empowers us to rise above the details, illusions, truths, and biases of the current moment into a broader plane of comprehension. This is genius and inspiration. This is discovery and revelation. We can't know everything. We can't currently create machines that will be able to grow, evolve, and learn, because these qualities are an effect and not a cause. They are the effect of consciousness itself, riddled with mystery that itself is the energy and means for true transformation. (*See* "Spiraling into Infinity.") Another way of saying this is that we are part of a living system whose roots, boundaries, processes, and facets will always be larger than our comprehension. One reason for this is that the system itself is growing, evolving, and learning. To believe that we can bestow consciousness onto something else is very egotistical. To contend that we may deliberately or inadvertently (by mistake) foster the conditions under which some new form of consciousness arises is another matter. We can't judge the ultimate mysteries of life with absolute certainty.

Self-consciousness appears to be a function of living organisms with well-developed brains. We cannot be sure that our prime assumptions are correct. There are long-standing cultural traditions backed up by sound and valid intellectual reflection that advocate (stand for, espouse) a vastly different view of consciousness. For those who advocate these traditions, consciousness is not a function (by-product or effect) of a brain. Some of these people believe that consciousness is a shared phenomenon distributed between living beings. Others believe that consciousness is sewn into the fabric of the universe itself. For them, a more rudimentary (basic) level of inquiry has to do with "what is life?" For them, there are meaningful ways of understanding life that are not limited to the biological forms. For others, there is the belief or prime assumption that consciousness is the substratum (root) from which the fabric of manifest (observable) life emerges.

If you've followed all of this stuff about information, data, artificial intelligence, consciousness, growth, evolution, learning, genius, and life, then try a really big and interesting question: when your pet is looking at you directly in the eye, is it wondering about something? Is it imagining (in a vein of humor) that you, the human subject, possess intelligence? Might the pet be wondering if you can apply genius in the form of the fusion of diverse experiences and insights and the capacity to leap beyond all prime presumption in a creative manner to organizational, professional, or personal challenge?

Extensions

What kinds of phenomena in nature happen in these little parcels (segments or pieces) of time? What kinds of phenomena in nature happen during long periods of time? There are cycles of nature that take moments, and there are rhythms and cycles that take an hour, a day, twenty-eight days, a month, a year, or many years. What are some of the longest periods of time? Hint: first we have to discern the presence of patterns. Try to define as many of these phenomena as possible. (*See* "Circadian Rhythms.") Could something be a pattern that only occurs once, occurs irregularly, occurs only if we are unaware of it, or occurs regularly based on a totally unanticipated regulating mechanism?

OBSERVATION AND JUDGMENT

Somewhere along the way, I picked up the insight and behavioral patterns related to withholding judgment of others so that I can deeply observe them and learn why others act as they do. I have no idea where it all began. This has allowed me to be around people who are vastly different from myself. Instead of being upset that the world doesn't match my criteria (mental list of what should be), I have been able to learn great lessons from those whom I could have simply cut off and erased from my memory. I've noticed that when my first impulse is to judge others, I fit them into a preconceived mold or box that I mentally carry around with me. If we consistently do this, we really don't see what is there. Rather, we only see what we expect to be there. Try this out for yourself. There is an amazing world out there and within us if we can learn to observe with detachment.

Observe yourself and your reactions when you have significant judgments about others. What goes on inside of you? If you learn to observe yourself in this manner, you will learn to see others in a way that can amaze you. We carry around with us mental frameworks that can serve us very well. It is also the case that some of these frameworks prevent a fuller comprehension of the meaning of evolving circumstances, if we cling to them or automatically revert to them. Flexibility and adaptability are two vitally needed skills in our rapidly changing world. (*See* "Remembering, Anticipating, or Just Being Creative?")

Extensions

Recently, while I was stopped at a red light, the person in the car next to me suddenly threw open the door and began leaning out. When you train yourself to observe deeply, you are aware of so much that is occurring around you. I didn't get concerned, but I did keep my eye on what was developing next to me. Mental frameworks from the past serve us well when they provide us with an array (range) of possible scenarios. Frameworks from the past are only a burden if we stay stuck in one and won't let go of it (or if we don't admit in new possibilities and interpretations). This blinds and binds us. As it turned out, all the person was doing was spitting on the street. Being mindful of a vast array of mental frameworks means that we can be flexible, adaptable, and creative without prejudging circumstances. The unique and sometimes unexpected fusion of insights from these diverse frameworks can empower us to leap beyond the known and familiar. What kind of rapidly developing circumstances have you experienced in which a rich variety of interpretive frameworks were useful? Who knows, maybe they really aren't marking territory, but they are demonstrating an adaptive behavior that reflects demands and challenges in their environment. Maybe it's genetic in origin.

OCTAVE OF NOTES

There are eight notes in an octave along with the combinations of flats and sharps. Are these all the possible notes? Are there other possible notes for the piano? Hint: what can one do to the piano to create notes that sound differently? One standard way of looking at the issue is to image our possibilities only within the range of striking the keys. If we change our image and basic assumptions, other notes come flowing right out of that old box. What happens if we retune the strings? Then how many notes are possible from the piano?

Extensions

There are many different kinds of scales. Find out what they are. What do they sound like? What kinds of instruments can play these scales? What is the definition of a scale? Scales are a particular nomenclature and taxonomy. Are there alternative means of frameworks that can be used to describe the range of musical sounds?

ONE DAY'S COURSE

In the course of one day, we experience many different feelings. Sometimes we are not consciously aware that we are experiencing these feelings. Sometimes we know we are experiencing some deep feelings, but we can't name them. Slow down enough to be able to be aware of your feelings. One useful tool is to name or write down the feelings experienced in the course of a single day. As you write, you do not need to understand everything. Record your feelings and your ideas associated with these ideas. When you go back and read this material, patterns and new understandings may arise for you.

Extensions

It is possible to be aware of what we are thinking, feeling, sensing, imagining, and doing in every moment. Explore the innate (inborn) trait (skill) that allows us to monitor (observe) what we are up to in the present moment. This is one of the greatest gifts in life. Some call this gift self-awareness. Becoming mindful of this gift is a true beginning point to wisdom and creativity.

ONLY ME

In a group, have you ever been the only one of your gender, race, religion, sexual orientation, ethnic identity, or nationality? How did it feel? Did you act any differently? Do these experiences cause you to learn anything about your assumptions of others?

Extensions

How do you think others feel in a group when they are the only one of their gender, race, religion, sexual orientation, ethnic identity, or nationality? Can we all be more aware and sensitive as to what it is like for others to be in a minority? Do we tend to associate with others who are like us? Why? Is this a way to reinforce our assumptions of what is normal, regular, and good? Can we benefit from diversity?

I recall my first day in college. I was dropped off at my dorm in a city far from where I was raised. I was going to go to what was called "freshmen camp." I thought about the fact that I did not know a single person on the entire campus. As I reflected back on the experience, I realized that I had presumed that most people would know other people. Within a few minutes of joining the large group assembled to go on the retreat, I realized that almost everybody was trying to meet new friends because most people didn't know the others. It was a perfect situation! I noticed the tendency that larger groups tend to break into smaller groups of people who hold some kind of affinity (identification that makes us feel comfortable).

Imagine what the world would be like if our curiosity and love of learning were a persistent counterbalance to our impulse for security and comfort. Imagine groups in which people deliberately made efforts to relate to others who, in some ways, are significantly different. Imagine the impact if we naturally felt refreshed in the presence of diverse people. Lifelong learning would certainly be enhanced. How does the culture reinforce what we call natural responses? In what ways can these cultural reinforcements of our individual and group responses be changed? For instance, if it is a common practice to boo at another team and shout mean things at them, what are ways that a community can alter its culturally reinforced behaviors? If someone of another race is having challenges settling into your neighborhood because of feelings of isolation and racism, what can you and the community do about this challenge?

OUR BIASES MAKE US BLIND

Scientists have discovered that human life emerged from Africa. How could any person not believe that Black is beautiful? (This comes from a person who is Swedish, French, and German).

Why do so many human beings persist in using race as a means to put other people down? Do you know what was the biggest mass slaughter of human beings by other human beings? It happened to the Africans as they were being sold into slavery. Learn as much as you can about this horrendous (terrible) piece of human history. What are other mass slaughters that have occurred in history? How can groups of people allow themselves to participate in such kinds of behavior? One of the current pieces of history that is a silent tragedy is what is happening to millions of baby girls in China and India. This is a complex issue. Look into the mystery of the missing baby girls. Why would boys be more valued by some people in some cultures? Join some discussion groups to talk about the effects of *sexism*. Is there such a thing as a cultural bias that is so pervasive (commonplace) that many people fail to see it at play in their lives?

Extensions

Is race a useful way to divide the human community? Why or why not? Who benefits from gender-based inequality? What happens to people when they start to raise issues related to cultural biases that many people do not want examined and questioned? What happens if nobody raises the issues because they are unwilling to assume the risks of backlash? If a community remains silent in the face of violence, it loses its soul (in a limited sense, soul is a metaphor for our human capacity to be creative, compassionate, responsive, and responsible). Is there a way to raise certain issues with a group of like-minded persons in such a manner that you personally do not have to lose all your security relative to that community? This silence is a terrible experience that inflicts untold and immeasurable unnecessary suffering. There are organizations that take great pride in their self-images as groups that deal with injustices and unnecessary suffering while remaining completely silent in the face of tremendous pervasive and ongoing violence occurring at the heart of their organizations. Is there such a thing as questioning the use of power, or confronting the violent and violating behaviors, the effects of prejudice, and the benefits of a more inclusive way of living without incurring wrath and anger from others who are being challenged by the very nature of the question? Can a loving presence be the example of the benefits of an inclusive way of living? When you challenge core cultural biases, personal behaviors, and group behavioral patterns, be wise in your ways. Continue to learn about how people act and react during times of transition.

OUR OWN SPACE

What is your favorite space? Is it your bedroom? It might be in a loft or cove. Is it some special place out in a park? What do you feel like when you are in this place?

Extensions

What happens to people when they don't have any place to call their own or a place with which they identify?

OUR PERFECT CHILD

Find out all you can about cloning. We often think of cloning as taking a special cell from one's own body and then deriving a perfect image of ourselves asexually. With the confluence (joining) of our knowledge of the human genome (genetic material), proteome (protein material and processes), biotechnology, and nanotechnology, our capacity to alter our biological future will grow tremendously.

The DNA from an ovum is removed. DNA from a somatic cell of any human (including the donar of the ovum) is inserted. There is also embryo cloning in which a single or multiple fertilized eggs could be cloned in the mother's womb, or implanted in a surrogate (replacement) mother's womb. Which traits do you think would be at the top of the list to eliminate or select? Is this use of technology inevitable (certain to occur)? Is it right? What might be some of the positive advantages of such a system? What are some of the disadvantages? Who would tend to benefit? Would all people be able to participate? What would this power of choosing a future life do to us? Beyond a concern for ourselves, how could this behavior affect evolution?

Extensions

Could there be the possibility of taking some human characteristics from another animal's genetic structure and input (insert) it into the human genome? Could we get better hearing and a wider range of colors? Which colors? Which characteristics might be preferable? Might we be able to insert plant-based genetic information into our human genome? Can you imagine humans synthesizing energy from the sun directly through the skin via photosynthesis? It may be impossible given our technology at the current time, but such ideas will be seriously considered by researchers who someday might be able to take some unexpected traits from animals or plants and get them successfully inserted into the human genome. Already there are successful examples of utilizing genetic information in transplants across the division between the plant and animal kingdoms. Always watch out for the word "impossible."

What would it mean to have a qualified acceptance of cloning? What would it mean to have a qualified resistance to cloning? Can it ever be stopped once we have created the technological means to use the knowledge? Look up the historical group called the Luddites. They resisted new forms of technology. Then there have been religious groups that have been against all sex. When it came to the propagation (continuance) of the faith and the community, they ran into some difficulties. None of them are around today. Which will be the groups and who will be the persons who contribute to our ethical understanding of how to use this cloning technology? It is here today. It will develop in new and unexpected ways. It will not go away. Would you like to turn your back on the developments and let others decide? Major decisions need to be made that will affect all our futures. It is a major responsibility.

OUTLASTING OTHERS

Certain things outlast other things. You will probably live longer than your pet. Name some animals that outlive most human beings. Some persons claim that certain communities have significant numbers of people living past 120 years of age. Is this accurate? Who are they? If it is accurate, what is different about these people? If you were the only friend and loved one to live to be 130 years old, would you want to do so? Find out the length of life expectancy for smokers and nonsmokers, children born into poverty and those born into financially secure families, or the relative expected life spans of men and women.

Extensions

This is a complex subject. Do not try to picture it all at once, but just read it through and get a feeling for it. Get a very general picture in your mind of what is happening. Get a sense of the patterns that are arising within the mass of details. Reread it and then start to develop a series of mental pictures that relate to each other. The art of picturing complex things can be of real use to you in many ways. You may want to draw actual pictures of what you sense are the patterns at play in the story.

Compare your likely life span to other things in your environment: How long will a tall office building be there? How long will a young tree be alive? The house you live in—how long will it be standing? How long will mountains last? If you are the Olympic gold medalist in a particular sport, how long will it be until somebody else emerges as being faster and better than you are? How long will this continent upon which you are standing be in its exact position? Will your house be standing for a longer period of time than the continent will be in its current location?

Think about a wooden house with a granite floor in one room. Which is going to last longer, the house or the floor? Compare the longevity (how long it will last) of a granite floor in an office building versus the steel that forms the building's frame. If the building is not ripped down by human beings over the course of time, what will degrade (fall apart) first in that same office building? Every bridge, office building, museum—every human-made structure—has an expected lifetime (given proper maintenance). Let's switch around a few variables. With any of these human-made structures, its life expectancy is based on continued maintenance and on the continuing presence of human beings.

Pretend all the human beings on the face of the Earth were to disappear all at once; then what would happen to that building over the course of time? Pretend that it is nighttime and the middle of a hot summer. The air conditioning is running. The lights are on. The computers are running, and these same computers are connected to the Internet, with many connections active and exchanging data. Some of these programs run projects inside the building. There are a massive number of gardens and water ponds. The water ponds contain many kinds of life. The gardens have many specimens (examples) of every kind of plant on the face of the Earth. There are secure rooms that are temperature-controlled so that the microorganisms that are being studied can continue to survive (some are hot and some are very cold—so that certain organisms can be held in suspended animation in a frozen state).

In some areas of the building, many lasers are pointed at one single point, holding a plasma reaction so that it can be held constantly heated to millions of degrees and held in perfect place by the force of lasers combined with magnetic fields. On the rooftop are solar collectors that are governed by computers (whether the covers for the solar collectors are open or closed).

Many of the rooms contain isolated populations of mammals, amphibians, reptiles, insects, and microorganisms of all kinds and birds of all kinds. In one room, there are many pieces of fractured amber that all have ancient remnants of mosquitoes that all have the genetic material of unknown animals in their digestive tract from the past. Different sets of genetic matter of all living beings are held in little dishes that are connected by little tubes. Little gateways keep the tubes closed. If the electricity is cut off, the gateways automatically open and all the kinds of genetic matter mix in different pools, in different ratios, at different temperatures, in different kinds of liquids.

All the windows of the building are hermetically sealed (airtight). They can only be opened if a sequence of codes is entered into a computer in the main office. Fresh air is circulated into the building by equipment run by the solar panels supplying electricity to the entire building. The interior doors to all individual rooms will automatically open if the electricity is cut off. All the unbreakable glass doors leading to the outside of the building are computer commanded to close and lock automatically if the electricity is cut off (the closing process would be governed by back-up batteries). These outside doors are hermetically sealed.

In the building is a population of primates that have recently experienced punctuated equilibrium (accelerated evolution). Their neocortices (neocortex is the top part of the human brain with resources for rational thought) are expanding rapidly with each generation. Their intelligence levels are rising rapidly. Only the left sides of their brains are developing. The porpoises, dolphins, and whales in the great number of interconnected tanks have experienced the same punctuated equilibrium. Their right sides of their brains are developing rapidly. The primates and the water mammals learn how to communicate with each other via musical sounds. Both the advancing primates and the advancing water mammals lack a deeper sensitivity to feeling connected to other life-forms.

All the plants in the building start to interact in one unified field of electromagnetic energy that carries information between plants. Once this occurs, the plants discover a self-awareness that emerges because of a field of life energy that is greater than mere electromagnetic energy. This self-awareness allows all the plants to feel connected and play together. Some of their play is to survive together. The plants learn that they can communicate this sense of unified life (being connected) to all the other animals that do not have a greatly developed neocortex. Both the underwater and the land-based plants begin to learn that they can help produce fresh air in abundance for everybody.

Certain of the insects begin to develop a capacity to share music with each other that communicates information. This music is also playful for them. Only some of the insects are able to determine which is playful and which music contains information necessary for survival. Some of the insects learn how to communicate with the music shared by the primates and porpoises, dolphins, and whales. Some of the plants listen to this music and imagine it to be useful and playful in the same way. Some insects are quite sensitive to the ecological balance of the place. They grow in their understanding of how to communicate this importance to the animals with developing neocortices. Some of these animals have grown to mistrust insects. One group of laughing hyenas learns how to listen to this music and alter it to confuse all other listeners. The laughing hyenas think this is really funny. Only the clams can keep the field of music from being confused by the humor of the hyenas. The clams can communicate to the whales only once every three years. Whales tend not to believe clams.

Some of the oysters learn how computers work. Oysters communicate regularly with some of the more responsible hyenas. The oysters stew (ruminate, grumble) over the fact that hyenas take so long to learn about computers. The oysters are still learning how to discern which of the hyenas are more trustworthy. The oysters finally discover that the real problem is not trustworthiness at all. The real problem is in the way some of the hyenas use their gifts. The ones who turn out to be the best learners and most consistent in behaviors that are good for everybody are those who evolve in their use of intelligence, imagination, and creativity. It took the oysters a while to figure this out. It turns out that certain hyenas are able to leap beyond many of their prime assumptions. The oysters are able to teach some of the hyenas the creative processes of reversing the flow of a set of assumptions, inverting some of the prime assumptions, enlarging the picture of the problem, extending logic beyond the current context, and applying a different kind of logic to any given issue. Only some of the hyenas that turned out to be trustworthy were able to comprehend what the oysters were teaching. The few who did understand this art became prime sources for communication across the lines of the species. They continued to laugh, but in a deeper way.

Gamma rays from outer space hit certain strains of microorganisms. They gained the capacity to metabolize (digest or eat) food sources that were not primarily organic (based on carbon, oxygen, hydrogen, and nitrogen). Some of these new food sources were based on compounds (combinations of chemicals) made out of iron, nickel, aluminum, zinc, copper, and silicon. These microorganisms began to get hungry. The metal and glass in the building became a food source for them.

What would happen to all the contents of the building over time, and what would happen to the building itself over time if all the human beings on the face of the Earth were to disappear instantly, all at once? Nothing else in the Earth's ecology is altered except that the humans are inexplicably and instantaneously gone. The building is not located in a flood plain. No earthquakes have ever hit this area. Create a time line and describe what you think would happen. Create a picture of the complex environment. Do you know how to web complex phenomena? Start with a circle of something. Then create circles of all the other things. Draw connections to the other circles and write the relationship between the two circles on the lines. Picture the whole process in your mind. Get a feeling for the process. Try to determine the primary dynamics at play. What are the secondary dynamics? Try to envision the process of what occurs within and to the building over the course of one day, one week, one year, ten years, a hundred years, and a thousand years. When the time frame (period) is long enough, the question of what happens inside and to the building becomes irrelevant. Why? Alter the framework of the story. Once the building becomes a totally open system, how would these creatures affect the environment?

If the humans were to disappear, what would your town look like one week later, one year later, one hundred years later, or one thousand years later? Which of our human artifacts (things that humans have made) would degenerate or disintegrate first? Which would last longer, and which would be the longest lasting artifacts? What would be the effect on the ecology of the planet? What species of animals has been most insensitive to the needs of the Earth's ecology?

Now imagine that human beings do not disappear but continue to grow in population at the rate that we are growing today. How long could we all last? Now try to picture how humans could become benign partners sharing the gift of life with all others in an ecologically sensitive, wise, and sound way. What would have to occur and how would we need to change in order for this radical transformation to actually happen?

OWNERSHIP

Are there certain things (such as intellectual property) that are so vital to the future of the entire human race that ownership of the rights to these things ought to be in the public trust (owned by us all for the benefit of us all)? Would the human genetic code be a candidate? What might be some examples you can come up with?

Extensions

What about the rights of individuals and groups who have put a lot of effort and resources into the discovery of such information? Is there a better way to mediate (take care of, balance) this tension between the rights of the whole human family and the rights of individuals and groups?

PARENTS

We all carry with us certain images of our parents. What are the many images and biases you have about your parents? Be really honest with yourself. Now try to imagine them as human beings who have (or had) many hurts, pains, broken and fulfilled dreams, hopes, and great love for you. When seen in this manner, can you relate to them differently?

Extensions

If you were going to surprise your parents, your children, or other persons for whom you have great concern with a totally unexpected act of compassion, what would it be? Would it be a one-time thing, or could you change the way you relate to them?

Many offspring infrequently or never experienced the love of one or both of their parents. That is neglect. Many others have suffered abuse from one or both of their parents (or other adults who were in a position of power or authority relative to the child). Since children can be extremely vulnerable, how is the wider community responsible for the well-being of vulnerable children in homes in which neglect and abuse are present? How is it possible for these children to find caring adults who will care for them? This is a most complex and challenging question. We desperately need to find some answers. Talk to others about these issues. Write a paper, read a report, get a book, or start a discussion group on the topic. Whatever we do for the good of life will be felt by some victim somewhere. Victims have a great need to know that some persons of conscience care for them. If a victim can have the minimal knowledge that somebody cares for her or him and is actively working with regard for the victim's well-being, this minimal piece of knowledge can make all the difference in the world. This caring provides the critical hope that can result in the tenacity, resilience, and courage to continue believing in the goodness of life and in one's capacity to persevere. Effective caring has a voice that is heard, and it is an action that often requires some risk. Too often, silence and the flight to a safe and secure place apart from the suffering of others comprise the well-practiced pattern. Then, countless people suffer silently in an isolated manner. This is a real loss of human potential, and it is completely unnecessary! Caring makes the difference for some people between hope and hopelessness. Some little thing you do may have significant life-altering consequences.

PATHETIC AND TRAGIC

There is a world of difference between a pathetic behavior and a situation in which something tragic occurs to a person. When something tragic happens, there is significant pain, suffering, loss, grief, and undesired change in one's life. To be pathetic means that a person is:

- not able to learn from the past
- not willing to let go of the past but actually lives in the past
- not willing to embrace his or her tragedies and then move on in life
- continuing to identify with some trauma or drama from the past as a means of avoiding responsibility for growth and engaging life in the present
- continually presenting him- or herself as a helpless victim who must be rescued by others consistently
- filled with so much fear of something that he or she fails to take risks in life
- unwilling to take any kind of stand on any issue
- unable to find the courage to define the most essential aspects of his or her self-identity
- unable to set boundaries between him- or herself and the demands of situations and other people

These are all learned behaviors and responses to the stresses and challenges of being alive. If they are learned, they can be unlearned.

Tragedies occur. None of us can avoid them. What we fashion and create is our greatest opportunity and contribution. To find the nerve to pursue goals, set limits, have principles, take any risks, or to engage the future are examples of us practicing fidelity (honesty of a most basic kind) to life. Tragedies do not force us to lose our capacity to be fully alive. Pathetic behaviors always prevent us from being fully alive and responsible for ourselves. What is the attraction of pathetic behaviors? Is there ever any good that comes out of tragedy? Do those who suffer tragedy deserve pity? Look up the relation between pity and something that is pathetic. What is the best response to those who have suffered tragedies? It certainly isn't pity.

Extensions

Look up *pathos* and *bathos*. What are the differences?

PENCILS: CORE

How do they get the lead into pencils?

Extensions

Think of other common objects we all use and ask how the object is made. Rubik's cubes—how do they work and how are they made? Think of others.

Find the answers. Have you ever tried to disassemble something that has no obvious place to begin the disassembly process?

PENINSULAS

Name the two states in the United States that are peninsulas. Alaska has a huge peninsula but the entire state is not basically a peninsula. Hint: one is near saltwater and the other is near freshwater. Are there other major peninsulas in the United States?

Extensions

There are many examples of certain words that most people assume mean one set thing, so they look for what is commonly expected. We assume that all rubber balls bounce. What would happen if we dropped a supercooled rubber ball onto a cement floor? Watch out when you want to respond to some challenge with an automatic answer that "everybody knows is right." Be the one who senses things that others miss. These anomalies (exceptions) can lead to vastly new insights.

PICTURES OF ATOMS

Certain microscopes can take pictures of very small objects. Some of the microscopes can create images of things as small as atoms. Look up some of these pictures. To see atoms! This is a stupendous gift. In these pictures, things appear to be bumps with fuzzy material around them. The fuzzy areas of the photographs are the electrons racing around the nucleus of the atoms.

Someday, might we be able to take pictures fast enough that we can actually get images of atoms with the electrons frozen in place? Investigate how these pictures of atoms are taken. What are the limitations? Are we able to create absolute-zero environments (no atomic motion)? Does this freeze the electrons—why or why not? If absolute zero is the temperature at which atoms do not move, might this still allow for the motion of electrons? If so, might there be a temperature colder than absolute zero? Be careful about the language being used. Thermal energy is directly related to atomic motion. Not all motion is directly related to thermal energy (there are moving particles in existence that are subatomic that are not affected by the thermal energy of atoms).

Extensions

Will we be able to get pictures of quarks someday? Is this impossible? Is it impossible given our present technology? Is it impossible given our present understanding of physics?

PLAYGROUND QUESTIONS

There are many things you talk about with certain groups and not in other groups. Given specific situations and groups of persons, what is it you feel comfortable talking about, and what is it you do not feel comfortable talking about?

Extensions

A degree of risk taking in life is necessary. Too much risk taking can put us in harm's way. What are the signals from other persons and groups that it is safe to open up and share ourselves? What are the signals that convey (communicate) to us that we need to be safeguarded around certain people and certain groups?

PLAYING WITH TIME

Some persons are usually late for engagements. Why are some persons persistently behind in their schedules? Does it really help to set your clock ten minutes or fifteen minutes ahead? What would be the effect of this game?

Extensions

Are all cultures like our dominant culture in terms of schedules, being punctual (starting on time), packing so many things into the course of one day, and what we expect of ourselves everyday in terms of being busy and productive? Is being busy the same thing as being productive? What are we missing in life by being so busy?

POLES OF THE EARTH—ALL FOUR

The Earth has two geographic poles (the North and South Poles) and two magnetic poles, one in the north and one in the south. Locate the northern magnetic pole and determine its distance from the North Pole. Next, can you locate the southern magnetic pole? How far is it from the South Pole?

What do you suppose would be the effect on a compass of being near the magnetic poles? Does your compass point in the direction of the magnetic poles or the geographic poles? Does this cause navigational problems? How do maps correct for this challenge? If you were directly at one of the magnetic poles, how would your compass act?

Extensions

Do the magnetic poles change their locations, or are they static and permanent? Are the geographic poles set forever in one place?

POPCORN'S MAGIC

Popcorn is a very old treat. Who do you think discovered it? How widespread was its use when European Americans discovered the continent? If popcorn was so widespread at the time of the discovery of the continent, how could the continent be discovered? Most of the corn used for popcorn is grown in one country; which one do you think it is? What is it inside the corn kernel that causes it to explode? When it explodes, why doesn't it just shatter into many little pieces? How many times the original size of the kernel is the final popped piece of popcorn? If you were in outer space and you managed to pop some popcorn in a pot suspended in outer space, what do you think the popcorn would look like? If you made a whole lot of this space popcorn and then dumped it out of your space vehicle, what do you suppose it would look like on radar screens back on Earth? How do you think they would interpret what they see on screen? Next time you're there in space, try it.

Extensions

What are some other materials that contain something inside that causes them to explode and take on unusual shapes (and not just explode into fragments)?

PRECESSION OF ELLIPTICAL ORBITS

The orbits of planets are not exactly stationary (set in the exact shape over time), nor are these orbits perfectly elliptical (a perfectly elongated circle). Precession means that the entire elliptical orbit rotates (precesses) very slowly in space due to the sum of the gravitational pulls of all the planets and sun. There is one rotation every 225,000 years. How can we know such things? When the period of the cycle is so long (225,000 years), how can we determine that this pattern exists?

Extensions

What are other patterns that have very long periods?

PREHISTORY

When we think about yesterday, we can accurately remember most of the major events in order. When we try to think about history that goes beyond our personal memory, it ceases to be personal history. When we try to read about history that goes beyond written history, we must go beyond the immediate evidence and make assumptions. Our judgments or assumptions are then said to be inferences; we infer from some evidence that some other process or phenomena occurred.

We have all read about the supercontinent from which the other continents emerged (Pangea was formed about 260 million years ago). Before Pangea, there were two supercontinents (Laurasia, which included North America, Australia, Antarctica, and India; and Gondwanaland, which included South America and Africa).

Now there is some evidence that some scientists say allows us to make further statements about the prehistory of continents. Apparently, there may have been a supercontinent some people call Rodinia that may have existed about 750 million years ago. Then all the continents drifted apart and regrouped into the two supercontinents of Laurasia and Gondwanaland about 422 million years ago.

Is there any evidence anywhere of supercontinents before Rodinia? Some scientists are beginning to theorize that the separation and joining together of continents goes on a cycle of about 400 to 500 million years. This raises the issue of where are we heading in the future. Is there any way to predict this future pattern of supercontinents from the present knowledge of the flow (vectors) of the various tectonic plates? Look up an article on this topic and have some fun in prehistory. Look up the vector lines (lines of force) of the present-day continents. Now draw a picture of what you think the continents will look like millions of years from now.

Extensions

What are some other areas in prehistory that would interest you? How do we infer from present information? What is the role of hunches and intuition?

Related topics: Is there a way to predict the future? Can we use the past to help us predict the future? Can we infer from present data or information likely or probable patterns for the future? Test this out on various processes (like pollution). Some people think they can predict the future of the stock market and get rich. What kind of predicting accuracy do our best mathematical models give us for various kinds of phenomena?

PREJUDICE AND BIAS

What is the difference (if any) between prejudice and bias? Bias means that we lean toward interpreting things in a certain manner. We learn to have certain biases from the earliest moments of our lives. As a very young child, we learn to develop feelings about whether the world is a friendly, loving, caring place or not. We learn to express ourselves in certain ways. We learn to view ourselves in a certain way.

Biases are tools we use to interpret the world. They are tendencies that seem so natural to us. It is not unusual to have biases. What is of importance is the degree to which we are aware of our biases. If we are not aware of our biases at all, this causes us to feel and think that our way of looking at life and the world is the only natural, intelligent, informed, good way to look at things. If we are unaware of our biases, we also can develop strong negative feelings and firm ideas about alternative views, cultures, and values that cause us to look down upon others who, in some ways, are significantly different from us.

Prejudice is a severe and extreme kind of bias. It is based on a fear of life and other people. Fear causes anxiety. Anxiety causes people to look for simplistic explanations of things. What is the difference between some explanation that is simple and one that is simplistic? When we are prejudiced, we are not willing to consider the life experiences of others or other alternative possible explanations for how life and the universe work. An indication of a prejudice is that we become upset, angry, defensive, hostile, hurt, or threatened by others who are different from us.

Not everything in life is good and supportive of life. Not all ideas are life-honoring or useful. What is of greatest value is what is good and supports life. This is a bias. We all need to develop our capacity for wise judgments about ourselves, other people, and the many challenges of life. These wise judgments reflect a certain set of values. This is necessary and good. Name a bias you hold. Is it healthful and fair? Might you have some prejudices?

Extensions

Are there any prejudices that are good and fair? Are there any that aren't good or fair but necessary? Why or why not?

PROMISE KEEPING

Are there limits to the belief that we should always keep a promise? Are there ever circumstances under which you'd feel obligated to break a former promise? For instance, what happens if the promise turns out later to be actually hurting somebody?

Extension:

Is there such a thing as circumstances so complex that you can't keep the promise exactly as stated, but you can carry on with the spirit or intent of the promise (as best as you are able to determine)?

QUESTIONS—ANSWERING

When somebody presents a question to you, it is framed in a certain way. The manner of this framing of the question often reflects cultural, scientific, historical, gender, religious, racial, or personal biases. Questions always reflect certain views and perspectives. They carry with them certain assumptions about how the world works, what is natural, and what is assumed real and important. The question may be deliberately phrased to be a trick question. The question may not reflect biases so much as limited understanding of a given topic.

When somebody asks you a question, must you answer it in the manner in which it is asked? Can you use your imagination and experience with creative leaps (genius sneaking out) to rephrase the question in a manner that broadens the context, enriches the depth, or makes it more useful? Can you rephrase it so that your response reflects a more valid view of the widest context in which the question emerges? For instance, if you were to touch a firefly when it is lit up, would it be warm or hot? The question about the firefly plays on the bias (assumptions based on experience of individuals and groups) of us expecting to have heat associated with luminescence (emitting light), such as occurs in fires or lightbulbs. Could there be such a thing as something that emits light but feels freezing cold?

Extensions

Many people are in the habit of answering another person's questions immediately. Some people feel that if someone doesn't answer quickly, they may not be quick-witted (intelligent). Is it OK for you to actually think about an answer before giving your response? It is extremely rare to observe others actually taking time to think through a response to a question. It is a joy to me to see this when it occurs.

For instance, it used to be thought that boys and men were more gifted in math than were girls and women. Then it was discovered that there was a cultural bias at play in the classroom. Teachers (male and female) had fallen into the behavior of responding quickly to those who would answer their questions quickly and assertively (trying to get the teacher's attention quickly or first). It turns out that it is more often that boys and men react this way in class situations. They are rewarded by teachers saying, "Yes, that is the answer, very good!" Then it was also discovered that girls and women could do just as well at math as boys and men, but girls and women more often like to process their answers before a quick response. It was also discovered that many girls and women like to cooperatively derive answers in group processes rather than as isolated competitive individuals. They do not, as a group, have the tendency to shoot their hands up as soon as they think they may have an answer. If these group differences are recognized and adjustments are made in the educational settings, then the math scores of girls and women are just as high as those of boys and men.

QUICK CARRYOUT RESTAURANTS

We have so many quick carryout restaurants available to us. Can you name twenty of them? Why are they so popular? Is the food served in these places the kind of stuff you like? Rate the quick carryout restaurants. What are your criteria (means of judging) for rating quick serve or quick carryout restaurants? What does "quality quick carryout food" mean to you? (Look up the word *oxymoron* sometime.) Can the word *quality* mean different things to a variety of persons? I still wait for the day when I can eat some food at a restaurant alongside a highway that tastes great (as though somebody put some personal attention and care into the preparation of the food).

Extensions

When did these kinds of quick serve and quick carryout restaurants become popular? Before they became popular, were there relatively unknown quick carryout restaurants? I recall as a child in New York City being at a restaurant that had all the food prepared in advance. Each dish was held behind a little glass door. You could pick whatever you wanted to eat and it was instantly available.

RADIO WAVES

How did anybody in the past even think that radio waves could carry information through the air? Did anybody think that information could be carried through the air before the discovery of the radio? Once the discovery was made it became obvious, but how did somebody come up with such an original idea? Was it really original?

Extensions

The role of genius is not just being highly intelligent. The role of genius has to do with being able to leap beyond what is given in the body of knowledge available at any one time. Also, genius has to do with uncovering what is there in the knowledge base that others do not see. Genius also has to do with being able to transmute and convert existing pieces of knowledge and insight into other forms that have relevance in new contexts. This new understanding can be used for new ends.

Identify several persons you consider to be geniuses. Why do you think they are geniuses? What do they all hold in common? Are there patterns at play that you can uncover? Do geniuses invent everything? Are they totally original? If they are not completely original in all things, what are the things they took from the existing body of knowledge, and what did they do with this preexisting knowledge? Do you think you might be capable of genius? Don't underestimate yourself! Remember, it is important how questions are asked. It is also important to recall that we tend to hear certain kinds of questions in certain ways that match our preexisting biases. Leap beyond these biases and open your eyes to another whole world of creativity.

RAILROAD GAUGES AND OUR LIFE ASSUMPTIONS

The U.S. standard railroad gauge is 4 feet, 8.5 inches. That's an exceedingly odd number. Why was that gauge used? Because that's the way they built them in England. People with training in England helped the English build the U.S. railroads.

Why did the English people build them like that? Because the first rail lines were built by the same people who built the prerailroad tramways, and that's the gauge they used. Why did "they" use that gauge then? Because the people who built the tramways used the same jigs and tools that they used for building wagons, which used that wheel spacing. Why did the wagons use that odd wheel spacing? Well, if they tried to use any other spacing, the wagons would break on some of the old, long-distance roads, because that's the spacing of the old wheel ruts. So who built these old rutted roads? Imperial Rome, for the benefit of their legions, built the first long-distance roads in Europe. The roads have been used ever since. And the ruts? Roman war chariots first made the initial ruts, which everyone else had to match for fear of destroying their wagons. Since the chariots were made for or by Imperial Rome, they were alike in the matter of wheel spacing. (This material is from an e-mail [computer network message] with unknown original authorship. Many of us receive many e-mail lists of quirky unusual things. This was by far the most insightful and original. It's the only one I've used in the book. Who has time to write and who has time to read all these lengthy stories that somebody keeps cranking out? Might they all be from one person?)

We all get into ruts. We have ways of channeling our lives on a daily basis. We come to assume the natural necessity of so many of our well-practiced patterns. This deeply affects all senses of who we are and who others are. We are, in fact, composing our lives persistently. In the act of composing our own lives, we are greatly affecting what is possible for us in the life of the wider community as well.

How we measure our lives and the lives of others is of utmost importance. There are certain ruts that become so commonplace that few persons question why they seem to be so necessary. No matter how odd or peculiar some of these ruts may be, they persist because they are interpreted as being deep necessities. What are some ruts in your life? What are some ruts in your circle of friends, community, or culture? Does it make us feel secure and safe if we are preoccupied with and absorbed in the mundane and given routines of life?

Extensions

Different vehicles have different sizes of tires and wheels. What is the advantage of smaller tires? What are the advantages of larger tires (we are speaking of diameter)? Tractors out in the farm fields have huge tires. Why? Some cars have very small tires (small diameter). See what you can find. Is there any advantage to tires that are wide versus the tires that are narrower (distance across the tread)? Is there any advantage or disadvantage to tires that have a narrow distance between the wheel rim and the edge of the tire tread? Why do round tires come in so many different shapes?

RAIN AND SALT

Many of the clouds that dump rain on us formed over the oceans by absorbing huge quantities of water. The oceans are composed of saltwater. Ever wonder why the rain isn't salty?

Extensions

How much could clouds really suck up into the air? Do clouds really "suck up" anything? Might some clouds actually create forces that pull things off the ground or out of the water? There are stories about frozen fish falling from the sky. Do you believe any of these kinds of stories? A waterspout is a tornado over the water. Is a tornado a special kind of cloud? Could this special kind of cloud really suck up an entire house and drop it in some far-off land?

RAINDROPS

Raindrops are interesting things. Take a careful look at them. Study them. You may see more than you expect.

Are they transparent? If a drop of water allows all light to pass through, might it be possible to imagine an invisible raindrop? In order to see that it is a raindrop, you need to see its borders or you need to see that its presence affects how light is reaching your eye. Look into a raindrop (one that may be dangling from a tip of branch). Try to see through it to the other side. Are images distorted? Is light refracted (separated into separate colors)?

If you are observing a raindrop and you are concentrating on its inner portions to avoid its outer edges, for a moment, you may be able to concentrate on seeing only the inner region of the raindrop. This is far easier if the raindrop is about three feet across. If you look only at the exact center point where light is not bent, could you experience it as a raindrop and see it as being invisible at the same time? Is it possible to hold two different things in your attention, beholding them as one thing just for an instant? Could we view a beautiful sunset and be concentrated on the fact that Earth is spinning around the sun at the same instant that we are simply enjoying the appearance of the sun moving around our fixed position?

What we can't do is have two contradictory primary reference frameworks of the same thing at once. We can have two (or more) contradictory primary frameworks of the same process, person, thing, or relationship, but what occurs is that we flip-flop back and forth between them. This happens all the time in our lives. One common example is ambivalence. We flip-flop because we don't want to make a choice (for many reasons).

One way that we can hold seemingly different things in conscious attention at the same time is if we discover a greater or wider comprehension of an underlying unity. When we hold at least two different perspectives in conscious view simultaneously, it is because our field of understanding is greater than the contexts for these frameworks that define them as being different. If we are struggling with a particular issue, or if we are dealing with a fundamental question of life, we must have courage, strength, and resolve to find a way to a resolution. As we remain focused on the issue or question, something happens within us that is rather mysterious. For the toughest of our issues, questions, or quests, the resolution occurs in a surprising manner. Something inherent to our deep capacities wells up. There is a sudden moment of convergence of that which had been separate and dissonant. Instead of struggle, confusion, proliferating problems, multiplying vexing riddles, and ever-deepening intellectual complexity, there suddenly is a simplicity that breaks old dividing walls of incomprehension.

When we discover an aspect of our humanity that directly experiences a breakthrough, expansion, or piercing light of comprehension, we find ourselves instantaneously in a vastly greater field of fullness. We literally see what appeared not to be present in the preceding instant. If we identify with this lucid (clear) moment, we can then be surprised with the wisdom that flows through us. One of the amazing things is that the unexpected is revealed, and it is always more encompassing than we ever could have suspected. If we are focused on a narrow issue, the "answer" may appear in an unexpected form. There has to be a leap of comprehension to grasp that an "answer" has emerged that we need to recognize. Ironically, the "answer" enlarges the initiating question, and often the original question becomes obsolete or irrelevant. The "answer" often points to yet greater questions. So, when we experience an unexpected answer to a narrowly defined question, challenge, or issue, we ourselves become enlarged. Our prior personal, social, and cultural conditioning didn't prepare us for this leap of comprehension. If we respond to such moments and learn to identify with this expanded sense of self, then we realize we can focus our attention, concentration, and reflection on more expansive and inclusive concerns. This is the mystery and secret of genius at play through our lives. As the domain of human concerns enlarges and becomes more inclusive, we may realize that this leap of comprehension is not the exception. It no longer emerges only in snatches, broken moments, dreams, and rare odd moments. As we focus on the widest and greatest of human concerns, we realize that this enlarged view of life is the foreground and norm of our lives.

The first mystery of genius has to do with some initial bursts or leaps of comprehension that allow us to directly experience these lucid moments. A deep layer of the mystery emerges when we realize the relationship between an enlarged concern and focus and a more stable centering in this way of existing. A deeper layer of the mystery emerges when we comprehend that we can remain open to the impelling force that causes this inclusive awareness to appear. We can continue to be open to its possibilities. Now this widest comprehension is becoming our stable foreground of awareness. Most of us would reject this condition as an impossibility. Therefore, we miss the next deeper mystery.

We are able to identify with what we are opening ourselves to. With us concentrating on the greatest life issues, this opening up and entrusting of ourselves become our way of living. We begin to resonate with deep currents of mysterious creativity, and we begin to associate with greatly diverse cues and clues of emergent patterns that possess an indescribably integrated fullness that is always surprising. We identify, resonate, and associate with an unfolding creative process that is greater than our mere intellect. We become identified with a process whose outcomes can never be predicted in advance. This sensitivity to the effects and consequences of our leaps of comprehension on ourselves and others emerges as a core dynamic in our lives. We discover that we are becoming increasingly responsive to the needs of others and more responsible in our thoughts, feelings, actions, and the selection of what we choose to concentrate our lives upon. This process leads us to an astounding insight.

We begin to see a pattern and a deep desire arising within us that is related to our attentiveness to what is best for all others. Something mysterious blossoms inside us that leads us into the presence of others. Our greatest concerns become focused on the most inclusive and most encompassing of all contexts. Genius is for the sake of all! The Hollywood image of a genius being a quirky weird person pursuing some narrow and often dangerous and self-centered goal is only a very limited portrayal of genius at play in our lives. The attention related to the greatest issues reveals the greatest contexts, which in turn reveal the greatest outcome—sharing and the enhancement of life itself.

If we entirely concentrate our lives on narrow and limited challenges, questions, or issues, we may experience what is called genius. When we don't continue to open ourselves to the wider implications of the outcomes of this kind of genius, we severely truncate (limit) ourselves, our growth, and our evolution of comprehension. Most important, if we fail to open ourselves to and identify with wider contexts emerging through these leaps of comprehension, we fail to experience the interconnections between the limited narrow domain of a particular leap of comprehension and the wider implications of this leap of comprehension. If we remain narrow in focus, we will remain largely oblivious to the effects and consequences of our leap of comprehension on others. We will remain oblivious to the potential within us of opening and identifying with the greatest context and comprehension related to sharing life responsibly with all others. Remaining identified with this narrow and limited vein of concerns, questions, and issues can be dangerous. We may, in fact, become ingenious at things that are highly detrimental (bad) to us and to many others.

Becoming open to these more encompassing fields of comprehension is not ordinary problem solving. There is nothing ordinary about an experience like this or living in this manner. This is the moment of genius (the fusion of all our capacities that results in an insight or comprehension of something much greater than what we had expected). We experience something occurring through us. In an ordinary sense of self, it is no longer we who are making this process happen. When we have tapped into this part of our humanity, something much greater is at play in our lives.

This wisdom allows a strange and new coupling of feeling, intuition, imagination, logic, memory, and intelligence. We are then able to be aware of many different frameworks of understanding that coexist within a wider field of comprehension. We discover the tremendous creative potential in the capacity to place our attention, concentration, and reflection in any of these frameworks. Once we have experienced and identified with this indescribable opening to the widest field that includes all other frameworks, we realize we didn't create the resolution. There is something more at play than our mere intellect, emotions, intuition, logic, and memory. This is an aspect of genius—to experience what unifies or integrates what is seen as a process while others only experience scattered, separate, and contradictory frameworks of experience.

One way to view our life journey is in terms of wisdom. The wider the field of comprehension, the greater our capacity to understand how multiple frameworks that on the surface seem to be inconsistent are actually unified in a wider field of comprehension. Find as many examples of this kind of wisdom in your life. As we learn to suspect the presence of the unexpected, we may learn to discipline our lives to be focused on a continual process of opening to something that will always be greater than our comprehension. If you are actually in the process of comprehending and realizing what is being talked about in this section, you will never look at raindrops the same way again!

Extensions

Frameworks for understanding are like windows. Windows have a border that offers a view of something we are focused on. Sometimes borders and particular views increase our wisdom and comprehension, while sometimes borders and particular views can act as filters (conscious and unconscious biases) that limit us. Certain windows warp (bend) or filter the light. Thus, the picture we are focused on is distorted. Our windows of understanding affect how we see reality (of anything). What are the filters or windows through which you see the following things?

- You are at a sports game in which you intensely want "your" team to win, but your team is losing because of bad refereeing or inept (bad) play on your team or great play on the part of the other team or bad luck. Do you see the whole game as it is actually being played? Are you seeing all the dynamics of the game "objectively"?
- Your best friend is receiving criticism from a whole group of people. Your friend is obviously emotionally hurt by the criticism. What are

your automatic impulses? What are your filters and views through which you interpret the situation?

- You are in a situation in which you are totally expecting one thing and an absolutely unexpected thing emerges or happens. For instance, when I was a little boy, I was fishing with my grandfather. Something bit my lure. When the "fish" came to the surface out of the dark waters, there, right in front of my face and close to my hand, was a creature from the depths unlike anything I had ever seen or heard of. It looked like a snake with four weird legs and feet. I was shocked. As it slithered across the surface of the water, I was horrified. My grandfather took care of the situation for me. He was relaxed. I was shocked. The frameworks and filters through which we observed the situation were the only differences between the two of us.
- You are in a group situation in which all the other persons are different in culture, race, religion, gender, and age. You're it. There is nobody else with your background. You're talking about how to be sensitive to each other's needs. Do you think all the people in the group would use the same examples and see things in the same way?

Our filters are pervasive (widespread) and persistent. Learn to see these filters at play. We can learn to observe our filtering, but only if we open ourselves to a larger comprehension of the significance of being aware in the current moment. It is amazing as we start to see how we are all so deeply affected by this filtering process. It is a royal opportunity to experience creativity that we've never imagined possible. There is an observing that arises that is amazing. It is a timeless, detached stillness in which we see with indescribable clarity. We've all experienced tidbits of this dynamic stillness. We can learn to identify, resonate, and associate with this direct experience free of our normal filters. In the absence of our fragmenting smallness, an astounding world of splendor and wonder bursts open within and around us. This is seeing with fresh eyes!

RAIN FORESTS

So many people are deeply concerned about the rain forests being cut down at such great rates. Find out how many acres of tropical rain forest are destroyed every day. What is impelling (driving) this deforestation (cutting down the trees)? What are the effects on the planet of this massive deforestation? Where are the rain forests of the world that are not tropical?

Extensions

Was the Asian landmass also deforested like North America? Why? What were the effects?

REALLY BASIC NEEDS

What are your basic needs in life? List as many things as you can.

Extensions

One way of doing this task is to simply randomly list any need that comes to you. You can do this entire process by yourself. It is a great means for reflection. You can also participate in a most interesting group process. An advantage to randomly listing needs is that you encourage passionate involvement in the process. Naming our core and vital needs is not a logical rational process. Needs are felt in the heart, which is our seat of passion, sensitivity, intuition, and wisdom. You might have several people doing this project independently. Afterward, the assembled group can compare the items listed. What kinds of patterns do you observe? You could do this process by imposing some logical categories in advance and then fill in the categories. This presupposes that we know in advance the ways to analyze our human situation. Don't presuppose so much. Learn to see emergent patterns in direct, fresh, spontaneous, and heartfelt responses. The entire group could sense together the patterns and natural associations and groupings. Through the group interaction, a deeper comprehension of our human situation arises. Once the entire listing is displayed, review everything with the entire group. The group could split into different groups and see what groupings they notice and sense in the random listing of human needs. Then all the group members could reassemble and compare their experience of the groupings and associations they saw and felt in the listings.

REALLY ORIGINAL

What are some examples of original thoughts or inventions? Create a list. Look at this list and see if you can see any patterns of things that preceded these original insights or inventions, or creations that made the genius, inventor, or artist able to create the idea or product.

For example, the Wright brothers with their airplane—what preceded them that helped them create the first successful powered flight at Kitty Hawk? They weren't the first ones to conceive of powered flight for humans. How old is this dream of flying? What are some examples of ancient ideas of human flight?

Extensions

Are there any original inventions? Is there anything new under the sun?

REFERENCE POINTS—PRIME

When one is examining some complex system, it is critically important to have some reference point from which one can determine the position of other elements relative to this prime point.

If you are traveling around in the United States and you wish to know where you are located, you would need to find out the distance from where you are and some known point. Every point of the country is relative to other points. We actually have many main reference points. Some examples of main reference points might be the location of a river, state border, major city, big hill, important bridge, or other well-known place.

A challenge with having a local main reference point is that you have a difficult time telling relative position and distances to points that are beyond a familiar area. One way to solve this issue is to create a grid (many equally spaced lines used for measuring distance). The challenge with this is how one grid relates to another grid. If everyone is using a different grid, the place where they intersect will not translate into terms consistent with to the other grid. Also, the scale used for one grid may be too small when you start to piece together a large number of grids. This would be like trying to measure the distance between the Earth and the moon in terms of inches. If the area you are examining is miles across, the grid will be in terms of miles. If the area being examined were light-years across, the grid lines would be measured in terms of light-years (or parsecs).

What is needed is an appropriate grid to begin with to measure the entire area. For the world, this is done with measurements of latitude and longitude. With this large-scale grid system, any position on Earth can be calculated in terms of degrees, minutes, and seconds of a particular position. Look up what degrees, minutes, and seconds are, when used in terms of longitude and latitude. (*See* "Latitude and Longitude.") If the area you are examining is that of a microscopic cell (say, a cell from a cow's liver), what kind of grid and what kind of measurement would be appropriate?

For the Earth, what is the prime reference point? In terms of longitude (east-west measurements of relative position), there is the prime meridian that runs through Greenwich, England. In terms of north-south relative positions, there are the equator and the mathematical points called the North and South Poles. These are the prime reference points from which all else is measured.

One thing you may want to figure out is how sailors and maritime folk can figure out exactly where they are located. When you are in the middle of the night in an area of a large lake or ocean that is covered with dense fog, how can somebody know exactly where he or she is located? Historically, what was used was an astrolabe; in later years, people used what is called a sextant. Find out how these instruments worked. Hint: they could only work when you saw the stars. Sailors can now tell precisely where they are located, even at night in a heavy fog. Look up navigational systems and specifically locate information on Lorenz systems and the global positioning system (GPS).

Everything we have talked about in terms of relative positions on the Earth assumes that everything is static (meaning holding steady or still). What happens if everything is moving; then how do you determine relative position?

For instance, the surface of the Earth is moving (it is dynamic and not static). This is called plate tectonics. If all the plates are moving relative to each other, how can it be determined how much any one plate is moving relative to any other particular plate? Greenwich at the prime meridian is moving not necessarily at the same rate at which other plates are moving. Nor is its plate necessarily moving in the same direction as other plates. Therefore, the prime reference point doesn't hold still relative to the position of other points on the globe.

This is very complex stuff. Therefore, what is needed is a model or picture of the process. Pretend you are a skin diver, and you are diving under the ocean. All around you are swirling currents of water and moving fish. How would you determine from your position the relative positions of the fish? The fish are moving. The water currents are moving you (the prime reference point) while you are seeking to measure distances and determine relative positions. Sometimes divers lose their sense of which way is up or down. What is needed in this picture or model is a fixed reference point that is not dynamic. Under the water you might find a fixed point like a rock or fixed plant that does not move. Pilots can experience the same problem in terms of the location of the horizontal plane parallel with the Earth's surface. In steep and rapid twists, turns, inversions, and flips, pilots can lose their orientation.

Back to plate tectonics—the limitation of this model of longitude and latitude is that when we are looking at the Earth, its moving plates mean that there are no fixed points from within the system or grid (or at least it appears this way). When entire continents move small distances in a year, it becomes even more difficult to track and measure such minuscule (small) movements given such a large scale as continents. How can it be done? To find out the answer, you must consult something written by geophysicists or go and talk to a geophysicist. They can actually be quite pleasant people.

Before you do this, use your skills at logic and reasoning to determine in advance some likely or possible answers. One possible solution might be to have a reference point outside of the system—like bouncing radio waves off one specific position on the moon and then bouncing them back to Earth. Sounds crazy? See what you can come up with.

Hint: might there be fixed points on the Earth that don't move? (*See* "Reference Points When All Things Are Moving.") Always pay attention to how a question is framed. Does the motion of the continents actually affect the relative position of the prime reference points of the equator, North Pole, and the South Pole (could this movement deform the shape of the entire planet)? What about the prime meridian? If it is defined as being a north-south line running through one geographic location that is located on a tectonic plate, don't we have more than just a little problem here? Look up what is called a uniform world geodetic system. The prime reference points are all embedded in a mathematical model that is imposed on the complex dynamic Earth. The prime reference point is an idea, not a fixed physical place. Extend this metaphor. Our primary reference point is not necessarily any obvious external thing; rather, it can be an inner sense, insight, or truth!

Extensions

Want to tackle an even bigger challenge? If all the galaxies in the universe appear to be moving away from each other at a uniform rate (look up something called Hubble's constant), how can we determine the relative position of any galaxy to other galaxies? Might the answer be to track all the galaxies back (reverse vector) to their common point of origin (assuming that there is a common point of origin)? Then you could measure the distance each galaxy is from this single point. Has this ever been done? Keep in mind that there was once that person named Einstein who taught us a thing or three about space-time. One of the implications of his theories is that the universe is expanding. Galaxies are not flying away from each other from a common point. This is not an issue of velocity as much as it is a mystery of space-time itself expanding. Talk to an astrophysicist. If you can't find a local astrophysicist, you may be able to locate a regular physicist (sometimes they look different). A best friend for researching original questions is a really astute and curious reference librarian. Treat him or her very nicely. Another possible ally in the search for unusual answers to original questions is to find a person at a college, university, or other school who is willing to help direct you to resources. Remember that some people really appreciate originality and intelligence while others are threatened or bothered by such stuff. Of course, you can always use search engines on the World Wide Web. If you really want an interesting way of solving a problem, use the method of changing your focus away from the direct problem, issue, challenge, or question, while at the same time making a deep commitment to hold a certain kind of attentiveness to this issue. This sounds impossible, but it is not absurd or unrealizable. What it requires is that we become mindful of the possibility of seeing connections, patterns, and associations we or others have not experienced before. Being mindful, in this manner, is the same thing as being committed to a continuing process of opening ourselves to more inclusive and encompassing contexts for comprehending our issues, questions, problems, challenges, issues, and concerns. (*See* "Raindrops.")

REFERENCE POINTS WHEN ALL THINGS ARE MOVING

The surface of the Earth is moving in many directions at once due to plate tectonics (and ocean, sea, lake, and river currents). What are other examples of significant movements of the Earth's surface? What are examples of fixed points on the Earth's surface? How is it that they are fixed if everything else is moving? Hint: look up Hawaii and the geysers at Yellowstone National Park.

Extensions

Where will Hawaii and Yellowstone National Park be in the future (thousands and millions of years from now—geologic time)? The question about Hawaii is an ambiguous one. There are many islands in this chain of islands. Try to determine what is moving and what is stationary within that system we call the island chain. Once you derive an answer to this question, you can know the answer to the question as to whether or not there are fixed reference points on the Earth's surface. (*See* "Reference Points—Prime.")

REGENERATING SOMETHING THAT IS LOST

Different animals that are simple in form can regenerate a part of the body that has been lost. Look up which animals can regenerate lost parts. The word *vestigial* refers to some trait that is left over from the past. We humans are mammals that carry with us some vestigial traces of this capacity to regenerate lost parts. What is regenerated in our bodies (start with skin)? What doesn't get regenerated (start with lost limbs)? Why do some animals regenerate major sections of their bodies while humans can't do the same? The simple answer is to say that we are too complex, but might there be a hidden or undiscovered gene that if it were turned on could enable us to regenerate organs, limbs, or digits (fingers)?

Extensions

How is it that humans can have a limb removed and years later actually feel pain in that missing limb?

RELATIVISM—VALUES

Is everything relative? This is often taken to mean that you can believe anything you want and behave any way you want because all things in life are relative (meaning that they are of equal value or equally without value).

This idea has ancient roots, but one of the modern sources is Albert Einstein. His big theory that changed our way of looking at the universe is called his general theory of relativity. Einstein firmly believed in what is called cause and effect. Certain events cause other things to happen. These other things are related in a coherent way. What happens as a result of some event is called the effect. Another way of saying this is that Einstein envisioned (saw, believed in) a universe in which laws governed nature. He believed these laws could be understood. There is a basis or foundation for what we observe in the universe.

He spent his last years until the very night he died looking for a unified set of formulas that would explain the underlying unity of all the forces of nature. Look up some things about his struggles with the physicists who defended quantum mechanics.

In common parlance (language), relativity is taken to mean that no thing, set of values, way of viewing life, or way of behaving is of greater or lesser value than any other. It's all relative. In this kind of social universe (the life we share together with other people), consequences of thoughts, feelings, and behaviors are of no importance, because everything is of equal value. If one person believes something and another person believes something very different, does this mean that anything anybody believes is without foundation? Is there a way to allow for a variance (differences) in human values and behaviors while also not falling into the trap of pure relativism?

Extensions

Look up the term *multicultural*. We live in a world that is very much multicultural. Many different cultures contribute to the larger whole. Some people are very upset that their own culture is dominated by other cultures. In the schools and in the wider communities, how are the issues related to multiculturalism being played out? One example in the United States is the issue of whether English is the official and only language for the country. There are many other issues related to multiculturalism. Identify them. How do you feel about these issues?

RELATIVITY—ACCELERATION ELEVATOR

If you were on an elevator accelerating upward and a ball fell out of your pocket and it hit the floor, would if fall at a rate faster than 32 ft./sec.^{2} (the terminal velocity of free-falling objects)?

If there were no outside references, would you be able to tell the difference between being on another planet versus being on a rising elevator? The effects of acceleration and gravity are the same. Guess who came up with this insight.

Extensions

If you were traveling at the speed of light and you threw a ball straight ahead as hard as you could, would the ball be going faster than the speed of light? Assume you are traveling at the speed of light and you shot a laser beam straight ahead. How fast would that laser-generated light be traveling? What would occur if you shot this same light ninety degrees relative to your trajectory? Would it be a curtain of light (a scattered laser beam)? What would occur if you shot this same laser light directly in the opposite direction relative to your trajectory? Would the light be standing still (static waves and photons with no motion)? Assume somebody else is looking at you from a stationary position (standing still, no motion). You are passing this person at the speed of light. Just before you pass this stationary person, you throw the ball straight ahead (in the direction of your travel) as hard as you can. The instant you pass the observer, the ball has already passed the person and is accelerating in front of you. Assume this outside stationary observer saw you shooting the laser beams in the previously described directions. What would they observe?

Now assume that you have a flashlight. Just before you pass the person (at the speed of light), you turn on the flashlight that has red light only. This red light is streaming away from you at the speed of light. How fast is the red light traveling relative to the observer? What would the observer experience in terms of color if the flashlight were shined directly at the observer or if the red light where shined directly away from the observer?

Now try the possibility of this same person traveling at the speed of light, and just as the traveler passes the observer, the traveler shines a blue light straight ahead. Would this make any difference to the observer? Now assume this blue light was shined directly at or directly away from the observer. There are the two related issues of the speed of any luminous (light-emitting) object relative to an observer. As this luminous object is moving away from the observer, there is a shift in the color spectrum toward red colors. As the object is moving toward the observer, there is a shift toward blue light. So what occurs if previously red shifted light is either moving away or toward the observer and previously blue shifted light is moving toward or away from the observer?

RELATIVITY—ACCELERATION ON MOON

If you were on the Earth and you dropped a rubber ball and a heavy steel ball from the same height, which would hit the ground first? Now assume that you release a feather and the same steel ball at exactly the same time, which one would hit the Earth first? Why did you choose one over the other?

If you were on the moon and you dropped a feather and a heavy tool from the same height, which would hit the ground first?

What does this have to do with Galileo Galilei and his famous experiment performed on the Leaning Tower of Pisa? (Remember when he dropped two objects at the same time?) What keeps that tower from toppling over? What caused it to start leaning in the first place?

Extensions

Would you expect that this feather and the heavy tool would fall as fast on the moon as they would have on the Earth? Earth's gravity is greater than that of the moon. The free-fall acceleration rate (assuming there is no air resistance) on Earth is 32 ft./sec.^{2}. Find out what it is on the moon. Is it different? If so, why? Are there any planets with no atmosphere that are larger than the Earth? How does atmosphere on any planet or moon get there? Might there be an atmosphere associated with our sun?

RELATIVITY—SPEED APPROACHING

Assume two spaceships were approaching each other at the speed of light, signified by the lowercase letter *c* (c = 299,792,458 m/s [meters per second]). Assume that you are flying one of the spaceships and you were looking directly at the approaching spaceship. Also assume that another pilot was flying a helicopter in a stationary position and that pilot was directly observing the approach of the opposite spaceship. From the perspectives of all three pilots, what would be the rate of their approach to each other? Is this a simple arithmetic problem? Our frame of reference is extremely important.

Extensions

Have you ever had the experience of something flying directly at you at a much faster rate than expected? How did you react? What did it feel like? Although it happened quickly, did it feel like it was happening quickly when you were inside the circumstances? Sometimes when things happen very quickly in very demanding circumstances, does it seem as though time slows down and your concentration is instantaneously greatly enhanced?

RELATIVITY—TIME CLOCKS

We have two identical clocks. One is at the top of the Empire State Building in New York City and the other is in the basement of the Empire State Building. Are they running at the same speed? Why? Is there such a thing as universal time? If you live at or near ocean level, be careful when you make an appointment with somebody living up in the mountains.

Extensions

If you were traveling in outer space at nearly the speed of light, would you be able to tell if your clocks were running at a different speed than those used by others who were not traveling with you? Do you think radio communication could be established between you and the Earth base? If you think it could be established, what would the words from the Earth base sound like to the people flying at nearly the speed of light? What would the words sound like projected from the hurtling vehicle to the people at the Earth base? If they were to be reporting time to each other, what would the comparisons indicate?

REMEMBERING, ANTICIPATING, OR JUST BEING CREATIVE?

Many people over many years have shared their experiences called déjà vu. This is an experience of apparently remembering that the current events that are happening have already occurred in the past. When this happens to me, the present moment is always stopped and I realize that I am intimately familiar with what is happening. It is a fascinating form of awareness. It is so familiar that it seems that I've already experienced it. Has this ever happened to you? Could there be an explanation? Does this mean that some set of events has already happened in the past? Are there other explanations? Is there an opposite of déjà vu?

Do some reading on how the mind works (that alone could take several lifetimes). More simply and more directly, become an acute (sharp) observer of your own mind. Be very focused on how the mind deals with time frameworks. We create frameworks of understanding within which we comprehend what is happening in our world. The mind works with awesome speed. It might be the case that sometimes in certain circumstances the frameworks and pictures the mind creates and what we see with our eyes and sense with our other senses emerge faster than our comprehension of their meaning. Often, we can be looking at something and not really seeing it fully.

We can have some set of circumstances transpiring (happening) around us, but it is not until later that we fully comprehend the meaning of what is occurring. This is something like a blind person who suddenly sees everything but comprehends very little of the meaning of what is being seen at first. We may be used to seeing only in a surface manner. Suddenly we see with utter clarity and depth. Then it may appear as though things have already happened by the time we comprehend the meaning or integrity of these frameworks. In a sense, they have happened in the past. There may be some deeper part of us that does in fact comprehend the meaning and depth of what we are experiencing, but this remains largely an unconscious experience. The instant we realize the preexisting unconscious comprehension, it seems like we've been here before.

It is also possible that we carry with us unconscious separate groupings of various barely grasped experiences that for some reason spark through an astounding fusion process that seems to be instantaneous into a more defined shape with character or definition, which causes a conscious emergence of an arresting and startling experience of clarity and depth. (*See* "Genius.") We barely know how consciousness works. Perhaps we need some critical clarity and then instantaneously our consciousness leaps into an entirely new framework of comprehension. This may occur instantaneously because we've leapt beyond all frameworks that have had the effect of squelching consciousness within a fragmenting smallness. In terms of the creative process, we carry with us unending arrays of semidefined primal images, intimations, insights, intuition, and senses. One or a few of these suddenly gain shape and definition. This unconscious experience literally crystallizes other nascent (yet to be born) insights, intuitions, and senses. Suddenly and instantaneously, an entire complex of unified focused experience results in a process (seemingly instantaneous) of enlarging comprehension. It appears as if this enlarging process is out of nowhere. Utter clarity and depth are the main impression of this emerging experience. It can strongly seem as though we have been here before. (*See* "Raindrops.")

For most people, the meaning or fuller understanding of a set of circumstances is usually delayed, unconscious, and gradual. This explains why these experiences are relatively infrequent. Thus, we do not have a déjà vu experience. For déjà vu to occur, there needs to be sufficient intensity and disparity (discrepancy or difference) between our usual sense of time and the sense of time within a déjà vu occurrence. There needs to be a surprising and arresting (captures our attention) sense of utter reality to the experience. Its influence is the sheer power of startling surprise. It is almost always totally unexpected. These can be lasting and powerful impressions. Especially when we reflect afterward on such experiences, they seem to be special because somehow we've violated a basic principle of time itself. This is taken to be messing around with Mother Nature, and that is always amazing and a little disconcerting (mildly alarming). Messing with Mother Nature would be something that totally violates all natural expectations (like waking up dead or suddenly being in two places at once). Internal alarm bells tend to go off when we sense we are dealing with a highly unusual set of circumstances. Déjà vu qualifies as being an unusual experience. We can be startled by its presence. We haven't broken any laws of nature. The mind works this way. It is natural. Mother Nature is fully intact. It's her breath that animates these experiences.

The metaphor of Mother Nature is a most interesting one. It can mean everything we take to be expected in life based on our experience. There is an entirely different rendition (version) of what the metaphor of Mother Nature actually refers to. Consider that we cannot know everything. (*See* "Numbers Large and Small.") Our consciousness itself is riddled with gaps in conscious knowledge. All this means is that the field in which all life takes place is vastly greater than the contexts in which our conscious knowledge is based. Our sense cannot grasp what anything is in and of itself. We don't see what light looks like independent of our five senses. What do life, the universe, and broccoli look like independent of our five senses? If there were no human being present in the universe, life, the universe, and broccoli would still exist, but they might not be composed the same as what our five senses and our brains construct. Mother Nature in this sense is not what we believe is natural based on our experience. Mother Nature in this sense is what life is without our presumptions, assumptions, interpretations, needs, desires, attachments, and aversions. Of course, there is a paradox involved in all of this: everything that exists is part of nature. We humans exist; therefore, what we experience is part of nature. There is a resolution to this conundrum but not at the level at which the conundrum is described. Now back to déjà vu and its first cousin that is its inverse, prescience.

Sometimes we get a clear internal sense of things before our five senses detect—and our minds define—a clear picture of a set of circumstances. If this were so, we wouldn't label this as déjà vu but as a case of prescience. To be prescient is to possess foreknowledge or foresight of things before they happen. Is this magic? Is this supernatural? Many people would say yes. There are alternative understandings.

Might it be the case that sometimes, under certain circumstances, the meaning of an emerging framework or set of circumstances comes into focus before the mind creates a well-defined conscious picture, image, or framework? On one level, we need a rational framework that helps us fit the current experience into a more encompassing framework of all prior and future expected frameworks. On another level, the meaning of a particular experience is something that runs much deeper. The meaning ascribed (given) to an experience touches and is related to all our other deep connections of the subconscious mind, heart, and intuitions. This level of consciousness is primal. As we resonate, identify, and associate with a direct experience of these deep currents of awareness, we see what is not normally seen. Time is a cognitive construct rooted in our discursive thinking that is itself rooted in the split between subject and object and between past and future. We can experience life apart from these bounds. The same laws of logic and rationality do not govern what is real in this part of our humanity, because everything we associate with being logical or rational is embedded in defined frameworks.

Prescience can be defined as a process of meaning preceding the well-formed definition of the experience. As an individual or as a group, we are prescient when we deeply grasp something prior to our rational grasp of a set of circumstances. We've been talking about déjà vu and prescience in terms of individual mental processes. When déjà vu and prescience emerge in groups, fascinating things begin to occur. The only things I'll mention about this astounding process is that most often these emerging dynamics are discounted as being anomalies that don't fit in with the regular consciously affirmed flow of attention. If two or three persons sense what is happening, they may choose to talk about it afterward. The reason for this is as follows: what appears to one or a few persons to be marvelous and astounding connections, revelations, and leaps of comprehension may appear to others as confusing gaps, interruptions, and diversions. (Look up the story of the self-taught Indian genius mathematician named Srinivasa Ramanujan. At first, the most advanced mathematicians could not figure out his methods because of so many gaps and interruptions in his theorems. Finally, it was recognized that he was continually making leaps of comprehension that couldn't be tracked in a linear fashion. Genius was the only possible explanation.)

If you ever have the privilege of talking about these experiences with others, avoid the urge to speed up and get very excited. Instead, slow down (hopefully keeping your excitement in a slightly cooler fashion). Passion is a good thing. It is a fundamental energy that impels adventure, exploration, and discovery. Too much of it causes us to actually experience diminished awareness. Sense what is occurring with great depth and openness. If we speed things up, our energy becomes magnified in such a way that we reinforce prior associations rather than a radically new and shared wonderful comprehension of experiences revealing themselves through us. We may become aware that others are aware of some vastly deeper process at play by the energy that is in their eyes, voice, or body language. Most often, some mysterious inner connection becomes apparent between two people that cannot be explained based on logic and rationality. Sometimes this is caused by a sense that allows us to experience a tangible synchrony between others and ourselves. This sense is not one of our five senses, and it manifests itself before our rational mind controls the moment.

Deep structure meaning might in some instances precede (come before) the full rational and conscious grasp or mental visualization of the phenomenon. Sometimes individuals "get it" before a group "gets it." Sometimes the subconscious, intuitions, or heart "gets it" prior to our intellectual (idea-driven) conscious mind. These are the *Aha!* experiences that always are problematical because it's like you're in a time warp. The insight, sense, deep feeling, and wisdom can't be directly comprehended by ourselves or relayed to and shared with others until there is sufficient conscious clarity of what it is that we are experiencing (alone or with others).

Experiencing prescience is living outside the boundaries of the expected. This could cause us to feel that the future has already occurred. This, of course, would be slightly problematical. Prescience empowers us to be able to sense what is happening in our environment prior to the full disclosure of the outer features of these events. Prescience allows us to see with our heart or intuition prior to seeing what our eyes see and our rational minds understand. Many people tend to call real that which we see with our eyes, our five senses, or our rational understanding. The stuff of our heart, intuitions, and wisdom is often labeled as being less real or fantasy. Research the historical reasons for this bias.

This research can lead you into the deepest and most profound brain research and into research on social structures as well. We often have a sense of things prior to their becoming apparent in our sense-based field and clear rational understanding. We receive intimations of things that we feel but don't fully understand. If we learn to observe and sense these intimations, we can grow in our understanding of them. We can learn to respond to them in a manner that reflects that these intimations are a natural and integrated part of our lives. We can learn to give these intimations more credibility, and we can learn to respond to them as sources of wisdom that we need to listen to. Our response time to these intimations can be vastly decreased, meaning that we can learn to move freely, spontaneously, and gracefully with these emergent insights. Instead of viewing them as being anomalies, we can learn to view them as interesting revealing aspects of our humanity that are vitally important.

Extensions

Once we learn how to be open to the experience of déjà vu and prescience, even more amazing things can begin to emerge in our conscious attention. We become aware of the much greater field of awareness in which we exist. Déjà vu and prescience are not supernatural, paranormal, or psychic experiences; they are anomalous and exceptional only from the perspective of our culturally reinforced ways of living. What people popularly label as supernatural, paranormal, or psychic experiences are actually very natural but little understood facets of our human capacities. In the greatest context or scope of understanding, there is only one unified dimension in which all life transpires. (*See* "Dimensions—How Many?") These particular experiences of déjà vu and prescience are associated with a vastly greater array of experiences that rises into our conscious attention and which adds tremendous depth and richness to our lives. There are many examples of this wide array of associated experiences that results in a discernible fundamental shift in our life orientation:

- We discern the presence of unexpected patterns completely outside our previous experience base.
- We sense repeated and persistent coincidences that are unexplainable and meaningful.
- Suddenly we see a completely surprising and previously unknown extension of some previously known process (or we see the solution to a complex problem with no apparent explanation as to how we arrived at the solution).
- We see the association between patterns or processes that usually are experienced as having no apparent or inherent connection.
- We experience a surprising transformation in what had been a gap in our understanding and awareness, which suddenly becomes a source of comprehension, continuity, and unity.
- We become aware of the arising of a different and more inclusive field, in which we are aware of the unity and interrelated nature of all life.
- We no longer take life for granted. We are amazed by the proliferating diverse expressions of our astounding gift of Life! This sense of being amazed abides with us, affecting everything in our lives.

- We comprehend Life! in a manner that exceeds our capacity to communicate it to others with words. We learn to allow ourselves to become expressions of this comprehension. These expressions are enacted but not necessarily verbally expressed.
- We see entire complex processes as one integrated and whole image.
- We discover that a mysterious creative process is occurring through us instead of it being defined as the product of something we willed into existence or take credit for creating (specifically, the mysterious quality that we call Life! and its discernible energy).
- We sense the energy within ourselves and in others that precedes our cognitive and affective processes. We recognize the process of imposing our impressions, feelings, senses, reactions, projections, filtering, and ideas on this energy.
- We realize how to focus this energy for the sake of Life! itself. We learn to live beyond the compulsive self-absorption and self-importance that only delude us. This energy is for the purpose of extending, enhancing, and honoring Life! We experience ourselves as the means of its expression.
- We experience senses other than our traditional five senses. (*See* "Senses—Imagine Some More.")
- We discern a path we consciously choose that reflects our intention and ultimate concerns in life. Among the many contradictory and enticing options, we choose the few that resonate with our deepest values and wisdom. This is evolving into our true self.
- We discover what it means to be authentic. We respond to, identify with, and remain in the place of deepest comprehension and compassion.
- We become aware that in every moment we take what is essentially a living, whole, interrelated unity (in which we are fully alive) and split it up into segmented objects that we define based on our attachments and aversions. This creates a context of our own making in which we exist in a persistent state of self-absorption and self-concern. We create a worldview that filters all objects based on our interpretation and needs.
- We realize that we are constantly setting contexts within which we interpret and symbolize all the objects we hold in consciousness.
- In certain moments, we can directly see this process at play. These moments allow us to experience a state of utter clarity, stillness, astounding freedom, and the awareness of being fully alive in the current moment.
- While experiencing such lucid insight, we intuitively see that at the core of every conscious moment is a crystallizing influence that we create. This crystallizing influence is rooted in our attachments and aversions. Our tendency is to reshape the endlessly evolving, living, whole, and interrelated unity (womb, matrix, and life web) that gives us life. We tend to reshape it into a controlled and familiar context in which we practice the habit of making everything into separate objects that we interpret,

name, symbolize, and categorize. All of these prior inclinations become unconscious presumptions that influence us at the core and root of every emerging moment. These crystallizing influences form and shape our basic view of life. These crystallizing influences deeply affect the context in which all relationships emerge.

- We see the energy that impels these ongoing crystallizing influences only when we are perfectly attentive to and directly experiencing a moment of sheer clarity and utter comprehension. This moment is free from the bounds, tendencies, and filters of our need to hold life within a context rooted in our attachments and aversions.
- The most amazing discovery is that we don't know our Life! background (stage, source, and substratum) through our conscious mind. The mind is controlled by the drive to interpret and symbolize everything through the lens of our personal divided context. In this moment of sheer clarity, stillness, and utter comprehension, we see that the heart is an eye that sees. The heart is the place of passion, fundamental life energy, basic life orientation, and affirmation of what is real. In a moment of being clear and sage (wise), we awaken to the primal experience of our true condition, which is that we are free to live in this marvelous, undivided, fully alive, and interrelated whole (womb or matrix) that we call Life!
- In such a moment, Life! is not an object we hold in our consciousness (within a context that we construct). As we open ourselves from our heart, we see an entirely different environment. This is seeing through our heart. It is astounding, and we become speechless.
- We then see that we have been constantly identified with complexity, ambiguity, miscues, misinterpretations, and false presumptions. From within a moment of sheer clarity, stillness, and utter comprehension, we directly experience Life! in such a way that we see the wellspring within every moment that gives us Life! It is simple and profound. It is vastly different from the crystallizing influences that cause us to distort our orientation to life and which cause us to live in a fundamentally divided condition. We cease creating massive and unnecessary complexity. We know that we are at the beginning place of all creativity, compassion, and intellect. We feel rooted in life material that is very significant. This emergence of genius is a genesis point of wisdom that exceeds our grasp. This beginning point is the source for any genius that manifests the capacity to leap beyond what is given in life. Only then do we realize why things aren't set and given.
- From within a moment rooted in this sheer clarity, stillness, and utter comprehension, we see that fate is a real force but only in a most limited and specific way. We are fated to live out the consequences of our behaviors, values, interpretations, habits, and tendencies until or unless we realize the presence of these moments of sheer clarity, stillness, and utter

comprehension. Only then do the chains of fate (the sense that life is a given context that must not be challenged or questioned) cease controlling us. The chain is broken. This means that we are able to live with an undistorted and undivided orientation to life. We can also see the process of these habits becoming almost totally unconscious. We see the effect of this process of the habits becoming unconscious, which is that we come to presume the necessity of our dividing, confusing, complex, and ambiguous personal context. This presumption causes us to remain stuck in an illusory condition. What appears to be natural and necessary isn't merely given. We see the deep irony that to those given to such a broken and misleading way of living, fate (the sense of things necessarily and naturally being the way they are) is a given in life. It really is given and true within the context that most people take to be the only option.

- As a result of this presumption of life being something that is given, we see so many people manifesting resigned spirit, muffled voice, constrained range of interests, tethered vitality, limited imagination, narrow involvements, reactive impulses, diminished trust in others and life, and cynical outlooks. If all is given, then the willingness to take risks for a future that could be more life affirming is less likely. From within a moment of sheer clarity, stillness, and utter comprehension, we experience the renewing and encouraging sense that all is not given and that many things are possible that we cannot imagine. What are unconscious presumptions rise into conscious awareness.
- We are able to take imaginative and intuitive leaps of comprehension. We become able to experience Life!'s greatness and potential. We are also able to see that things are far worse than most people can imagine as they remain stuck in ruts of presuming that life is basically something given to us. We gain the capacity to see that things are far worse in the current moment than most people imagine and that the seeds for creative and life-affirming transformation are entirely intact and present for every individual and for every collective challenge facing us today. We see the greatness of the challenge and the marvel of the opportunity.
- Realizing the presence and stunning wisdom yielded only within these moments of sheer clarity, stillness, and utter comprehension allows us to persistently focus on root issues, the actual crystallizing influences, and the most central presumptions. The focusing is through the direct experience of this wellspring of clarity, stillness, and comprehension. We then realize the importance of attention, concentration, and reflection. What we focus upon matters. How we focus upon what we pay attention to matters. Being aware of how we are focusing ultimately matters. What we focus upon becomes real, substantial, and material. Our focusing process either sets us free to express creativity, compassion, and genius or it imprisons us in ways that we become unconscious of.

- We directly experience that we are the only ones in the universe who are responsible for our focusing process (what we focus upon, how we manifest this quality of focusing, and cultivating the awareness of this responsibility).
- We realize that we are part of nature. Our interpretations, perceptions, feelings, senses, intuitions, and primal images (our fundamental picture of life that serves as the root of our consciousness) can only find their fullest expression when we are directly experiencing Life! as it truly is (apart from and beyond our illusions). The illusion is the mistaken notion and prime presumption that it is natural and necessary to live within the confines of our limiting and confusing context that we fill with supposedly separate objects that we define (and thus to some degree control). The paradox is that we can't know of the illusion until we experience a lucid moment in which we see the mostly unconscious process of dependence on self-created and self-sustained contexts.
- We hold in creative tension the simultaneous wisdom that we are capable of understanding that our senses and minds are filters for what is actually there, that we live with constructed accounts of what we interpret to be real, and that we are able to experience an awareness through which we become lucid, fully alive, directly observing, and discerning Life! in a nondistorted manner.
- Most people experience this simultaneous wisdom of apparently paradoxical capacities only in a fragmentary and ambiguous manner.
- We accept that there are always gaps in our understanding and that these gaps provide the basis for persistent learning and growth.
- We experience a depth and acuity (sharp focus) of concentration that allow us to see extraordinary aspects of our outward environment. We may be able to observe things at the periphery of our consciousness that usually disappear when we attempt to turn our conscious attention to them. We may be able to see processes slowed down or sped up and thus see emergent facets of our environment that had been hidden. We may be able to concentrate on either the network of relationships or one quality of our relationships and hold it in our attention to learn from it. (*See* "Sight—To See the Unseen.")
- We experience a depth of attentiveness that allow us to see extraordinary aspects of our inward awareness. The most extraordinary aspect is our capacity to observe ourselves moment by moment experiencing emergent feelings, ideas, relationships, challenges, opportunities, and patterns.
- We realize that distinctions between what is labeled inward and outward are no longer prime organizing metaphors in this greater condition of clarity and comprehension.
- A gripping question arises: What is this mysterious process of observation, attention, and consciousness?
- We may become surprised by the tenacity (persistence) of our capacity to stay with one single, mediating, greatly important question.

- We discover an interesting capacity to place a mediating or central question or need into the background of our consciousness while we focus on other concerns. We may experience a sudden burst of resolution in which an entire, well-formed, refined, and new solution or insight arises as if out of nowhere.
- We experience an amazing shift and transformation of our fundamental awareness. We shift away from defining ourselves as a separate object relating to other objects that are out there beyond us. Instead, we focus on a radically different kind of awareness that is not rooted in the filtering presumption that life is basically composed of separate objects attempting to relate to each other.
- We observe ourselves in real time (current time) from a place of complete attention and utter detachment from the presumptions that have impelled, limited, and distorted us.
- We become amazed at how we can be perfectly attentive and detached while being more fully involved in life's relationships and challenges than ever before.
- We experience a lucid (utterly clear) observing that is not just a deeper extension of what we normally call great concentration. It is a mysterious and astounding process occurring through us that is fundamental to us being alive in every moment. This lucid observing becomes the bedrock source of creativity, compassion, intellect, and genius. There is the insight that it is not a special unique talent of one separate individual. Its quality is sewn into the rudiments (basics) of all our lives in every moment. It begins to dawn on us that this capacity for lucid observing is the mainspring from which our vitality flows.
- We experience being fully alive, alert, and aware.
- We realize a capacity to give everything of our energy and commitment to Life! We are not consumed, because the fully alive, alert, aware, and creative capacity is an ever-replenishing resource. This capacity is not to be mistaken for the illusion that we can deny our physical or mental health needs.
- We experience lucid moments both in our waking and sleeping states.
- We realize that this still, dynamic, creative, detached, involved, and observing aspect of our lives is always steadily present in a perfectly unbroken fullness and wholeness.
- We learn to live with paradox (simultaneously holding in an awareness of what most people consider to be exclusive things, like being involved and detached, still and dynamic, creative and logical, feeling and thinking, strong and sensitive).
- We realize how to live with and sense the presence of paradox that allows us to experience a leap of awareness into greater comprehension in which opposites unite. We experience Life! as a web or relationship in which we

are always being urged to open ourselves to greater diverse expressions of an abiding underlying unity.

- We become aware of an arresting, amazing, direct, and immediate experience (beholding) of everything being magnificent, astounding, right, ignited from within, a fullness that is in everything, and a certain and specific brightness.
- We become arrested by an experience of "This is my Life!" This insight reveals itself when we take full responsibility for our reaction to everything that has ever happened to us and for everything we manifest in life, when we are mindful of the great nature of the gift of being alive, by being alert to the importance of sharing one's own unique combination of gifts; by comprehending and savoring the insight that everything we've experienced (the good and the bad) has resulted in our current wisdom (capacity to give of oneself in an life-affirming way); by an acceptance of all that has caused us grief, confusion, or fear as being part of a larger context for a life that is good; by an obvious excitement to dive into life with an indescribable self-assuredness and creativity; by an acceptance of who we are; by an acknowledgment that we can't know what lies ahead of us; by a willingness to treat all of life as an ever-unfolding mysterious adventure; and by an emergent curiosity and impelling attraction to experience yet greater depths of involvement, comprehension, and gratitude. We cease identifying with our wounds, limitations, sorrows, grievances, hurts, and pains in life. We commence being attentive to what we can do with our lives and how we can contribute to the betterment of our shared condition. What is given in life eventually becomes a part of what we have to give back to life.

REMEMBRANCE

How is it that the brain remembers anything? There are those who believe that the brain also remembers everything. Some people while in deep states of attentiveness are able to recall certain incidents in startling details. Assume that one had at one time looked at a vase filled with flowers. In a deep state of attentiveness, some people are able to remember back and from within that frame of reference from the past. They are able to change their focus of attention and recall other things that were not originally consciously remembered. This means that there is some unconscious remembrance at play. For instance, instead of recalling the vase with the flowers in it, you might change your focus of attention from within that frame of reference and begin to focus upon the cat in the corner of the room. Then you might be able to notice the insect on the edge of the left ear of the cat. From there, you may even notice that it's time for lunch. How does this unconscious memory work? Try it on yourself.

Recall some vivid experience. Start with your initial picture of the event. Become attentive to a greater context. See if you can alter your focus of attention.

Extensions

Does the brain remember more than we are aware of in any present moment? What happens to the brain when people begin to lose their memory?

REPRODUCING

There are both sexual and asexual forms of reproduction. Look up information on both. What are the simplest forms of life that reproduce sexually? What are the most complex forms of life that reproduce asexually?

Extensions

Are there any forms of life that reproduce both sexually and asexually? Hint: this could be a mixture of the sexual and asexual means of reproduction in one organism's multistage reproductive process, or it could be in a species alternating between sexual and asexual reproduction. What are the adaptive advantages of having both sexual and asexual reproductive methods available? Look up the biological term *schizogamy*. Don't get it mixed up with the term *schizogony*.

RESEARCH IN CONTROVERSIAL AREAS

Are there areas of research that we ought not to investigate? Are there areas of human knowledge that are too dangerous for us? Read the book *Frankenstein*. If we could make identical people out of genetic material (clones), ought we research how to do this? If we could make these clones do all the nasty boring work for us, couldn't we be masters of our fates? If the lives of people in North America and Europe could be saved by doing human research on human beings in the poorest areas of the world, ought we be doing this? An example might be testing drugs in poor areas of the world to see if they are safe for us here in North America. What are other possible areas of research that would be controversial?

Extensions

There have been tests run on people who had nuclear materials injected into their bodies without the knowledge or consent of the patients (victims, test subjects). Members of the military have been marched into areas that had just been ground zero for nuclear explosions. There was one famous experiment done over the course of many years that involved a pool of volunteers who were primarily African American males. The government knew that they had venereal disease. For years, the patients thought they were being treated for the disease. The government was actually simply observing what happens to people whose venereal disease goes untreated. Were they really patients? Does the government owe anything to these persons? Our president has apologized to the victims. Is this enough? What else do you feel that our country should apologize for? Should we make reparation payments to any group of people for certain actions? Is money the proper vehicle for the expression of regret? Besides words and money, what are other means of reconciling ourselves with past acts of violence and gross insensitivity?

RIDDLE—DIMPLED WHACKEE

An organization has ruled that the items under its control that fly (technically, glide) must not travel over 250 feet per second. (There are examples of ones flying faster, and the ones that do fly faster make the sender look very good, but he or she is considered to be cheating.) Traditionally, there have been 336 dimples on the surface of these items. They can be no larger than 1.68 inches in diameter and no heavier than 1.62 ounces. Now there are many manufacturers claiming that their item goes farther with more dimples. Some claim their product goes further with fewer dimples, some claim their product goes further with larger dimples, and some claim their product goes further with smaller dimples.

What is the object? When do you use the word *further* and when do you use the word *farther*?

Extensions

Hint: the ruling organization is the U.S.G.A. What do dimples do to the flight of these little round things? Would it travel further if it were heavier, lighter, smaller, or larger? Would it fly faster and further if it had different material at its core? What are most of these little round things made of?

RIVER—LARGEST IN THE WORLD

What is the largest river in the world? Try determining your answer by looking at a map. Which rivers look the biggest? How is it determined which is the biggest river? If a river is very shallow, it could be very wide and long and not carry as much water as a river that is much deeper, shorter, and more narrow. Is volume the main factor in determining the "bigness" of a river? Always be careful about how questions are asked. Might it be possible for a certain river to have slightly greater volume but another river is "bigger" because the water has a higher velocity (flows faster)? Listen carefully to the format or form of the question. Might the "bigness" of a river be determined by how much land it drains? Is it a good question with a potential for rich answers? Might it be a good question with one weak link, such as an ambiguous (fuzzy) word that isn't very useful? If so, seek to clarify (make clearer) the term that is weak or ambiguous.

Extensions

Do all rivers flow at the same speed? If so, why? If not, what would account for the differences? When a question is asked, learn how to picture the question in your mind. Then once you have a picture of it, alter the picture. Change the framework of the question. Test for assumptions you are making about the question (look up *implication* and *inference*). For the first question of this section, would you believe that the biggest river "in the world" is up in the sky? The river flows over the Andes Mountains, flows southward, and veers across the Atlantic Ocean toward Africa. It pumps more water per second than the Amazon does. Amazing! Find out all you can about rivers of water up in the sky. Are there other major rivers up in the sky? Where does this one go? How would you like to live at the end of it? Imagine looking up into the sky seeing this great cascade of water plummeting downward at you. Might there be significant rivers under the ground? Look up some information on aquifers. Some rivers flow under the ground and then pop up and start to flow aboveground. For one very wide river, look up information on the Florida Everglades. Are there other places in the world like the running waters in the Florida Everglades? How about deltas? The greatest river in the world may be the ice flows on the Antarctic landmass. Another candidate might be the massive ocean currents impelled by thermal differentials. Do some research.

Another challenge: Did you assume that the term *river* meant flowing water? Are there other materials (that aren't water) "in the world" that are in a liquid state that flow? Are there other forms of matter that flow that aren't liquid? (*See* "Liquids—What Is This Stuff?") Does the term *river* always refer to material in a liquid state? Now what kind of answers do you get for the question? What about a river with material in a gaseous state? What about plasma state rivers? Who says the rivers must be composed of matter? Recently, it was discovered that there is a huge stream or river of antimatter flowing from the center of our Milky Way galaxy. What about a river of time? What about a river of particles above the Earth that are the current that catches particles from the bursts of the sun's energy and the effect is the Northern and Southern Lights? What is this current or belt? Is it flowing? What about the current between our North Magnetic Pole and our South Magnetic Pole?

Do not expect that every person in your life is going to appreciate and value such ways of responding to questions. Most people assume that the way in which questions are asked ought to be received in precisely the manner that the questioner implied. Look at a court trial sometime and observe how questions are being asked. What are other circumstances in which it is encouraged and welcomed to challenge questions? Get to know the difference between such circumstances. You'll avoid many problems knowing this distinction between circumstances when it is OK to question and when it is not. If you're in Army boot camp, leave this book in your bag (real deep inside the bag).

When you learn this technique of responding to questions with deep creativity and your personal stamp of genius, you may have to remain silent sometimes because others may not want you to be questioning their questions, intent, motives, meaning, or points of view. What is the difference between a friendly, affirming, and encouraging challenge versus an abrasive and disrupting challenge? Learn when and where not to challenge others. Always challenge yourself. In short, be aware of connotations, denotations, what is being implied, what you are inferring, and how the question is being asked, and be able to alter the framework of the question, expand the framework, reverse the order of the question, invert prime assumptions, extend the logic used, alter the logic used, and test for ambiguous terms.

Be aware that some people love challenging all authority. They enjoy getting people upset. What I am talking about is very different. These are ways of challenging our entire base of human knowledge with the intention of expanding what is possible for us to know. We do this by learning how to liberate our own genius and creativity while honoring that same spark and presence in all others. So where is the biggest river? Just give me the simple answer!

RIVERS OF LIFE

Rivers all over the world are sources of life. Without their water, crops are not raised, people are not fed, and entire communities would be dislocated. Tremendous pressures are being exerted on our Earth because of a combination of population increase and increased demand for natural resources. Fresh clean water is becoming a most valuable resource. Four major river systems already do not make it to the oceans at least for part of the year. These are the Ganges, Nile, Yellow, and Colorado River systems. What is the quality of this water as it does reach the ocean (if any)? What are the many factors leading to water depletion?

Extensions

The population explosion is one major factor in the story of us causing harm to the Earth. What are the demonstrated relationships between the empowerment and education of women worldwide and the lowering of the rate at which the population is rising? Why do so many men in so many regions of our world resist any educational processes designed to empower women?

ROOT MESSAGES AND PRIME REFERENCE POINTS

There are some messages we carry around inside us that affect all aspects of our lives. These messages are like prime reference points. All other things are understood through these lenses or windows of interpretation. For instance, there are many "I" messages we all have. I am this or I am that. I am too tall or too short. I am too lean or too fat. I am bright or I am not very bright. I am good at going into social situations in which I don't know many people. I am a klutz at social circumstances unless I know everybody. I need to control. I need to have somebody else control things and make decisions for me. I am lovable. I am not acceptable for who I am.

A few minutes ago, I was playing basketball with my son and some of his friends. One of them is a talented bass and piano player. He says to me that he couldn't sink a free throw if his life depended upon it. I told him that he can easily find all those keys on the piano, so if he practiced shooting baskets he might be a whole lot better in basketball than what he suspects. He stepped up and immediately sank a perfect free-throw shot! These kinds of messages emerge at different times in different circumstances. What are the messages you carry around inside of you that affect, limit, or enhance (make better) your life?

Extensions

What can we do about these root messages? Are we stuck with them for the rest of our lives? Where do they come from? The really core messages are the most important ones. They are the most difficult to see and change. Who gives them credibility? Of course, we do it to ourselves! The social environment conditions us with many different kinds of messages, but ultimately it is we who ardently (with great passion) preserve, nurture, and cultivate these core internal "I" messages. Why do we reinforce messages that don't foster (encourage) our well-being? Then, of course, there are those messages that encourage our well-being. Does the society support these messages? What are these "I" messages that are very good for us? One set of research results indicates that too much unearned praise is detrimental (not good) for people. What do you think is the reason?

ROOTS AND BRANCHES

Of the deciduous trees (the ones that generally drop their leaves in the fall), do you think that the roots are roughly equal in size to the branches? Is there a relation between the size of the tree, the age of the tree, and the relative size of its branches versus the roots? Look up the bristlecone pine trees (the oldest trees in the world), the redwoods (the tallest trees in the world), and the sequoias (the biggest trees in the world). Which single state has all three varieties of trees? Look up information on the environments that support such trees. Then find out about their branches and roots. What is the most common tree in the world?

Extensions

What are other things that you see very often but you only see part of the structure? Ever wonder what those portions of the whole structure look like?

ROPE IN SPACE

Take a rope that is one inch in diameter and ten thousand miles long. Attach it to a rocket that goes straight up into outer space. When it becomes tightly outstretched and vertical, the rocket releases the rope. What would happen to the rope if it were attached to the Earth at its base? Would it make a difference if the rope were not attached to the Earth? Would it float straight up in our atmosphere? Would it tumble back to Earth? What do you think? Why? Vary the length of the rope—would this make any difference? If this rope were a very strong tube, would air rush up toward outer space (because there is a vacuum at the other end)? Hot air rises, so wouldn't this also provide energy for impelling air to move upward? If you were to cover the Earth's end of the tube with your ear, what would you hear? Might you hear the ocean? Why? What would occur if you got sucked up into the tube?

Extensions

How far can the effects of Earth's gravity be felt?

ROUND SQUARES?

Are there such things as round squares? Remember to switch and alter the frameworks within which questions are asked.

If you draw a square on a flat piece of paper, it is impossible to create a round square. If you alter your context, different things are quite possible. Imagine drawing a square on a transparent sphere (like a perfectly round balloon). Draw it in such a manner that all four corners touch. Is it round? Is it three-dimensional? Might it be a two-dimensional surface protruding through several planes?

Before, we were assuming that attempting to draw a round square must be done in two dimensions (length and width). We have now assumed that it can be done in three dimensions (depending upon your interpretation). Now try to imagine what it would look like in four dimensions. If space-time is curved, pretend that there is some mass present causing a warping of space-time. This requires a special kind of creative thinking. Einstein himself needed to go consult with a mathematician who could teach him the complex math related to curved surfaces. So don't feel bad that the job is demanding. Really, think about this challenge. Try to visualize it.

We need to project, reconstruct, or portray ways that approximate the experience of other interpretive frameworks (such as seeing the fourth dimension). In a TV series on how the brain works, the commentator was describing what it must be like for a woman who had suffered a brain stroke that left her without the ability to see motion. It is very difficult for us to understand and visualize how she must see life. The TV series showed her trying to cross the street in London, England. Then it showed what it must look like to her. They showed still picture shots of the video that was taken as she was crossing the street. Then they took one frame per few seconds and cast them up onto the screen. If she is seeing one frame at a time, a bus that is one block off is seen in the second still picture as being right in front of you. In the third frame, the bus may be fifty feet in the opposite direction. In the fourth frame, the bus may be one hundred feet in the opposite direction. This would be shocking and dangerous for all of us to suddenly start seeing motion in this manner. She might also be seeing several of these still pictures all at once or not in the proper order or sequence. This would be totally confusing.

The TV version of what it might be like for this woman who suffered from this stroke is an example of portraying a way of realizing that there are other ways to visualize, experience, or think about realities that most of us assume are absolutely set and unchangeable. This kind of stroke was dangerous and tragic for this one person. Another kind of stroke (the stroke of genius) can be a gift to us and to our wider community, but this can only happen if we are liberated to leap beyond the bounds set for us by ourselves and by our social/intellectual environment. You can do it. Now try to challenge yourself with the question of what a square would like in four dimensions. Just because most people assume it is impossible, don't let this discourage you. Let your genius play. Follow its trail. See the gardens to which it will lead you.

Remember to combine both logic and creativity. The creative leaps of imagination are great, but you also need a plan to help sustain your creative processes. In this case, study everything you can get your hands on related to the fourth dimension. Talk to artists. Talk to scientists. Gather all your pieces together and reflect on them. Be careful to watch and record your dreams. This is often where your genius will leap into view. Frequently, this is only after you have deeply worked on a challenge for a protracted (long) period of time, concentrated on the issues related to the problem, been attentive to greater and more inclusive contexts and reflected on the insights gained from your efforts. Be playful in your work and projects. Learning ought to be enjoyable.

Imagined reality can be powerful stuff because it teaches us to look at what most people call reality in fresh and creative manners. It also teaches us lessons about one of the most startling insights, which is "reality is not set." We *Homo sapiens* interact with our environment. In this act of relating to it, we are affecting many aspects of what is called reality.

Extensions

Many people believe that all people are motivated primarily by selfishness. You can meet many people who are driven by self-gain. Then you might meet somebody who loves others and life in such a generous and self-giving manner that the old assumption needs to be changed. Reality ceases to be defined in terms of groups of people all acting out of selfish reasons. Life can be founded in another manner. We can't change other people directly and immediately, but we can live according to our own version and vision of life. In this way, we affect our environment. What would you like to change in the world? What and who can you change? What can be changed if enough people become willing to participate in change?

ROUTINES IN LIFE

What are the many routines you practice? Different routines have different frequencies (how often they occur) and amplitude (how much energy we commit to each of them). Try to list the ones that you do every day, every week, every year, or only a few times since you were born. Why do you practice these routines?

Extensions

Try to uncover routines that you practice that you are not aware of. How can this be done? One way is to observe other people and the routines you think they are not aware of. Another way is to practice the art of becoming ever more self-aware of how and why you do things. This requires tremendous discipline. We can learn to observe ourselves in every lived moment. (*See* "Remembering, Anticipating, or Just Being Creative?") We can observe our feelings, intuitions, ideas, emerging senses, and evolving comprehension of life issues. When you become aware of something, take note of it. See if there is a pattern at play in your life of which you were previously unaware.

Once, when my mother-in-law was staying with my family, I noticed that she talked to herself. One night while falling asleep, I mentioned this to my wife. She immediately responded that I do the same thing! "Impossible!" I replied. Yet the next day, sure enough, there I was talking up a verbal storm to myself without anybody else present. How do we learn to become more self-aware? It is something like learning not to wet your bed. You commit yourself to something, and then the mind goes to work on the challenge. Things work out.

ROYAL ISLAND

Isle Royale is a national park located in Lake Superior right off the shoreline from Minnesota. There are many wolves and moose on the island. Park naturalists tell hikers and backpackers that the wolves and moose got over to the island mostly on the ice in the wintertime and that some of the moose swam over. There is only one little problem with this theory. The distance between the shoreline of the mainland and the island is about twenty miles. Moose are powerful swimmers—but twenty miles? Even twenty miles on treacherous ice is almost unbelievable. Ever tried to walk on uneven ice whose depth is unknown? Where there is a will, there is a way. Do you think that moose and wolves could swim for twenty miles in water that is almost as cold as ice water (even in the middle of the summer)? How often does it get cold enough for the ice to form twenty miles out from shore in a deep enough fashion to accommodate moose and wolves?

Extensions

If it were relatively rare for such animals to successfully get across the expanse of water, wouldn't you think that genetic tests would confirm that the wolves and moose are from a relatively few animals that originally made it across?

Why are so many people afraid of wolves? A wild-game biologist once told a group I was in that the only recorded instances of wolves killing human beings are when people domesticate wolves. The speaker had just come from a home where the owner's half-wolf attacked their six-year-old son. Over a hundred stitches were necessary. There used to be a person two miles from our home who had signs in front of his home advertising puppies for sale: wolves crossed with Doberman pinschers and wolves crossed with rottweilers. These are two breeds of dogs that many people judge to be potentially vicious (along with pit bull terriers). Why would anybody want to do this? Is this crossbreeding ethical? Should it be legal? Are certain breeds of dogs naturally vicious or do human beings train them to be vicious? Might it be that certain breeds of dogs have certain tendencies that predispose them to be "trainable" as attack or fighting dogs?

RUSHED ALONG

What do you feel like when you are rushed? What do you notice in your behaviors when you are rushed? Do certain kinds of things tend to happen when you are rushed? What are the usual reasons for being rushed? When you have many things to do in a limited period of time, do you prefer to get the big jobs done first, or do you like to get all the little messy jobs done first and then concentrate on the really big ones? How comfortable are you with having tasks interrupted (where you are forced to move on to other tasks before finishing the first one)? How good are you at keeping track of multiple tasks that are in various stages of completion? What are various means of keeping track of incomplete tasks for which we are responsible? How comfortable are you with leaving messes behind you (interrelated tasks that cause further complications if they are not completed)? How good are you at limiting the number and kinds of things for which you and others hold you responsible? Do you get overinvolved? Are you undercommitted in terms of being a responsible person in the wider community? What are you learning in terms of how to hold the importance of being involved and the necessity of having time and space in which to pursue those things that refresh you in creative ways?

Extensions

When we are rushing through our tasks and day, how often is it that you try to do more than one thing at a time? In computer language, this is known as multitasking. Many people believe that this is a very efficient and effective way of dealing with stressful, high-demand jobs or situations. Is it really more efficient and effective? What are examples of you trying to be concentrated on more than one thing at a time? Examine your behaviors very closely and you might be quite surprised as to what is actually occurring. Be aware of the possibility that you are never really concentrating on more than one thing at a time consciously. What you are doing is segmenting different tasks into smaller units, and you are processing multiple large and complex tasks in the same time frame (not the same instant of conscious attention). When the complexity and intensity of the demands we place upon ourselves or that are placed upon us become very concentrated in short bursts of time, there are definite things that begin to happen to our intellectual and emotional capacities. In addition, things clearly begin to happen to our body. How aware are you of your body and its reactions and signals?

SAVING FACE

When you are in a group and you have a conflict or disagreement with another person, is it possible to deal with the issues without hurting the other person and getting hurt yourself? Is it possible to find common ground, make peace, or learn to live with each other? One little piece of wisdom that frequently works well is to recognize the need of every person to be accepted for who he or she is. In a conflict situation, try to learn how to save the face of the other person (their sense of self-identity). Instead of challenging them in terms of them being jerks, idiots, blind, insensitive, racist, bigoted, sexist, or unfair, try finding something positive in their lives to which you can relate. This doesn't work all the time but keep it in mind. When certain persons are engaged in violence of any kind, your first ethical responsibility is not to understand the person but to stop the violence. What are various forms of violence that people inflict on others? What happens when a community does not want to deal with emerging forms of violence? What are your options? What effect does silence have on aggressive people who are determined to hurt others?

Extensions

Do we have to be nice to everybody all the time? What does it mean to be nice? Might compassion be different from being nice?

SECOND LARGEST LAKE IN THE WORLD

Lake Victoria is the world's second largest freshwater lake, after Lake Superior, based on surface area. What is the third largest freshwater lake as measured by surface area?

Extensions

What is the largest volume freshwater lake in the world? As measured by volume, what is the second largest freshwater lake in the world?

SEEING INSIDE

Some things about ourselves we cannot explain. For my entire life, I have loved seeing the insides of things. Driving around, if I see some interesting object being thrown out and waiting on the street to be picked up, I'll take it home, get out the goggles and tools, and go to work. If you choose to do anything like this, be sure you've checked out the possibility of any dangerous materials (nuclear, vacuum tubes, chemicals, gases, etc.). Always be extremely safe. Consult with others before you get into trouble that you might not expect. Almost anything can be interesting: washing machines, cardboard, old computers, radios, TVs, engines, motors, gauges, and the vascular system of large plants pulled out of the garden in the fall.

Extensions

Twice in my life, I've had surgery. Each time, I've asked the doctor, in advance, if it would be OK to view my own surgery. Both times, they have been very surprised but said it was OK. It was awesome seeing inside my own body. Think of other ways that you can look inside of things that aren't usually seen. Is there any way to see the xylem and phloem (vascular system for transporting liquids and food) in a plant rise and fall with new nanotechnology? Could this be recorded digitally? Look at some films of blood flowing through vessels, substances being exchanged across permeable membrane walls of cells, and neurons in the head firing. From the inside, observe nature. Could you get to the inside of an atom? Be creative. See where it gets you. Just don't land in prison because you read this book and became curious about how to get inside a safe illegally.

SEEING UPSIDE DOWN

What would it look like to hold your breath and go down under the surface of water and look up at the blue sky? If the surface of the water were perfectly still, do you think that you could see the vapor trail of a jet overhead? If it was nighttime, do you think you could see the moon or stars? Only do this in a safe way (with others)!

Extensions

Seek out ways to safely view nature and other people from perspectives that allow you to see life creatively. Could you imagine being the first person to succeed in photographing the trail of moonlight on still water from underneath the water?

SEEING YOUR TWIN

Is it possible to see someone who looks exactly like you more than once in life and each time it is a different person? How would you know it is a different person? Investigate how artists draw faces. Talk to an artist about the types of faces. There are only so many combinations.

Extensions

Could somebody else have your exact same voice? Look up what voiceprints are. There is a whole science related to graphing the prints of people's voices. Could there be two people with the same fingerprints? Could there be two people with the same genetic structure?

SEICHE

What is a seiche? How do they occur? Hint: they are unusual phenomena that occur on large bodies of water. They can happen quite quickly.

Extensions

What are some other forms of unusual phenomena that occur with lakes, rivers, seas, or oceans? The governments of Russia and the United States have released data related to their secret military research on the regions under the polar ice cap. Some very unusual things have been discovered. You might read some interesting firsthand accounts of unusual events on and in the waters, from rogue waves to rivers running backward. Just as a passing note: if a mirage is an optical illusion in which it appears as though there is water where none really exists, then what would the illusion be called if you were on the water and it appeared as though land exists where none really was located? If this were actually to occur, what would it look like from under the water? One candidate might be a fata morgana. Look it up.

SENSES—IMAGINE SOME MORE

We have been taught that we have five senses. Try to imagine what it would be like to have more than five senses. Maybe we do have more than five senses and we don't know about them yet!

Imagine what other senses might be like. How about a sense of deep and lucid dreaming in which truths and wisdom emerge?

Another sense might be the ability to see things in a way that is different from others. For instance, everybody was saying that gravity is necessary to explain why things drop toward the center of the Earth or any other body with mass. Then along came Albert Einstein who developed a greater and wider realm of comprehension of the fundamental forces at play in the universe that helped explain phenomena like gravity in a way that enriches us. He saw the world in a different manner.

Another sense might be the capacity (ability) to be deeply attuned (listening to or aware of) to the feelings, values, life perspectives, worldviews, and sentiments of others. We become so encapsulated (held within the shell) in our own ways that we become defensive in response to the ways and experiences of others.

Another sense might be the passion (life energy), compassion, and wisdom for seeing what is necessary to foster (encourage, engender) life. One sense that you could develop over your life might be the gift of being able to see the damage that others are doing to life's interrelated web. We are all interrelated. We are all interdependent. Develop the sense of being able to see what is harming or limiting the life net or web. Also, develop the sense of what it is that is necessary to enhance (make more likely to thrive and live well) the life web. It is one thing to see what is wrong with something. It is another form of the gift to be able to sense and name what is needed and envision a practical means to accomplish this end.

Another sense is the capacity to envision (to see) alternatives for the future and imagine models that could crystallize communal energy related to transformation and growth. These models become avenues and ways of getting to that future. Combine a vision, a model, and inspiring energy and then alternative futures become actualized. This sense is the gift of taking dreams and providing the opportunities for human beings to make them real.

Another sense is that of seeing the need and means (how to) to live with all other forms of life instead of trying to control all other forms of life and the planet itself for our own ends, desires, and supposedly critical needs. What is it that can make us caring and responsible beings living cooperatively with all other life-forms on the planet? A sense of valuing life in all of its forms might be an emergent critical gift of humanity.

Another sense is the gift of being able to see things as a whole. Many people go around in life only seeing separate chunks of a larger whole. Then what we do is to say that this little piece of the whole is separate from the other pieces, and we try to defend it. This sense allows us to experience a larger framework in which we no longer have to believe that we are separate individuals in competition with each other, needing to use aggressive power as the primary means of surviving. See the wider, fuller picture of all life being interdependent. This sense could lead us into a new future.

Another sense is that of being able to see into the lives of other people (both those who appear to be similar and dissimilar to us) and to sense what we all have in common. A great gift is to be able to deeply sense the most profound (great) material and energy that we share in common. We all share diverse and wonderful things. With this sense of deep awareness of our common life, do we need to fear our diversity?

Another sense is to be able to intuit (deeply feel) the beauty and worth of human lives, ideas, sentiments, life experiences, feelings, and worldviews of those who are beyond the walls of our given community, culture, or society. These are the ones who not only live elsewhere, they live in each of our communities. They are the outcasts. They are the ones whom most people do not understand or accept. This is a sense that allows us to see vast realms of possibilities by living in a manner that has no need for the walls of fear and prejudice. Create further lists of other senses that are vital and important.

Extensions

Can you imagine that we human beings are just beginning to develop our capacities? One reason why peace and justice in the world are good things is that if the world were more stable and fair, more people would be able to experience the wonder of expanding human potential. This benefits the entire human community. As we give support to forms of deeply ingrained violence and as we deemphasize the importance of justice, we become unstable, we could annihilate the human race, and do even more damage to the Earth's ecology. Then our potential wouldn't have much of a chance to emerge. Compassion is the source for peace and justice. This peace and justice can give us the possibility of discovering the wider and greater realms of what is possible in life. One aspect of this compassion is the capacity to work toward more stable and life-affirming patterns of coexisting. Imagine all the people of the world being able to focus on their creativity and genius rather than survival. What could our world be like? Make note of the many things you believe we, as a human race, are capable of if we were to liberate our human spirits by making the world a more safe and secure place for all people.

SHAME

Have you ever felt ashamed? Usually this occurs because of something we've done that relates to something we believe about ourselves. I stole a billfold from a store when I was very young. I'm sure I didn't think of it as stealing. Perhaps I had seen too many Robin Hood movies. I simply acted on an impulse that I wanted something. When I got home, my Dad asked me where I got the billfold. I told him the truth because I felt so ashamed about having stolen something and I didn't want to start heaping lies upon lies. The larger values to which I compared this behavior were the values of honesty and integrity. I felt shame. Is shame always good? Is it always bad?

Extensions

What are the destructive forms of shame? Do some people use shame as a means of gaining power and authority over and against others? Is there a form of shame that doesn't have to do with something that we've done but has to do with a sense of whom we are? Might some people feel ashamed of being themselves because of destructive messages given to them by others or a persistent (constant) sense of being powerless? Be mindful of the ways that shame is used and be aware of its consequences.

SHAPE RETENTION

When things are stretched and they return to their original shape, what gives them the capacity to go back to their original shape? For instance, a balloon will go back to its original shape.

Extensions

What are examples of things that return to their shape when stretched within certain limits but when stretched too much they fail to return to their original shape? How are springs made? What gives things this quality of elasticity?

SHE'S ALIVE?

Is the Earth itself living? Look up the definitions of what qualities constitute life. (*See* "Life—What Makes the Difference?") Does the Earth match these criteria? Look up the word *Gaia*. Some persons have named the Earth Gaia for the belief that the Earth is a living organism.

Extensions

Is the universe alive? We had better stop there. Your encyclopedia may not cover this topic. Tell your librarian that you believe that the universe breathes. The person will be glad to help you to the door out of the library. If you can't find such answers in standard libraries, where are the nonstandard libraries of the world? They exist! What is another name of library? Where are alternative databases, sources of information, and wisdom? Never judge a librarian by the person's cover. One of them might be just the perfect person to help you find the rate of the heartbeat of the universe and how often it breathes. Find a research expert who is great with metaphors. Learn to cultivate awareness and use of metaphors.

One reason for this is because your use of the language will be more effective. Another reason is that metaphors are a means of experiencing larger fields of comprehension, wisdom, and insight. Those who are fluid in their use of metaphors and highly adaptive in their comprehension of the place of metaphors are the ones who are able to be conversant with many different frameworks of understanding. This person is most likely to be very flexible and adaptable.

SHINING LIGHTS OF THE COMMUNITY

Think of all the people you've known who have selflessly given so much of their time in service to others. These people have sacrificed so that the lives of others can be better. Years after I had gone to college and moved on in life and career, I thought about the choir director in my church. My parents had communicated to me that she was quite ill. I decided to write her a letter and tell her all that she meant to me. She wrote back one of the most beautiful letters that was filled with gratitude that I had remembered her. She soon died. I was thankful and always will be thankful that I took the time to thank her and express my gratitude for her countless hours and years of service. Who are the shining lights in your community who help make the life of the community better?

Extensions

Take the time to express your thanks today to somebody who has given of him- or herself and made a difference in the lives of others. Don't wait. Do it now. Follow your heart and really let him or her know what you feel. You may be the first person to thank him or her from the heart. Formal recognition events are one thing. Plaques are nice. A personal thanks is worth its weight in gold.

SHOCK WAVES

How fast do shock waves travel under the water? Do the waves we see on top of the water travel at the same rate as the waves under the water? Can you see the waves moving through the water from underneath the surface? If you were in perfectly clear and still water, could you see an approaching shock wave? What do you imagine it would look like?

Extensions

Does the bulk of the actual water of the wave on the surface move? If it does move, in which directions do you think it moves? Because some of the water may move in a certain direction that is easy to see, do we assume that the bulk of the water is moving in the same direction? If the water is not flowing, what is flowing? What is it that is moving? Could you weigh or measure the stuff that is flowing? Could you have five pounds of it or one cup of it?

SIGHT—TO SEE THE UNSEEN

Imagine yourself to have the power to make your vision microscopic. You can now choose any power of magnification. Zoom down to the size of hairs, then tiny little fragments of things like the small particle on the back of a dust mite. Then zoom down to molecules. Then of course go to atoms. Does the entire scene look like what we imagine the universe looks like? Then zoom into the nuclei of the atoms. There are quarks. Oh oh, are there things smaller than quarks? You can zoom into the heart of infinity. What do you find there? It is something much different than we normally imagine.

Imagine being able to change to any magnitude of vision. What would be the opposite of microscopic vision? If you could see macroscopically, imagine seeing your entire county all at once. Next, imagine seeing your entire state at once. You could watch the entire continent at once. You could see the whole world from one point of view. You could see the entire solar system, or galaxy, or entire universe at once. If you could see the entire universe at once, where would you be located—in space or beyond space? If you could see infinity, could you find your way home again? Now imagine switching your point of view instantly back to the infinitely small view. Would there be a huge difference?

Now imagine that you can slow time down or speed time up. If you slow time down, you'd begin to notice patterns that you had never seen before, things that normally might occur frequently or regularly but very quickly might take on an appearance. It would appear as though these patterns came right out of nowhere. If you increase the speed of time, things that don't move would suddenly take on life, motion, and character. How would fast-moving things appear? Might there be some interesting patterns arising in the blur of the superfast-moving objects? These would be the things that occur slowly, irregularly, and infrequently. Maybe we'd begin to see some things in the blur that actually appear to be standing still. These might be patterns that occur all the time, but our senses and technical equipment can't detect these patterns.

Now imagine that you can see things from one or as many points of view as you want at the same time. Three-dimensional stuff is boring after this experience. Take any one object like the Earth and try to imagine seeing it from all angles at once. Now imagine seeing the entire universe from all angles at once.

Now, for the real treat. Imagine seeing with any of these combinations of gifts: time slowed down macroscopically from a hundred points of view; Time speeded up with microscopic view from an infinity of views.

Now imagine that you can sense the presence of all of these things without vision. You can sense growth, changes in texture, color, sound, ideas, feelings, smell, taste, thermal differences, and motion on all levels from the infinitely small to the infinitely large.

Extensions

Have interesting dreams tonight. Try to remember them. After you've finished a dream inspired by such thoughts, get up and write it down. Even if this occurs at 2:38 A.M., get up and write it down. If somebody just happens to ask what you were doing at 2:38 A.M., just tell them you're letting your genius out. They'll fully understand.

SIGNALS—BEAMING IN ONE DIRECTION

Wherever you live, assume that you have a radio transmitter capable of sending signals around the world. If your signal is a low enough frequency, it bounces your signal up against the ionosphere and it bounces back to Earth. This bouncing process continues until the energy of the signal transmission is dissipated (spent, worn out, runs out of energy, or goes kaput). If your frequency is high enough, the signal is sent straight out. It doesn't bounce off the ionosphere or the Earth, it just keeps going. You want your signal to be sent from the highest place available, with the greatest power, at a low angle relative to the horizon.

Have you ever had the experience of AM radio stations coming in from great distances at nighttime? AM radio transmissions are bounced off the ionosphere and the Earth. The conditions are optimal (best) at nighttime. Research this issue. Why is this so? What is in the ionosphere that allows for radio signals to bounce off it? How do they bounce off the Earth? Research the dynamics of reflection for any electromagnetic wave. Specifically, be looking for the angle of incidence and the angle of reflection to begin with.

Now assume that from your point of origin you wish to send your signal to some point of reception due east. Look at a flat map and pick any city or place on the same latitude as your own. Then look at a globe. If you send the signal directly at the city, will it get there? There are 360° (degrees) in a complete circle. Assume that 0° is due north, 90° is due east, 180° is due south, and 270° is due west. Assume you send your radio signal due 90°. Select a site at least a quarter of the way around the world.

Look out your window and look what is 90° from your present position. That signal keeps bouncing up and down in a straight line at precisely 90°. If you sent your signal at exactly 90° on a flat surface, the destination would be precisely where you pointed.

Now look at a globe of the Earth. The Earth is curved (curvilinear). It is handy to notice such things as the curvature of the Earth if you are traveling long distances. Will your signal get to your destination if it is sent at exactly

90°? Look carefully at a globe and trace your finger on the course described above. See what happens. If your signal sent originally at 90° remains traveling in a precise straight line (while bouncing up and down off the Earth and the ionosphere), this line is straight relative to a flat plane. Everything on the Earth is curving away from the projected line. Hold a pencil with the eraser located at the point of origin of the signal. It points exactly 90° east. The Earth keeps curving away from the line demarcated (described) by the pencil. This line of latitude that runs through your present location is following the curved surface of the Earth. Your pencil is not following this same path. How are radio signals directed so that they get someplace that appears to be 90° from your location? Hint: there are special maps for sending radio transmissions. Find out what kind of maps they are. Who else uses these kinds of maps other than radio signal senders? With the aid of these maps (or databases), if you want to send a signal to a location due east (or any other direction), you can't send it on the path the needle of the compass points to. You have to make adjustments for the curvature of the Earth.

Extensions

There are many places on the Earth from where you could send a radio signal due west or due east and it would get to your location precisely at 90°(east) or precisely at 270° (west). These places are located on land and water.

From the geographic North Pole, could you send a signal north, east, or west? From the geographic South Pole, could you send a signal south, east, or west? If you were to move one foot from either pole, could you send a signal east, west, north, or south?

SILENT OBSERVER—OUR BEST FRIEND

One of the most startling insights of my life took place right after I had gotten my finger smashed by a closing door. Up until that moment, as a youngster, I assumed that if I were to be physically hurt, the natural and only reaction was to be angry and upset. As the pain was beginning to rise, there was a serene (peaceful) insight that arose within me which gently, clearly, and with great power revealed, "Your body is experiencing pain. You are at peace. Be still." It was like it was out of nowhere! It was so real that I remember it clearly now in my middle years.

This was my first encounter with this silent observing within us. This is not magic, psychic, or supernatural. It is a simple and natural presence within each of us. Call it pure awareness. We are in touch with our environment (internal feelings and ideas) and exterior world of others and nature in an immediate spontaneous way. Our core essential self is always serene, focused, concentrated, and observant. It is our internal teacher. This is our deepest and truest self. It can be stunning when we first encounter this deeper layer of identity.

How could there be something at peace within us when the world around us is so frenetic (fast paced) and demanding?

We often mask this still, silent observing by implanting within ourselves different impressions based on prior experience. Often these impressions are things told to us by others who are important to us. Sometimes these impressions are associated with strong feeling tones. They can become very convincing. We can start to interpret every present moment in light of these past impressions.

These can be impressions of self-confidence that make us feel able to meet the challenges of living, or they can also be impressions that make us feel small, unimportant, or not able to meet the challenges of life.

What happens is that these impressions rise up within us before we have time to really examine them. In circumstances that are related in some manner to past experiences, we cultivate (encourage) these impressions:

- I can do this.
- I can't do this.
- I feel great about myself.
- I feel terrible about myself.
- I feel curious about these interesting and intriguing circumstances.
- I feel overwhelmed by this situation.
- I understand this challenge, and I am confident enough to engage the challenge.
- I don't understand everything about these things that are being talked about so I feel stupid.
- What the other person is communicating is complex, and if I concentrate, I will get it.
- I will shut down and not listen anymore because I am feeling anxious and insecure.
- What I don't understand will be an area of interesting inquiry.
- What I don't understand is stupid anyway.
- I know who I am and I love who I am.
- Others are calling me names and they must be right.

These impressions are constantly swelling up within us. We react to them. This reactive energy prevents us from directly experiencing this inner still part of our humanity that is always in all things and always observing with great clarity. It is the source of all creativity. These impressions are the result of our conditioning. They are our habits and tendencies to which we become attached and even dependent. When we experience them, we are often not even aware that we are labeling ourselves and limiting our options. We can train ourselves to be aware when these kinds of impressions are affecting us. In order to deal with them, we need an inner core sense of self that is not dependent upon these impressions.

There is a deeper and truer self. It can be called the center of conscience, intuition, reflection, true voice, inner voice, deepest and most important self, or your best friend. It is always with you. It is still and quiet. You need to learn to listen for it. Once you do learn to be aware of it, your life will forever be richer and more complete. You can learn to become more aware of your deepest resources for creativity and self-confidence. This still, quiet observing gives you endless power to see the play of your feelings, ideas, perceptions, values, intuitions, conditioning, prime assumptions, and life priorities.

Just as important, this still, quiet observing allows us the possibility of creative transformation (change). No matter what has occurred in our lives, nothing—absolutely nothing—keeps us locked into our past. Vast intention, creativity, intelligence, and compassion arise from this astounding center of our lives. What is amazing is that we can miss it entirely and so easily be ignorant of its presence by being absorbed in our conditioning, habits, tendencies, reactions, and attachment to the past. Through this center of awareness, we can become attuned to (mindful of) what it is that we are attached to, dependent upon, absorbed in, associated with, resonating with, and identified with. In any moment, we can observe how we are engaging life. This amazing discovery allows us to deal with the fundamental assumptions of our lives.

A power to be fully alive and responsible for what we do with our lives is released and made available to us. This capacity ought to astonish us. We can never get tired of this gift. Don't try slamming a door on your finger in order to have this experience! Simply learn to observe your inner workings, movements of thought and feeling, and actions. There will come a moment in which you discover this place within yourself that is always absolutely still and alert. You are able to directly experience this amazing gift.

When these various impressions arise inside of you telling you what is real, you have another source of strength and creativity—this is your deepest peaceful self. As you are saying things to others, have you ever wished you had said things differently? As we become more aware of ourselves, we can see ourselves in a new way. If you're feeling bored in a class or meeting, you can observe yourself being bored and change your perceptions, how you value the situation, or how you are defining the circumstances. If you are beginning to get angry, you can see yourself becoming angry and eventually come to know why you are becoming angry. If you are becoming very creative, you can be aware that you need to become attentive and believe in yourself (have the self-confidence to explore new things).

A clear awareness of these impressions and the presence of the deepest self can add to our flexibility and adaptability in life. Little things we tell ourselves can convince us that we are capable or incapable of meeting the challenges of the moment. Little impressions that sneak up on us can tell us that we are good or bad, bright or dumb, likable or unlikable, lovable or unlovable, attractive or unattractive, happy or sad, loving or hateful, and curious or bored. What is important is the capacity to see ourselves reacting to these various impressions.

Then when we are aware of them, we can act on them. We can then commence (begin) to be proactive (acting in creative and productive ways). We can see that we are able to respond to all life challenges from this place of inner stillness and creativity. This response is vastly different from the fearful reactions that all too often engulf and govern our lives.

The deepest inner self watches what we are telling ourselves. It is an undisturbed observation of what is growing, changing, and evolving in the present moment. We become deeply self-aware.

The little voices are things we tell ourselves that are habits we fall into and then come to depend upon. They convince us that things are a certain way. The deepest peaceful self simply offers us the gift of freshness, intention, spontaneity, creativity, compassion, and deep resources of human energy. Rise to the challenge of becoming more aware of the many and constant messages we experience about who we are and what our place in the world is. Wisdom will be revealed to you. Enjoy the presence of your deepest self that is beautiful and creative. Playfully enjoy the peaceful way of existing. It is liberating to be free from the massive load of reactive energy.

Extensions

List circumstances in which you are becoming aware of the presence of different kinds of impressions that result in messages about who you are. Keep a journal relating to the experiences of this inner, still, silent power of observation.

SIMPLISTIC AND SIMPLE

Have your ever listened to somebody explain something and it seemed childish or too simple for you? For instance, if you ask somebody how babies come into the world and somebody talks about a stork delivering them to the house, you might feel as though you are receiving an explanation that is too simplistic (or sarcastic).

As we become aware of the presence of wisdom, we come to value and appreciate thoughtful and heartfelt explanations of things that are beautiful, attractive, widely applicable (having relevance to a wide variety of life circumstances), and simple. Some explanations get so complicated that they begin to fall apart, cease to have explanatory power, or cease to have attractiveness or usefulness.

We can develop the art of looking for simple explanations. Some people have a tendency to look for unlikely and complicated explanations for everything. Keep the basics simple so you have the ability to put simple building blocks together later and assemble models and views that help you understand things that are more complex. Think of something that is quite complex and come up with a simple description of it (graphic, verbal, poetry, song—any way you can describe it). See how many relatively simple ways you can describe the same complex thing. This is a great challenge that takes much insight into the dynamics of communication. Simplifying something without making it simplistic is an art. As you learn to succeed in this venture, you may discover that you are more able to:

- understand complex issues in an integrated fashion
- effectively explore areas of detail because you can locate the right questions to ask and identify the domain (area) of issues you need to explore
- identify groupings of issues and how they interrelate
- comprehend the subtleties (nuances, less obvious important qualities) and distinctions more clearly
- explore side issues without getting lost in a forest of details with no map as to how to get back home (too many bright and creative people get lost in endless tangents—side trips)
- foster (create) a learning environment in which distinctions can be made between what is simplistic and misleading versus what is simplified and enlightening
- have greater access to a wider range of complex challenges
- more effectively communicate among members of a group working on a multidimensional project that requires people from many discipline areas working in synchrony (coordinated)
- reach a wider audience more effectively and efficiently
- effectively use persuasion because others are more able to see and identify with what you are talking about
- participate in the creation of group consensus because communication is enhanced
- help others absorb material in such a manner that their learning process is enhanced, encouraged, and internalized with decreased dependence upon you qua (as) interpreter

Extensions

Try to figure out how to describe something to somebody who has never had the capacity to experience this thing directly—like trying to describe a lightbulb emitting light to a person who has been blind from birth, or music to a person who has been deaf from birth. What are some other examples similar to these two? What are things you've never experienced that might be difficult for somebody to describe to you? I recall one time when some cousins of mine came to visit us and I was shocked that they had never seen snow before. There are things in our experience base that can help us relate to descriptions of new experiences.

SIZES OF STUFF

Have some fun with creating images of the comparative size of things:

- If an atom were the size of a pea, a baseball would be the size of . . .

- If the Milky Way galaxy were the size of a grapefruit, the universe would be the size of . . .
- If the sun were the size of an inflated beach ball, the Earth would be the size of . . .
- If the time elapsed for the age of the universe were equal to one hour, Earth's existence would be . . .
- If the time elapsed for all living creatures were one hour, the length of time since the emergence of the first creature with sight would be . . .

Extensions

What are other units of measurement that can be compared to each other? Try weight, density, friction, mass (not the same as weight), visual acuity, color discrimination, speed, acceleration, velocity, momentum, taste, smell, touch, sound, sight, happiness, peace, hate, love, fear, or courage. A unit is something that can be measured. How could nonmathematical human experiences (nonquantifiable experiences) like courage be compared with other experiences? There are examples of persons who have one sense absent in their lives, but they adjust by increasing their sensitivity in other realms. In addition, these people report that they can imagine the missing sense impression in different ways.

SLANG WORDS

All people use slang terms of some kind. What is slang? Watch any movie and list the slang words used. List as many slang terms as you can. Which of these are "foreign words?" Have you ever heard of the following words and phrases: that's just jim-dandy, everything's hunky-dory, that's jiffy, double whammy, kibosh, kit and caboodle, off-kilter, noggin, kaput, okeydokey, the road takes a dog leg? List the slang words that you can think of. Is there such a thing as standard slang and nonstandard slang?

Extensions

What is the difference between words that are jargon, slang, obscene, vulgar, and profane? If somebody becomes upset with me asking such a question, please remember that our children and youth are exposed and immersed in all these forms of language whether we like it or not. No matter how shielded adults try to make their offspring, all these forms of language emerge in the shared words of our youth. This happens in every culture throughout the ages. Sometimes the most highly shielded children and youth are the best versed in such words without their parents finding out. These are real-world language terms and knowing the differences can empower us all. (Knowing the distinctions is not the same thing as attempting to cultivate and use all the terms.) Also, knowing the distinctions can allow us to use language that reflects our values in life.

SMOOTH EARTH

Because the Earth spins at approximately one thousand miles per hour at the equator, do you think this might affect the directions of the winds? Learn about the prevailing winds in different sections of the world.

Extensions

Where are the jet streams located? How do they fluctuate? How does the jet stream change course, and how does its speed affect the weather?

SOAP

Soap is a dispersant (disperses things on any given surface). How does it work? It is made of material with long chains of carbon atoms. One end of the chain binds to water and the other end bind to oils. Thus, bodies are cleaned. Look up *surfactant*.

Extensions

What is the difference between a soap and detergent? When so many of the detergents claim to be concentrated (more value per unit of the product), is there a practical easy way to test these claims? If three different detergents come in half-gallon containers, how do we know which one is the most concentrated one? This is important because the prices vary so much between the products. Is concentration directly related to the effectiveness of the product? If we are examining various liquid detergents, are the ones that pour more slowly (more viscous, or greater viscosity) necessarily more concentrated and more effective?

Ever notice the difference between various brands of shampoos? Some lather up real well with just a little shampoo. Others require much more shampoo in order to get the right amount of lather. What is lather?

SOFT DRINKS

Coca-Cola did not start out as a soft drink marketed just for its flavor! In May 1886, Atlanta druggist and former Confederate officer John S. Pemberton created a mixture of stuff in a brass kettle. He cooked it over a backyard fire. He wanted to create a nonalcoholic tonic. It was called "Intellectual Beverage and Temperance Drink." It was marketed as a medicine that was able to cure headaches. It was a brain and nerve tonic that would cure "all nervous afflictions—Headache, Neuralgia, Hysteria, Melancholy, Etc." It came in a green, pint-sized bottle of syrup. It was supposed to be mixed with water. It included the African kola nut and coca leaves—both stimulants. It contained a trace of cocaine that was then a legal drug. It was considered a substitute for alcohol.

By 1903, they stopped using cocaine. A clerk mixed the syrup with soda water and it caught on.

Extensions

Look up some other popular drinks and see if any of them started out as "medicines."

SOMEBODY LIVES HERE

Have members of your family ever referred to "somebody" when they are wondering where something is? For example: Somebody used up the sugar! Somebody put the keys someplace! Somebody didn't put the orange juice away last night! Somebody is in trouble over this mess! Usually a person is looking at someone else, when this term *somebody* is used. Does somebody live in your home?

Extensions

Is it usually easier to blame somebody else than to take responsibility for our actions? Is it easier to blame others for something we participated in (even if it was just a minor little squeaky-clean role)?

One time when I was in the attic of our house, I reached up and into a recess where the roof met the top of the vertical wall of the house. I pulled out a book. Somebody had left it there about forty years before when this other somebody was a child like me roaming around a large house exploring. This somebody was my father. So sometimes things happen because somebody did something a long time ago. There may be a somebody in your house.

SPECIAL TERRITORIES?

Is there any land within the United States of America that is not located in one of the fifty states? Before you glance down for an answer, try to imagine some body of land within the borders of the United States that is outside of the normal geopolitical boundaries. Look up protectorates, territories, and Washington D.C.

Extensions

Are there any kingdoms or have there ever been any kingdoms with in the United States of America since its birth as a nation?

Yes—the Kingdom of Fulton located in Missouri. Also, look up what happened on Beaver Island in Lake Michigan. Just because a kingdom was declared, does that make it a kingdom? There may have been more kingdoms. Find them.

SPECKS THAT MATTER

A scientist claims that he has found the first speck (small piece) of the asteroid that hit the Earth 65 million years ago and destroyed up to 70 percent of the species of plants and animals on the Earth that time. The asteroid was possibly about six miles in diameter. How could something so large hitting the Earth just disappear?

Extensions

If you could find a speck of something from the past, what would it be?

SPINNING WHEELS IN REVERSE

Look at the wheels of other moving cars as they pass you or as you pass them. Have you ever noticed that sometimes the wheels appear to be moving backward? Why?

Extensions

Our eyes report data to the brain. The brain processes these data and forms composite pictures of the scene being observed. Under what other conditions do things appear to be something, but out there in reality we know they are not actually what they appear to be? For example, mirages—are they what they appear to be? List as many experiences of illusion as you can think of. Get a group doing this project. How do we know that what appears to us is an illusion? Sometimes might a mirage be an unexpected real puddle?

Imagine a world in which oranges smelled like pumpkins, dogs sounded like cats, sandpaper felt like soft fur, what is right-side-up appeared upside-down, and milk tasted like orange pop. All these things can happen if certain neurological connections in our brain are not connected in a normal fashion. The brain is extremely complex. If the brain becomes deprived of oxygen, we start to see many kinds of hallucinations that seem totally real. Is the mountain in the distance at sunset purple? Is it purple because of the sunlight playing with the atmosphere? Is it purple because our brains tell us that it is purple? If we woke up in the morning and the mountain was still purple, would we think that we were in a dream? All we can do in life is to continue testing what is real and what is not real. If we see the mountain as purple, isn't it the case that the mountain absorbed all the other colors and reflects back only purple? Then isn't the mountain all the other colors except the one we see?

There is such a thing as shared reality, but we need to continually refine our perceptions and judgments. Reality is formed in part by our senses. Reality is also something we create by our social assumptions. For instance, if you were raised in a household in which it was taught that people of other races, religions, or economic circumstances were inferior or dangerous, would you have the courage to continue testing what reality truly is? List as many assumptions as you can that you hold about other people. Then question yourself about how you have ever tested these assumptions.

SPIRALING INTO INFINITY

The following section is composed of mostly factual material. Some of the material represents intellectual ruminations (reflective ideas that are beyond the territory of observable and proven phenomena).

Science fiction movies made in the 1950s and 1960s sometimes depicted (portrayed) time machines as devices hung on the wall that had large black-and-white spirals rotating around its center. The people would jump into the spiral and then be sucked into the center where the spiral's lines get tighter and smaller. Finally, the person reaches the black hole and is whisked away on a journey into time. Imagine that you jumped into one of these 1950s time machines and you are traveling inside a spiral. Of course, you might prefer a more modern version of a time machine so you could take along your headphones.

From the perspective of an observer back on Earth, the closer you get to the speed of light and the closer you get to the black hole, it appears as if time is slowing down. Thus, it appears to you as though you never ever get there. It appears as though your arc (light being bent because of the presence of a massive body) and your time never quite get to the event horizon (edge) of the black hole. It appears as though the closer to the speed of light you are, the greater your curvature and time progressively become slower. From the view of others in a nonaccelerated state, you never get there. They think you're stuck. What they observe is a process of you spreading out as you approach the event horizon (boundary) of the black hole. They start to get worried whether or not you're staying in good shape. Sit-ups and push-ups just don't help.

To the people in nonlight-accelerated positions, space appears to be noncurved but light seems to be arcing or curving, which violates a basic principle that light travels in straight lines. Since this violation can't be tolerated, certain geniuses created the explanation of curvilinear space. You have now discovered, from your perspective of an almost light-accelerated body, that light always travels the shortest distance between two points. The trajectory you're on is called your world line. This is not a line through space (as seen from the observer's perspective). This startles you greatly. Your world line is in space-time. From the perspective of the nonaccelerated observer, it appears as though you are traveling through space. You discover this is not the case. Your world line is a geodesic. This is a fancy term for the line you're traveling within space-time that is curved if there is any object with mass close by. You look around you and observe very astutely (keenly, intelligently) that there is a black hole right in front of you. From this observation, you brilliantly deduce that your world line may be slightly bent (relative to the perspective of those in nonlight-accelerated positions). You begin to comprehend space-time from this accelerated framework. It amazes you that bodies do not just fly through empty space. Space is not curvilinear from the light-accelerated perspective, because you are not in empty space. It is space-time that is curvilinear.

Your world line is a geodesic that is always the shortest distance between two points. Earth is the point of departure, and the point of singularity at the core of the black hole is your destination. Your world line is taking you there directly in the shortest possible geodesic. From your framework, you are approaching the event horizon of the black hole with great speed. You now have reached the event horizon.

Light continues to come at you from the outside, but it is severely distorted in terms of space and time. This space at the event horizon of the black hole extends in all directions in a two-dimensional space for infinity. What happened to the third dimension and to time? Your wristwatch begins to act a little weird. Then you start to get hungry, and you begin to wonder just how big your appetite is.

This event horizon is a boundary or limit. No light or information can proceed from the black hole beyond this "place." It is the surface through which light and information from the rest of the universe are absorbed. Boundaries and limits are like no other places. This particular limit or boundary can be thought of as expanding at the speed of light and as being stationary at the same time. It depends on how one constructs one's framework for understanding these nifty black holes. They are not like your familiar backyard. You are able to see the outside coming to you, but you only see it in a radically spatial and time-distorted form. This distortion is so great that, in essence, the outside is not another dimension from our perspective. At the event horizon, you are in a two-dimensional boundary situation.

If you were to telephone home and you were asked what kind of mess you were in, you'd have a difficult time explaining this one. Your cell phone doesn't work quite right here either. Your problems don't end there. As you turn around (if you can figure out how to squiggle around in two-dimensional space, especially as your mass is infinite), you will look in the other direction. You see nothing but a void or blackness because of the infinitely small and dense point of singularity at the core of the black hole acting on everything within the event horizon. You feel as though you've reached the limits of your understanding and patience. Both your ability to understand what is going on in this strange place and your willingness to stick around here are being stretched very thin.

Being at the limit or boundary place causes you to discover some more interesting things. This is not a place at all. From the perspective of an outside observer, it is a theoretical construct (a necessary idea) and has no real dimensionality. The boundary is a one-way portal. You can enter but you can't exit. This is the oddity of this limit or boundary. Outside the event horizon or boundary, light and information can escape from the black hole, but the closer a body is to the event horizon the more energy it takes to escape. Precisely at the event horizon, it would take infinite energy or speeds greater than the speed of light to escape the black hole.

This limit or boundary can't be three-dimensional. From the perspective of the outside observer, you can't ever quite get there (asymptotic—never converging). From the perspective of the black hole, information or light can never get out or beyond its own limits. You realize that this situation for you is worse than being caught between a rock and a hard place.

You are startled to discover that the boundary is both infinite and nonexistent. Space and time coordinates are severely deranged (upset). You can't see out. At this boundary, what is seen of the inside is a void (nothing). The implication of this insight boggles your mind. You change your mind and want to go home for some cookies, but you can't get there from here. You remember the smell of fresh-baked cookies. You only have one of them left. This one has become a real whopper! There are only two problems (relative to the issue of the all-important cookies). You can't go back where they are made, and you discover that these cookies have infinite mass (because they've accelerated to the speed of light). Now everyone knows that cookies with infinite mass taste different. That's for a cookbook that will be published later. A third problem arises. How do you eat a two-dimensional cookie with infinite mass?

Matter, energy, mass, space-time, light, and information outside the event horizon are completely governed by the four known forces in space-time (electromagnetism, weak, strong, and gravity). Once any of this matter, energy, mass, space-time, light, or information has reached the event horizon and passed through this boundary, then the same forces of space-time are still at play, but inevitably their influence is weakening. Any matter, energy, mass, space-time, light, or information inside the event horizon will absolutely be pulled toward and into the point of singularity at the core of the black hole. From outside the point of singularity, you assume that you will be pulled inside of it. It looks like you are racing toward it. Actually, you start to realize it is racing at you at the speed of light. Big surprises await you.

The distortion of space-time eventually becomes so pronounced that the coordinate t for time and the coordinate r for the radius (distance from the edge of a sphere to its center point) are transformed. The t coordinate is transformed to represent something spacelike and the r coordinate becomes timelike instead of representing the distance to the center. You look at your body and wonder what kind of diet you need to go on next. "Gotta" stop eating those cookies with almost infinite mass! Maybe it's just the butter. This ends that matter, but then again, in this black hole, all matter and matters are different.

While on this inevitable course toward the point of singularity, the matter, energy, mass, space-time, light, and information progressively become distorted and transformed by the laws governing the point of singularity. Even your belly button is acting a little strange in this place. You start getting used to having two very different frames of reference held in your mind at the same time: the point of singularity is being approached, and it is approaching you. It seems odd, but you are comfortable with this array of frameworks.

As we approach this point of singularity, we realize that nothing is static. We are changing dramatically. Space, time, and our own body are changing. Everything is changing so much that we begin to understand that space and time were the very qualities that encouraged us to assume that there are static structures upon which we can predicate (base) our sense of identity, security, and reality. With space and time changing so dramatically, it's as though covers have been removed from our eyes of understanding. We comprehend that all things are forever in all ways changing. Everything is an interconnected process of change. At first, this scares and confuses us very deeply. The great teachable "moment" arrives when we are inevitably confronted with the issue of the boundary of the point of singularity.

If we thought the event horizon or boundary was strange, the surface of the point of singularity is even stranger. The boundary of the point of singularity is not two-dimensional. There is no boundary! The point of singularity is a surface-surfaceless entity. It's really there, but it's not there at all! It is something substantial, yet it is a void. There is no sudden point of transition for any matter, energy, mass, space-time, light, or information any more. This point of singularity doesn't have its own event horizon. All things are in process, but there is a point at which you realize that no laws of the space-time continuum are affecting matter, energy, mass, space-time, light, or information. Then you become aware that not only are you in the domain of the point of singularity, but those things you once called matter, energy, mass, space-time, light, or information are all distorted so much that you can't identify any of them by their former names. This realization comes to you, but it was not because you've passed any point in time or space. You're on your own. This did not happen at one surface area. It didn't occur at one point. You wonder how you missed this transition.

If you're a body inside that event horizon of a black hole, nothing is going to survive the entry into the point of singularity. But then again, we really don't know that. Nobody has ever taken out a two-way ticket. Everything becomes infinitely transformed, dense, and different—we presume. At least pretend that you're still alive. Then you remember that some of our latest research indicates that information about you, oddly enough, is stored at the event horizon in some kind of weirdly preserved quantum field. Just when you are trying to remember what a quantum field is, your mind turns inevitably to food. It turns out that those cookies with infinite mass helped preserve your body as an exception to everything else in the universe. You tell yourself, "I can't believe it really wasn't the butter." Your parents always told you that you were an exceptional child. Now you have the proof, but there is nobody to share it with. Now exceptional means singular, without a second. You wish you had one more second back there out of this place. Since there is no time as conceived in the universe outside the event horizon of the black hole, you have no second. Now you really know what it means to be without a second. How exceptional! You continue onward. You might as well since you have no choice at this point but to continue.

You discover that the surface of the point of singularity is actually surfaceless. There never was a crossing point over and into this point of singularity. You realize there is no here and there inside the point of singularity. What is theorized to be a point of infinitely small space has nothing to do whatsoever with space as conceived from the space-time perspective. The forces of nature become inverted. Space-time and gravity no longer support matter, energy, or mass. Space-time and gravity become the hidden qualities. What are apparent are the superstrings, foam, bubbles, and knots of reality. Since this is the case, there is no outer limit to the point of singularity from the perspective of being inside of it. An inversion of the basic forces at play becomes apparent but there is no boundary. There is no "here" and there is no "now." Time and space become hidden qualities.

You are sensing you are still alive or at least you convince yourself you are still alive. Then you realize the meaning of the phrase "all dimensions are a unified whole." There aren't multiple dimensions whatsoever. This point of singularity is not separate and set apart from the space-time continuum. Then you really get surprised because you realize that these superstrings, foam, bubbles, and knots are connected to each other everywhere. Everywhere is nowhere relative to experience from within the space-time continuum.

These superstrings, foam, bubbles, and knots are the substratum (underlying qualities of the universe) that makes it possible for space-time, gravity, mass, matter, energy, and life to exist at all. These superstrings, foam, bubbles, and knots create the field within which space-time emerges. What appears to be an infinitely small point of singularity is the source for what manifests as the field within which space-time and all of its forces exist. They are the background source for the inexplicable appearance of virtual particles that race through space-time in such short time intervals that they do not violate the laws of space-time. You remember how you used to think that quarks were strange (or charmed, depending on which one you're thinking about). Oh, for the good old days!

Then you realize one of the most stunning insights: the universe is in harmony with itself. Harmony doesn't mean that there aren't major transformations. Harmony means that all aspects of the universe interact with each other. While these superstrings, foam, bubbles, and knots are the substratum for space-time, harmony indicates to us that space-time itself is the substratum for these superstrings, foam, bubbles, and knots. That insight blows you away, but since the power of the point of singularity is so great, you stay on course. Then you laugh out loud because you realize that the term "course" no longer has any meaning. From the perspective of these superstrings, foam, bubbles, and knots, space-time is infinitely small, infinitely large, or nonexistent. From the perspective of space-time, these superstrings, foam, bubbles, and knots are infinitely small, infinitely large, or nonexistent. From either perspective, the other domain is infinitely small because it is smaller than the smallest imaginable thing. The other domain is infinitely large because it is all interconnected and it is everywhere. The other domain is nonexistent because it can't be measured or detected directly. The apparent or surface-level reality (surface with tremendous depth) can't know its own substratum directly (on its own terms). You wish things could be different, but that doesn't change the way things are.

The boundaries of these two domains are twofold. There is an event horizon and then there is something equivalent to a point of singularity. The event horizon is where one of the domain's laws starts to take over. These are windowless boundaries because the distortions of one's domain are infinitely great from one perspective; toward the other "direction," there is a void. This is why the event horizons are forever two-dimensional, infinite in extent, and yet nowhere. "Beyond" the event horizon of each domain, there is something analogous (equivalent) to a point of singularity that is a surface-surfaceless entity. From either direction beyond the event horizon, inevitably one will be drawn into its own laws.

Each domain or realm has its own kind of event horizon within which the deeply interrelated but uniquely different laws progressively meld one into the other. From the perspective of each domain, it appears as though nothing escapes, once something has gone to the event horizon of the complementary domain. From the perspective of space-time, the event horizon of a black hole can never be crossed twice because nothing can go faster than the speed of light. From the perspective of the infinite domain composed of superstrings, foam, bubbles, and knots, the event horizon of space-time can never be crossed twice because once these superstrings, foam, bubbles, and knots cross the event horizon of space-time, they are transmitted as virtual particle pairs that almost always instantly annihilate each other. This self-annihilation is necessary because of the laws governing space-time. Occasionally, one of these pairs is separated because one of the pair is annihilated and the other escapes this fate. The two can never return to that time or space to be paired up again and jump across the event horizon of space-time and reenter the domain of superstrings, foam, bubbles, and knots. Also, this realm composed of and governed by superstrings, foam, bubbles, and knots causes the bulging of space-time itself. The expansion of space-time comes from nowhere relative to its own laws. This is something like the hidden mass of the universe, except that mass is not a reality in this domain. This nowhere is the complementary substratum. Only from a limited perspective do they appear to be separate domains. They are essentially interrelated because they are each the substratum to the other.

A great paradox emerges. Things really start to get interesting now. If these are one-way event horizons, how can the two domains be in an essential and ongoing interrelationship? This gets back to the point that the mind that tries to comprehend great things is always riddled. Riddles are paradoxes, conundrums (unanswered problems), and riddles are *scotomas* (Greek for holes in our understanding). These holes are the gateways into which we can take the leap of the genius. They are not shortcomings or limitations. They are opportunities. They appear, to those who need to stay inside certain boxes, to be limitations. The issue of one-way event horizons is an opportunity for somebody to explore. This is a great paradox. The greatest paradox is that we can safely presume that there will always be more riddles as soon as we turn our attention to great questions. Only when we are satisfied with our current box of existence do the riddles disappear. Riddles that have been resolved can be held in static suspension as long as we only deal with inconsequential or small riddles and questions. Leaps of comprehension can inevitably open us up to the existence of yet greater riddles in a wider plane of understanding.

The greatest quest is for the unending unfolding of wider and deeper truths. Where there are riddles, there is growth and the fullness of life. Where there are riddles, there is no perfect safety in the things in which we find security. Any new discovery will place all other assumptions of life and the universe into question. Life is a reflection of the universe. The entire universe is in process. All life is in process. Except in the realm of illusion, there are no stopping-off places. Life goes on. So does the universe. Realizing this greatest paradox related to unending riddles and growth allows us to become aware that the universe is more than a few surface-level laws. The universe is the substratum from which all life emerges. The universe has infinite depth and dynamics. The universe is the cosmos—the infinite unfolding of harmonious order. We need to learn how to fit into its order.

As it turns out, these points of singularity are not singular isolated events. They are like windows to a broader dimension (realm) of the single unified whole. Black holes exist all over the place in the space-time continuum. Black holes vary in size from the super large to the microscopic. From the perspective of space-time, only the large ones are detected because of what they do to other objects and what they do to the space-time continuum on the macro level. Black holes are all the covers for a point of singularity. The event horizon of a black hole is merely the preamble (introduction) to the hidden beauty of what appears to be an ominous (threatening) presence. The single point is not a dimensional singularity except from the perspective of the space-time continuum.

What is called a point of singularity is a window to the entire expanse of what exists; since there is no distance or time separating these superstrings, foam, bubbles, and knots, the point is the entire universe. That is the point of everything! There is a way to imagine leaping beyond the great paradox of the one-way event horizons for both space-time and superstrings, foam, bubbles, and knots. What is called a single point of singularity is the entire universe, and what is called the entire universe is a point of singularity. This is why both space-time and the realm of superstrings, foam, bubbles, and knots appear to be infinitely small, infinitely large, nonexistent, and essentially interrelated simultaneously. This is the grandparent of all paradoxes, and it is the most startling diamond of wisdom. All is One. Within a speck that appears to have no dimension, the whole exists. Everything essentially is a web of relationships.

There is no outer boundary to the point of singularity. There is no inside to it either. Since there is no inside or outside, there is no entering it. It has no surface because the point is the universe and the universe is the point. There are no divisions in this manifold (diverse) unity. From the outside, it makes sense to say it has a surface. From the "inside," it makes no sense to say that it has a surface or boundary. One of the most shocking discoveries for you is that from the perspective of the point of singularity what we call space-time has no dimensionality. From the perspective of space-time, the point of singularity has no dimensionality. There was no time in which you entered the point of singularity. There was no distance within it.

From "within" this point of singularity, matter, energy, mass, particles, space-time, and gravity are not the manifest basics of reality. Your eyes can't see anything because there are no photons. You do not weigh anything because there is no gravity. You can't feel anything because there is no time within which nerve impulses could transmit information. There is no lightbulb to turn on because there is no electricity. There are no pizzas because nobody can deliver them. Actually, nobody wants to deliver them because they know they can't go back home. This is the ultimately strange place. Then you remind yourself that it is no place at all, because there is no space here. Oh yeah, here there is no there, but then again, here there is no here either. In the present, there is no now. There is no past or future. If there are cookies in existence, you have no way of finding them because there is no smelling, allowed. There is a sign forbidding any smelling but you can't see it. This realm is truly beyond all names, forms, and senses.

Extensions

Investigate anything you can find on the topic of limits or boundaries—just don't get too close to your topic matter! (*See* "Dimensions—How Many?") The dimension "that into which the universe is expanding" is not a dimension out there beyond the present universe. It is an inner quality of the space-time continuum. The space-time continuum is an inner quality of the realm of superstrings, foam, bubbles, and knots. There is symmetry on a much finer and greater scale than ever imagined. The universe is balanced. Cataclysmic (violent or destructive) events such as the big bang or collapse of a star are not aberrations (anomalies or exceptions) that upset the way the universe works. These events, as seen from a much larger (or vastly smaller) scale, do not destroy life. They all make life possible in an ongoing and ever-changing manner. All things interact with all other things all the time.

From the limited perspective of the space-time continuum, there are no things that exceed (go past) the speed of light. If everything communicates with everything else instantaneously, we can realize that the speed of light being held as a constant in a vacuum and the law that nothing can go faster than light are an accurate and valid (true) set of principles for the limited phenomena being described (the space-time continuum). These principles are not mistaken. They are limited. There is fullness to what we call every little speck of space that is beyond our imaginations. Each of these specks of space is part of a field that bubbles up into time because of the vast realm you have just discovered. If it really is beyond our imagination, how can we speculate or know about this finer and greater realm of the universe?

The mind is riddled (meaning that our capacities to comprehend life and the universe in its totality are limited, and therefore there will always be blank spots or holes in our understanding of ourselves, life, and the universe). At first, this may paint a bleak (not pleasing) picture of our human prospects. Eureka! (Aha!) It is the existence of these very holes in our understanding that provides the possibility for continual learning. Each of these holes of our understanding is not an impossible barrier entombing (sealing) our fate as restricted creatures in a forever-limited little box without windows. Rather, these holes of our understanding are each a window of opportunity. They are the source of curiosity, imagination, and genius. As we peer through the windows based on our past understanding, needs, attachments, aversions, fears, and biases, all we see is the blackness of the void. When we leap through the window's gateway, what appeared to be a void becomes a whole new aspect of the universe and life. These windows of opportunity forever appear as an enigmatic void until we take this leap.

Holes in our understanding permeate and suffuse (present everywhere) our current knowledge. There are some interesting metaphors about our holes of understanding. When a Korean jet (flight number 007) was shot down over Russian waters by Russian jet fighters, our American intelligence agencies had the data of the jet veering off course into dangerous territory being recorded in real (current) time in their computers. Given the massive databanks of raw data in our intelligence (spy) computers at that moment, nobody was able to discern (discriminate) that there was a pattern developing that ought to receive attention. We presume that our intelligence officers did not know what was occurring in real (current) time. Therefore, we presume that this unfolding event was not seen in real time. It was in our memory banks but not in our comprehension. This is like a hole in our understanding. It is potentially available to us if and only if we leap in and see what's there.

There are other events that are seen in real time, but they are so far out of the realm of comprehension that they go unreported to our conscious awareness. For instance, the first wave of Japanese fighter planes approaching Pearl Harbor on December 7, 1941, was, in fact, detected on radar. They were not reported to the highest central command. Why? Possibly, because they were expected to be an American bomber squadron. The idea of Japanese bombers on a beautiful Sunday morning was so improbable that it wasn't given a second thought. There are holes in our understanding for many reasons. We don't see what we don't expect. Two of the most common reasons for these holes in our understanding are that we can't interpret all new data in real time (actual lived time), and when something is so far from the ordinary we fail to comprehend its meaning. (*See* "Remembering, Anticipating, or Just Being Creative?")

There are many other reasons for the existence of the holes in our understanding, including the realization that what exists is vaster than our neurological system can process. There will always be the interplay between our rational logical knowledge of things and processes held in creative tension with our capacities to comprehend, intuit, feel, and sense the meaning of anything of which we are a part. These are all reasons why the holes in our understanding exist in such a way as to provide hope, opportunity, and renewal for the human family and for all living beings. (*See* "Normal and Necessary.") I sense that the universe is not here for human beings only but that everywhere life is evolving in unimaginable ways. So it would be very wise to take the opportunity presented to us by these holes in our understanding and continue to evolve also.

Genius is leaping beyond. Genius takes what is known, senses what is potentially knowable, and then leaps beyond all given and potential patterns. Genius thrives with the existence of these holes of awareness and understanding. This is why geniuses appear to snatch new insight out of nowhere. The geniuses may be dying to tell others, but unless others have taken a similar leap, they can't expect or comprehend that which the genius speaks, enacts, or intimates. Usually with great resistance, the insights of the geniuses are received and given credit for being something real. Geniuses jump into these holes of understanding. See the story of Tom Sawyer and Becky in the huge cave. This is a perfect metaphor for what occurs when the genius goes beyond the current boundaries and into the depths of the unknown. These people become a living Rosetta stone (look up *Rosetta stone* in a history book).

Genius is never threatened by what it doesn't know. The genius leaps into the hole and survives the leap. The genius experiences things that do not relate neatly to the body of knowledge that others intelligently safeguard. To the one who doesn't ever leap, these holes are guessed to be present but are deemed (judged) to be of no importance, or they are held to be scary irruptions (upswellings) from the messy area of the subconscious mind, or they are thought to be nonexistent. These holes in our understanding are neglected, denied, neutralized, and pushed to the periphery of our attention. An interesting irony is that those who feel comfortable with the incompleteness of their knowledge are the very ones who are able to leap beyond the confines of the known. Those who leap beyond threaten the ones who invest greatly in the assumption that they know so much. Go figure that out!

The most amazing discovery could be that our growth and learning have no limits because the universe is infinitely rich. For instance, we can expand our picture of reality by including gravity in with space-time. Then we figure out that the theorized gravitons (the carrier particles and waves of gravity) are actually not what create gravity. Gravitons are the presenting cause of the emergence of space-time. Gravitons may not be the carrier waves for gravity, but they may be the carrier particles' waves of space-time itself! Who knows, gravitons may also turn out to be the source of what we call mass. If so, then the gravitons would create space-time, and the gravitons in another form would create mass, which is responsible for curving space-time and the appearance of what most people call gravity. Then again, what is warping, renewing, transforming, and maintaining the space-time fabric may actually turn out to be the substratum that is the fundamental field in which space-time emerges. Gravitons may reflect this substratum. Space-time gravitons provide the field within which all other forces and particles play themselves out. Thus, we discover that the basic relation in the universe is between space-time gravitons and superstrings, foam, bubbles, and knots. Another way of saying this is to use the term *equivalence*. Space-time gravitons and superstrings, foam, bubbles, and knots are equivalent sides of an equation (just like energy and mass are equivalents in $E = mc^2$). They are not different things. Equivalence of energy/mass, space/time, gravitons/substratum are all reminders of the depth of interplay and relationship that exists between all things. Since life is a reflection of the universe, we can realize that all life is deeply interrelated. To understand anything about life, it is necessary to experience the nature of the basic relationships between ourselves and all other things.

Then we realize that this fundamental relationship or interplay is not the fullest explanation of the universe. These temporary holding bins (constructs) will be useful until some genius leaps into another hole of human understanding. This is not to say that our brains as presently constituted are capable of comprehending the entire universe. This would be hubris (a very overinflated ego). We know from careful observation that an overinflated ego is both delicate and dangerous. Always look out for those who ferociously or ever-so-sweetly control and guard some domain (little box) of human turf. They are both delicate and dangerous.

As we continue to challenge our brains, we will continue to evolve. In other words, as we all discover our genius, we are encouraging our evolution in very desirable manners. No one can predict the outcome of such a great adventure. Also, we are just beginning to discover an entirely new (and in some ways very ancient) wisdom related to the mind not merely being a large collection of cell-based electrochemical reactions. As we learn to study consciousness itself, we are beginning to come to wisdom related to what is pure awareness. This is not the book to be discussing this in full detail, but the existence of this quality within the realm of our experience suggests that we are capable of greater things than our rational mind alone admits to itself (another hole). This is a metaphor (among many) that there is a great beyond that is not separate from us. The entire universe is rooted in a web of intimate and evolving relationships. There is no beyond. There is no venturing outside any limiting box. There is only unfolding richness, depth, and yet greater fields of comprehension in which to savor what we call Life!

STANDARD ENGLISH

Standard English is a term that describes what many people feel is the norm for language in the United States. Is this norm set, or is it changing all the time? Try to find out how different groups of persons arriving in North America have contributed to what is called Standard English. There are countless examples of contributions from many cultures. Most of our words and language patterns come from European cultural roots. Pick some major groups, such as African Americans, Hispanic Americans, Native Americans, Asian Americans, or Pacific Americans, and try to find what their contributions have been to what some call Standard English. Now try to find what other groups who have fewer people in our country (aboriginal or native peoples from around the world, persons from ethnic groups that have been suppressed by conquering nations such as the Kurds in Iraq and Turkey) and discover their contributions.

Extensions

Find as many words as you can that people challenge as not being Standard English but that are very commonly used.

STAR COUNT

Is it possible to count the number of stars in the sky? Remember that we are only counting the stars we can see. How many stars can we see that are from another galaxy? There are challenges to counting the stars that appear to us:

1. Stars are continually coming into existence.
2. The light from the stars travels at the speed of light, which is very fast, but it still takes many years for this light to get to us. Therefore, as the

light reaches us, it may be the case that this particular star is no longer in existence.

If we only count the stars that appear to our eyes or to other instruments like telescopes, how would we count the stars? Try to imagine several different methods (means) to accomplish this task.

If you are listening to somebody give a possible solution to a challenge (like counting the stars), remember that it is only one possibility. Too often, we are pulled into a way of seeing the world and we become limited. What are other ways to count the stars?

Extensions

People say that there are an infinite number, of stars in the universe. What is the concept of infinity? Is it a number, or is it a concept standing for a set (any grouping) of things that we assume can't be counted because the members of the set of things go on forever?

If infinity means that something goes on forever, what does forever mean? For instance, do the stars go on forever? This gets us back to the big bang theory of the origins of the universe. We are told that the universe is expanding. If this is so, then it appears as though there must be an edge to the universe (this would be the current outer edge as it is expanding). This is something like a balloon expanding. The balloon itself would be the edge. If this is so, then the stars do not go on forever. If the edge of the expansion of the universe is the limit (an end of some process or set of things), the part of the universe that has stars in it is contained within a definite limited (finite) space. This portion (part) of the universe then could not contain an infinite number of stars, because if the number of stars were infinite, they would not be able to be contained within a limited space. This is a case for a finite number of stars based upon considerations of space.

Another way to deal with this issue is to say that at any one point in time the stars that are in existence are there. If there were to be a large bowl completely filled with marbles and this bowl extended for a hundred miles down and across, we would be tempted to say that there are an infinite number of marbles in the infinitely great bowl. The reality is that there are a certain number of marbles in the bowl, but we are unable to count them. If space is something like this great big bowl, there are a definite number of stars in the universe, but we can't count them all. Just because we can't count them, ought we to call this infinity? If stars are coming into and going out of existence continually, then we could say that in any given instant the stars that exist are all that there are. This means that there is some definite set number of stars in any given instant. What is, is in that moment. There aren't any more. Since there aren't any more than what actually exists, this indicates again that there is a vastly great number of a limited number of stars.

STARS IN THE DAYTIME?

Can one see stars only at twilight and nighttime? Might they be seen during the day also? Under what conditions could you see the star during the daytime? Hint: do you think it would be possible to see any stars (or planets of the solar system) during a full solar eclipse? Could there ever be a full solar eclipse when the sun is just on the horizon (at sunrise or sunset)?

Extensions

When you look up at the night sky, far from any other light source, why is it that the entire sky is not filled with stars if the universe is infinite and if there are galaxies in all direction? We assume that the universe is homogeneous (the same everywhere). We also assume that the universe is isotropic (the same in every direction from one's point of view). This principle would hold true of any observer any place at the same time in the universe. If we look on large enough scales, these assumptions of the universe seeming to be homogeneous and isotropic are valid. If our scale were large enough, the patterns of galaxies, clusters, superclusters, and maybe walls and filaments of galactic material would appear to be homogeneous and isotropic.

Try to find information on Olber's Paradox. This paradox deals with the issue of why we don't see stars everywhere. Hint: is time infinite? The universe is only about fifteen billion years old. So, beyond a certain point, there aren't stars. Also, consider the red shift phenomenon. As objects are receding away from the observer, visible light shifts toward the red end of the visible light spectrum. If this light from receding light-emitting objects is red shifted sufficiently, we will fail to see it. It will become infrared. We don't see infrared. Microwaves from all the electromagnetic emissions of objects moving away from us fill the universe. So a little piece of the issue of Olber's Paradox has to do with the fact that we are asking the wrong question. If we ask why is the sky not filled with visible light, we could be asking: Is the space above our sky filled with microwaves in all places? Then there is the issue of space-time expanding. If we are looking straight out at an object or area in space, between the object and us, there is much space in which the space-time continuum is expanding. This ought to add a little spice of complexity to Olber's Paradox. How is it that any light can come straight toward us from any other source if space-time is curved and if space-time is expanding? To further complicate this issue, some very recent research again brings up the delicate problem of some stars appearing to be older than the universe itself! Enjoy!

STORIES AND GENIUSES

Who are some story characters who display some characteristics that make you think they are geniuses? What is the difference between other people who are very intelligent and those who are geniuses?

Extensions

Look up the word *paradigm*. These are like models that we develop or accept that help us interpret reality. We become dependent upon them. One kind of genius is that of being able to see and describe new paradigms. Describe as many kinds of genius as you can think of.

STRANGE ARM

One night while sleeping on a bed in a train racing across Eastern Europe heading for the old Soviet Union, I was awakened in the middle of the dark night by the mysterious presence of a strange arm dangling over my head. I awakened my roommate who was in the upper bunk. He said it was not his arm. There was nobody else in the room. What was going on? Hint: the arm was asleep and I wasn't.

Extensions

What happens when various parts of our body go to sleep on us? Can an internal organ go to sleep on us?

STRATEGY FOR OTHERS

Have you ever found yourself using another person for your own personal benefit or gain? In a sports game, somebody outplays you, you get frustrated, and you do something to the other player for which you are never caught by referees. Some people make fun of others in order to be included in some desired group. In my junior high school, certain persons would take turns beating up a mentally challenged boy. They hit his glasses off his face. All these other boys would take turns after lunch beating him up while he was alone and without his glasses. In some way, have you ever used others and hurt others for your own ends?

Extensions

What risks are we willing to take when we see others being hurt? What are the options for us when we see emotional or physical abuse of others?

STRESS: PITFALLS OF IGNORANCE

Get to know about the effects of stress for the sake of leading a better life—starting right now. What does it do to us emotionally and physically? What is its impact on the body?

Extensions

Is stress always bad? Are there some forms of stress that are necessary (one example would be physical exercise)?

SUN—ROTATION

Does the Sun rotate?

Extensions

If the sun does rotate, could it be that the surface gases spin in an opposite direction as opposed to the core? Are there any planets in our solar system that do not rotate?

SUNSET RIDE

How fast would you have to drive a car heading due west precisely at sunset in order to stay exactly at the same angle to the sun? The particular angle of the sun doesn't matter; you might choose to have the sun directly overhead at 12:00 noon. What would be the necessary speed?

Extensions

How high would you have to fly straight up so that you always are able to see the sun? Look up an article on shadows that the sun casts on the opposite side of the Earth. You will learn some things about cones.

SUNTAN THROUGH GLASS

Can you get a suntan or sunburn through windows?

Extensions

How is it that certain rays are blocked and others aren't?

SUPERCONDUCTING MATERIALS

Look up anything you can find on superconducting materials. This stuff conducts electrical charges without practically any resistance. This avoids any significant loss of energy.

Extensions

Look up anything you can find on superconducting colliders. What forms of knowledge might we gain from research going on in these facilities?

TABLOIDS

Tabloids are those newspapers that sit on the racks of grocery stores and pharmacies that have huge headlines claiming such things as:

- B-17 [World War II bomber] Found in Crater of the Moon!
- Baby Born Pregnant!
- Predictions for the Future
- Mummy Comes to Life!
- Aliens Stole My Peanut Butter!

Few of the articles' claims can be verified (proven) or corroborated (supported by other credible [believable] sources). Specific locations and identification of individuals involved are not divulged. If it is not news, what is this form of communication? Who actually buys such tabloids? Have you ever seen somebody actually buy one?

Extensions

Are there any legal limits to lies and deceptive claims that people can publish? How many people actually believe what is published in these tabloids? Do our regular newspapers report totally objective and unbiased articles? What do *objective* and *unbiased* mean?

TAX ON NATURE

Do you agree with the idea that we should have an ecology tax? This would be a tax on any activities that cause environmental harm. Look up some stuff on this topic. What do you think about this idea? For instance, those people who pollute the air ought to pay a heavy tax. Anybody who purchases services or products from such providers would pay a considerably higher price. Why don't we institute this system worldwide immediately? Who would be against it? List all the advocates you can think of and list all the opponents you can think of. Try to figure out the case from either side.

Extensions

What would be done with the money? Who would collect the tax revenues (money taken in)?

TECHNOLOGY SAVE US?

There are many disaster movies showing on TV. In the end, most of them have some technological fix (nuclear missiles, laser beams, computers, jet fighters, or some new genetic discovery). With so much harm being done to the Earth by the effects of technology, do you feel that technology will save us? Is technology the problem? Are we becoming too advanced in our knowledge? Are we too powerful? Can our wisdom keep pace with our technology?

Is our current moral and intellectual substance or human spirit sufficient for:

- the burden of knowing how to create and manipulate life (the human genome project, cloning, and proteome knowledge)
- the knowledge of how to greatly affect the evolution of our human race, other life-forms, and other planets
- the burden of knowing how to split atoms (nuclear weapons)
- the challenge of technology and science creating the means to produce new weapons of mass destruction
- the burden of controlling massive accumulations of wealth (the disparity between the poor and the rich of the world)
- the burden of centrally controlled and widely disseminated (distributed) databases that possess vast and intimate knowledge of every person (medical, genetic, emotional, and financial data)

Extensions

Why do people love disaster movies so much? What is the attraction of horror stories and movies?

TEETH

When I was a boy, nobody used dental floss. We all used toothpaste to help keep our teeth healthy. When did effective toothpaste and toothbrushes start being used? Which one came first? What was used as toothpaste in the past? Would you put that material into your mouth now?

Extensions

Think of common things and practices (like having pets) and find out when these practices came into existence.

THAT SPECIAL SOMETHING

Certain people make us feel good. Certain situations make us feel contented and happy. Something happens and we feel that life is right. What are the things in your life that make you feel this way?

Extensions

Since everything changes, including all of our outward circumstances, wouldn't it be a good idea to find a source for contentment deep inside ourselves? Do we need to find certain truths within us and then live from those truths?

THE WORD *THE*

Why do we use the definite article preceding the following terms: the Florida Keys, the Northwest Territories, the Gulf of Mexico, the Pacific Ocean, the Ukraine (we used to say this), and the North Pole? Why do we not use the word *the* in front of Antarctica, Russia, Ontario, Pangea, and Mongolia? Why is it that suddenly nobody is using the word *the* in front of Ukraine?

Extensions

Who makes up the rules of grammar? Hint: are there people who sit around on Friday nights drinking weird concoctions (drinks) like carrot juice or prune juice and talk about new grammar rules that they are going to impose on others the next day? Do these rules reflect common usage already at play in the culture?

THE COMMON DENOMINATOR

What is racism, sexism, ageism, or classism? There is no agreement among all people everywhere on these definitions. These are controversial terms and realities in our social existence. What do racism, sexism, ageism, and classism have in common?

Extensions

In what ways do we put down others over whom we have some power or authority? What does it do to others and to ourselves? Does it make us feel powerful? Does it also cause us to be diminished as a human being while we diminish the humanity of others? For a moment of power or a lifestyle based on power over and against others, are we willing to hurt others? Do we become fragmented (torn apart) when we choose to hate consciously or practice behaviors and hold values that diminish (put down) others? Why do some people put so much energy into denying that there is any such thing as racism, sexism, ageism, or classism? What would you use as the name for biases against gays, lesbians, bisexuals, and transgendered persons?

THERE ARE QUESTIONS AND THEN THERE ARE QUESTIONS!

When a teacher, a parent, or somebody in authority asks a question, is there a way in which he or she asks the question that might predispose you to lying? For instance, a parent asks in a nice, nondemanding, nonthreatening tone of voice, "Did you take your shower last night?" Whether you did or didn't is only minimally consequential (nothing to worry about). It is just a fact that the person is asking about. If you didn't take the shower, they will simply ask you to take the shower.

Another day, your family is way behind schedule. Several things have happened in the last few minutes like the keys being lost, two siblings just had a real doozer of a fight, the car won't start, the dog ran off (not before piddling into the shoes that had just been purchased for this trip), and "somebody" used up all the milk the night before. Your family is running late to get to the airport for a special vacation. The parent turns to one of the children and asks in an upset manner with a loud, angry, and demanding voice, "Did you take your shower last night like I told you three times to do?" You know there will be consequences of some major kind. You didn't take the shower. In such circumstances, would you be inclined to lie? What are some other circumstances in which you might be tempted to lie?

Extensions

What are the differences and common features when people lie, deceive, are dishonest, make things up, bend the truth a little, tell a little lie, or tell a big lie? Are there ever any circumstances in which you would be tempted to lie?

How do people in authority treat you? Are the people in positions of power and authority in your life caring, loving people? Is power ever abused in your life? If power of any kind is being abused in your life, do you feel safe and secure in addressing the issue with the person who has some power and authority in your life? If you don't feel safe and secure addressing the issues you feel are important, are there others you can talk to?

How do we ask questions? How do we relate to others? Do we ever abuse power or authority? How can we learn to be more sensitive to the needs of others?

THEY ALMOST SOUND THE SAME

What is the difference between translation and transliteration? They both have to do with working with foreign languages. Is there one correct spelling of a transliterated word? Is there one correct spelling for *shish kebab*?

Extensions

Do all words translate perfectly into our language? Can we put together letter combinations from our own alphabet and make all the sounds from all other languages? Might other languages have sounds that we don't use?

If one is writing poetry with the sound of language being the most important element of the poem, might we be able to expand our realm of sounds in language by using foreign language sounds? If so, how would the poet communicate in writing to the reader how to pronounce certain words?

TIME—KINDS

When we ask what time is, we might pause to ask how many different kinds of time are there. Some examples might be:

- geological time
- biological time
- emotional time
- evolutionary time
- universe time
- imaginary time
- supertime (*See* "Galaxies in Collision.")

What are some other forms of time you can think of? What is time? How do the different kinds or forms of time relate to each other?

Extensions

Is there an objective time beyond our subjective senses? If this kind of objective time exists, how would we measure it?

Is time another sense beyond our five senses? Is time something we human beings made up in order to make sense of the universe? If we made it up, does it really exist? Look up the term *kairos* as another alternative kind of time (this term usually has religious meaning). Compare *kairos* to *chronos* as metaphors for time. Both of these terms are Greek in origin. Both of them are transliterations (English letter representing sounds from a word in a foreign language). One of them has found its way into our English language and the other has not been used widely in English. They both refer to time in very different ways. Are there other Greek words for time? Are there other terms denoting a variant definition of time from other foreign languages (ancient or modern)? You will need to have some foreign language resources to help you locate information on transliterations that are not widely used in English. Don't forget to research the experience of time as reflected in the languages of different aboriginal peoples around the world.

TIME—SYNCHRONY

How do we keep our clocks synchronized? Is there a single official time? If so, where is this clock located?

Extensions

Who is in charge of it? How does it work? What would happen if all the rest of the clocks in the world were in agreement with each other but not with the prime clock? Would we take two aspirins and go to sleep?

TIME ZONES

How many time zones are there? Are there official names that are universally accepted for each time zone? Does anybody have a system of names for all the time zones? Find a resource that names all twenty-four time zones.

Are there more than twenty-four time zones? If so, find them. Hint: there may be some intermediate time zones.

Extensions

How did people tell what time it was before a universal system of telling time? How did they determine what time it was a thousand miles away?

TOENAILS—WHY?

Everything has to have a top and a bottom, right? Therefore, our toenails are like lids on a jar. They are like caps on top of a bottle—they keep stuff in your toes. Do you have any better explanations? This assertion (belief) came from a very young child.

Extensions

Listen very carefully to children. They are seeing the world, others, and themselves in very creative ways. We must not forget the experiences and minds of young children. If we do, we all become old very quickly. Being old in our mind-sets (ways of looking at life) has little to do with our age. What makes us old in our mind-sets? Does this mean that a young person is good and an old person is bad? Don't we need the resiliency (adaptability) and creativity of young people while needing the wisdom of old persons? Can young persons have deep wisdom and can older persons have greatly novel (fresh) ways of experiencing life? After you have considered these simple little questions, go and hold a flashlight under a finger in a dark room. What color shows through? Now you really know why you have fingernails—for entertainment's sake!

TOO OBVIOUS

Have you ever realized something and then you see that it was so obvious before? How could you have missed it in the past? Working on a math problem, a spelling challenge, a relationship question (should I be cool or just be myself?), or some issue with learning how to dance—no matter the issue—once we know, see, feel, or "get" the solution, then it becomes so obvious. Have you ever had the experience of somebody trying to teach you something, and if you didn't get it right away, then the person trying to teach something said, "What don't you understand?" This is usually said in a slightly exasperated (frustrated) manner. Oftentimes, there is contempt (disgust) in the voice or look on the other person's face. In that moment, what is the person actually teaching?

We can be so close to an answer or a solution to some challenge and yet be so far away! Why is this so? List examples from your life related to being so close and not "getting it," and list examples of when you finally did "get it." Did you have to work hard for some of them? Did some of them come easily to you once you focused on the issue? List different kinds of growth or learning experiences (physical, intellectual, social, emotional, mechanical, etc.).

What are the circumstances that allow us to finally grasp that which we seek? What happens to us when we cross that line between not knowing and knowing?

Extensions

If we understand, know something, or "get it," how can we be helpful to others as they are trying to understand, know something, or "get it?" If a solution or answer or way of seeing things is so obvious to us, do we need to be patient and understand the inner workings of the other person? Do we need to remember that there was a time in which we didn't understand, know something, or "get it?" What role does fear play when we are at an emotional boundary of deciding if we have the capacity to meet a particular challenge? This is different than questioning if we have the will, time, or energy for the challenge. Sometimes we confuse the issues of will, time, and energy with courage and resolve. Has this ever happened to you? In what kind of circumstances has this happened to you?

TOP OF THE WORLD?

Where is the top of the world? Is it the North Pole? Why wouldn't the top of the world be right where you are standing? If you look outward toward all the horizons, the entire Earth drops away from you. Therefore, aren't you on top of the world right where you are?

Extensions

Wherever you are located, where is the bottom of the world? Is there a way of locating the opposite side of the world strictly "by the numbers?" Look up exactly where you are located in terms of latitude and longitude. With this information alone, given what you know about latitude and longitude, can you numerically work out the latitude and longitude of the opposite side of the world from your present location? If you wish to figure this one out, start with a simple location with easy numbers like the prime meridian at the equator. Look up the word *antipode*. Use it at supper tonight. See what happens.

TORNADOES—INVISIBLE?

The wind is invisible. We can only see the effects of the winds—like leaves quaking, branches bending, or the sound of the wind upon our homes. We can see debris, dust, and other suspended particles in the wind but not the wind itself. Therefore, would it ever be possible to have an invisible tornado? Under what conditions could this occur? Check with a meteorologist as to whether or not there are any recorded instances of this happening. Don't be surprised if the meteorologist has to figure out a way to look it up.

Extensions

Are there other examples of invisible things that pack a lot of power? One example might be the energy racing through the water creating waves.

TORNADOES—STRAW

How could a tornado drive a piece of straw into a tree?

Extensions

What are some other examples of things that look to be impossible yet they exist?

TRAVELER'S ENIGMA

Can you imagine a set of circumstances in which you've walked or run exactly one-eighth of a mile, but the real space covered is less or more than an eighth of a mile? Hint: you're on a long cruise ship that is heading south and you are walking north. Now try the same thing with you walking south while the ship is going in the same direction.

Extensions

Pretend that you are on a fast-moving train heading due west. Describe some interesting word problems. Pretend that you are traveling at the speed of light. What are some interesting word problems related to this scenario?

TREE FALLING IN THE WOODS

If a tree falls in the woods, does it make a sound if there are no animals or people in the area?

Extensions

This sounds like a riddle that can have no solution. Leap beyond the bounds of what is given to you in life. There are other ways of facing the challenge. The falling tree makes sound waves but not sound, because sound is created in the inner ear and brain of animals. Sound is a sensation experienced in a highly filtered manner by the ear and brain, while sound waves are the precipitating (initiating) outward cause of the sensation. How might other living creatures that do not have ears experience sound waves? What might be some organs in their bodies that allow them to detect sound waves? Are there ways of hearing sound without ears?

Another version of this kind of riddle has to do with images. If the tree falling in the woods is not witnessed by anybody, does the tree really fall? Even if we're standing right there to see the whole thing, has the tree really fallen? Obviously, on one level, the tree has fallen.

That which is falling we call a tree. This is an example of an object that we can define. We fill our mental universe with objects that we name. This allows us to see how the many different objects fit together coherently. In this manner, life makes sense to us. Redefine, review, repicture, rename, reconstruct, reconfigure, rearrange, and reimagine the objects in your mental universe that we all share. Envision them within a vastly different context. Are there other possible ways of experiencing our life contexts and ourselves?

Look up the term *semantics*. It has to do with the meaning of our words. Words are what we use to sculpt objects into shapes and textures, definitions and perspectives that are rationally understandable and useful to us. When we begin to look at the meaning of the objects we use to define reality, we are turning the light of our concentration upon our self-awareness. This is like turning a light back upon ourselves. This is looking at ourselves and our shared ways of looking at things in the deepest possible manner.

When we look at things (ideas, feelings, and objects), are they set for us? Do we participate in the creation of meaning for all these pieces of a larger whole? In a very real way, we are the context-setting source for life. What we set as the context and what we set as the definition of the interrelation of these things filling the context are all creative notions in our own heads (hopefully that have some pretty direct relationship to the world and the universe). These notions reflect life in a rational manner, but these are all representations of realities that are themselves vastly deeper and wider than our grasp. This ought to be humbling. What we set is a process that greatly exceeds all our boundaries and contexts. Thus, how things interrelate to each other is grander and more complex than we can imagine!

Life emerges from the universe. We humans are a small aspect of life. We have an ego-based filtering mechanism that encourages us to believe that we know what life and the universe are. Too often, we think in the following culturally acceptable terms:

- Life and the universe are the resources that we are entitled to utilize (use)—so we think.
- Life is to be molded into a form that supports our desires and attachments—so we act.
- We think we ought to control life and the universe—so we try.

This way of controlling and manipulating life falls apart when we begin to discern (become aware of) the humbling wisdom that teaches us that our separate ego-based filtering mechanism has its limits. We have tremendous power to name things and sense the existence of relationships. This is a paradoxical kind of power. If we take the gifts of life too seriously and in too self-centered a manner, the gifts become shackles. If we take the gifts of life humbly, these very gifts become gateways to wider realms of wonder, knowledge, wisdom, intuition, ideas, comprehension, knowledge, and insight. Life emerges from the universe.

Does the falling tree make a sound without anyone to hear it? Does the object we call a tree really fall down?

TRICKS

What are the best and funniest tricks that you've ever pulled on others? One form of tricks entails doing something that nobody ever figures out what exactly occurred.

The house in which I was raised was a big one. Above the attic was an additional little platform from which you could climb through a square hole in the top of the roof. Once outside, you were on another flat platform at the peak of the roof. One Halloween night I took a big flashlight up on the rooftop. I would shine the light right in front of groups of ghosts, Draculas, goblins, and witches. All of them were pretty startled, and none of them figured out the source of the light. Some of them spent quite a while looking up into the trees for the source of light. Whatever tricks you pull, make sure they never scare or hurt anybody in any way. Be imaginative and resourceful in your tricks. Tricks should be for the sake of humor—never anything else.

Extensions

How can we make our world a more humorous place? Learn to see the funny side of things.

UNEXPECTED AND UNWELCOMED BUGS

In the past, I've seen little creepy-looking bugs that manage to come up into the house from the sink drain. I usually flush them back down as soon as I possibly can. What are they? Where do they come from? What else is alive down there where our drain water goes? Do some research and find out what kinds of things live in our drainpipes. This kind of research you do not want to do firsthand. If nobody wants to do this kind of research, how would you get the information?

Extensions

What kind of critters live in our carpets, bedsheets, and clothes? Our homes are crawling with similar little critters. We are not the only living residents in our homes. Locate some photomicrographs of living organisms in our homes. Where else do living organisms live in our homes?

UNFULFILLED DREAMS

Two geniuses, Leonard Bernstein and Albert Einstein, both felt that they hadn't accomplished the great goals of their lives. Find out what they each felt was unfulfilled.

Extensions

How could a person's life that is so filled with so many great accomplishments feel unfulfilled to that person? How do different people deal with this issue? Some are broken souls while others continue to thrive in life. What is the difference? Look to the lives of entertainers, scientists, and leaders of all kinds. Examine the differences between the public image and the private lives of famous persons adulated (upheld) for being paragons (ultimate examples) of success.

UNUSUAL LAKES

There is a lake in North America that is big, round, and mostly filled with an island. Its shape is odd enough, but how it came to be a lake is most unusual. Hint: it is located in Canada in Quebec. Many maps show it. Locate it. Look up its name. Find out how this lake came into existence. Why is the island in the center of the lake? Are there other lakes that were created in this manner?

Extensions

Locate a lake near the West Coast of the United States that is round, very deep, a very extraordinary color of blue, and is located on top of a mountain.

UP AND DOWN IN THE UNIVERSE

What is up and down in the universe? Is there an up or down in the universe? Why do we say that north is up and south is down? If we lived in the Southern Hemisphere, would we call south up and north down? Hint: these are geopolitical terms established by the Europeans during their period of dominance and control while the maps of the world were being made.

Extensions

Up is the perception of being oriented in the opposite direction of the pull of gravity. Is this the simplest definition? Now answer the question: Is there an inner and outer dimension in space? We use the term *outer space*. What is the utility (usefulness) of these terms *inner* and *outer* in terms of the universe? Try to imagine that you are smaller than an atom. You are outside the nucleus and inside the orbits of the electrons. From that perspective, the space beyond you, all the way out to the great cloud of motion that is caused by the electrons in orbit around the nucleus, would be called outer space. Is the "outer" of the outer space of the stars any more "outer" than the space between the nucleus and the electrons?

We think our perceptions define nature and the universe. Life is fabulously more mysterious and more profound than our intellects and imaginations can conceive. How sure are we that life is exactly as we perceive it or define it to be?

Look up the difference between the terms *secular* and *religious*, *prosaic* and *poetic*, *factual* and *imaginary*, *literal* and *symbolic*, *nonfiction* and *fiction*, *history* and *myth*, and *logical* and *intuitive*. By analogy, each of these word pairs shares something in common. They are all part of our human knowledge base. Use all of these gifts as means to discover a way of experiencing life, other people, our planet, and the universe from as many perspectives as you can. None of them needs to be your primary perspective, but your repertoire (range) of means to comprehend the meaning and significance of life will be enhanced (extended) to the extent that you are familiar with all of these aspects of human knowledge and wisdom. This is one of the secrets for unleashing (releasing) your genius. Having a wide base of understanding is a beginning place for wisdom and genius.

Now, try to imagine again that you are outside the nucleus of an atom but inside its electrons. Do you surmise (guess or conjecture) that the electrons would be making a great noise as they race past you? Why or why not? Would there ever be a sunrise?

What are other word pairs like *up* and *down* or *inner* and *outer* that shape (affect) the way you experience yourself, life, and the universe?

URBAN MYTHS

There are certain stories that are circulated in our culture that aren't true, yet masses of people believe in them. These are like giant-sized rumors that gain a life of their own. They keep reproducing in different forms and times in varied contexts. Examples are: there are secret messages embedded in our television shows or advertisements; there are United Nation troops stationed inside North America who are poised and ready to take over our nations; all people of different religions, races, and cultures are dangerous; certain logos for different companies are evil symbols; supersecret organizations within the government are controlling us all; Elvis is alive and well; JFK is living out his natural span of years in a secret compound in Florida; and our government is already in contact with aliens from outer space. What are other examples of modern-day or urban myths? There are many myths in the countryside also. The best term may be *modern myths*.

Extensions

Do some reading on the term *myth*. Are all myths made up and untrue stories? Do many of the stories of mythology (modern and ancient) point to deeper aspects of our humanity? For instance, read different mythological stories related to the theme of going beyond the boundaries of one's own community and culture, and then returning a wiser person with gifts for the benefit of the community or culture. What are some examples of myths that are emerging from our current culture?

VACUUM FLUCTUATIONS—SOMETHING REALLY WEIRD IS UNDER MY BED AND IT'S REAL

Many children and more than just a few adults have had the experience of believing that something is under one's bed (in the attic, closet, or basement). The thing imagined is usually something like a monster or outer-space traveler. How do they get there? Of course, the answer is that we make up the idea and then give it credence (belief that something is real). Human beings do this all the time. This process is called reifying (taking an abstract idea or imagined concept and giving it the quality of real existence). Here are some examples:

- the ghost in the attic or closet
- the desire to believe that one is more powerful or gifted than others; thus one assumes that other persons of different races, religions, or the other gender are inferior in reality
- people who believe in spirits hanging around in deep dark forests
- a two-dimensional, four-sided triangle thought to be real

There are countless kinds of examples of ideas or fantasies being construed (interpreted) as real. A few years ago, a couple of people were going around various places in the West selling tickets. These weren't ordinary tickets. The sellers promised that whoever bought these tickets could, if they showed up at one place, time, and date, get a ride on a UFO that would take them away from Earth permanently. They finally got caught, but their scam (an illegal or unethical way of conducting business) netted (collected) a whole lot of very real dollars based on an idea that they portrayed as being real. There are some people who are quite expert at convincing others that something unreal is real. One phrase for this kind of deceitful (intending to lie to others) behavior is "scam artist." Look up the history of scams (frauds, swindles). It is fascinating to note how many different ways people accept what is untrue as being true. What are the signs of a scam? What are the signs of a gullible (easily swayed) person or group? Some people are like hawks with their very developed capacities to detect weaknesses and flaws in others. These same hawks know how to exploit these weaknesses and flaws for their own twisted ends. What are some examples of this kind of predatory (victimizing) behavior?

The more we know about our universe, the stranger and more wonderful it becomes. Sometimes there really is something under the bed. Right when we convince ourselves that there is nothing real under the bed, a mouse runs out. This kind of thing really helps parents who are dealing with fear-of-the-dark issues with an offspring.

We like to tell ourselves that what we see is real. Real things never come from nowhere. The term *where* refers to a place. This implies location in space. Things do come out of nowhere. Their origins are not discernible in spatial terms. It turns out that apparently particles really do appear out of nowhere. This is startling because it means the next time we hear a squeal, scrunch, or shrill scream from up in the scary attic at midnight, there might really be something there even though we tell ourselves it is impossible. The essential point is, who gets up to go take an actual look for what is making the unexpected and impossible sound? Most people bury their heads under the pillows. Sometimes, the impossible becomes real with surprising results. Some persons recognize the possible in the impossible. Actually, the sources of all these weird sounds are virtual particles having a little party. They like attics, basements, and locked rooms with no windows. To understand more about these mysterious virtual particles, let's reexamine the four basic forces of the universe.

There are four fundamental forces in the universe that we know of right now. The first three of them can be described as being interrelated in ways that physicists can now understand.

- Electromagnetism is the force that accounts for electricity, light, and magnetism.
- The weak force accounts for the nuclear breakdown of certain nuclei.
- The strong force holds the neutrons and protons together in the nucleus of atoms.
- Gravity keeps our feet on the ground, and it is what gets us back to Earth when we jump too high.

The model describing the relation between electromagnetism and the weak force is called the electroweak theory. The model describing the relation between the electroweak forces and the strong force is called the Standard Model. Gravity may someday be united with the other known three forces under what is called the Grand Unified Theory.

Each of these forces has to communicate itself somehow over the vast reaches of space. Three of the forces are known to have carrier or messenger particles. Electromagnetism is carried by photons. The weak force is carried by W and Z particles. The strong force is carried by gluons. Gravity may be carried by what is theorized to be gravitons. These messenger particles are strange. All interactions occur because of these carrier particles.

These virtual particles do not violate the known laws of physics if they only exist for an incredibly short period of time. Perhaps these messenger particles give matter the quality called mass. Mass is very difficult and almost impossible to explain. On one level, it is very simple to describe. On a deeper level, in terms of its origin and interaction with other forces, mass is a very mysterious quality of the universe. On this deeper level, it may be that space-time itself is an effect of gravitons. How's that for a weird idea—no gravitons, no space-time! Perhaps a deeper level of reality has to do with the interplay of the gravitational field (the weakest of all the known forces) and space-time. There are current theories that place the ultimate level of reality at a deeper layer than space-time and the gravitation field. (*See* "Spiraling into Infinity.")

The final or most primitive constituents (building blocks) of the universe may not be particles or fields but may be something like strings, foam, or knots. (*See* "Spiraling into Infinity.") Could it be that there are more than our four standard dimensions that account for what we see? (*See* "Dimensions—How Many?") This deepest layer of reality may forever remain strange and unknown to us (but it might still be there)! Try to find references that are written on the topic of the ultimate layers of reality. Look under such titles as superstring theory, space-time, Grand Unified Theory, or astrophysics. Come up with some of your own theories on how life and the universe work (and play).

The next time somebody tells you there is nothing real under the bed, ask him or her what he or she means by reality. If virtual particles can pop in and out of existence, maybe it's not such a surprise that a mouse really does run out from under the bed or out of the closet. At least it's not a virtual particle on the loose in your closet!

Extensions

Find out all you can about particles, fields, forces, antimatter, matter, mass, energy, virtual particles, knots, foam, superstrings, and dimensions. You may be amazed. Get up out of bed, go look in the attic or the basement or the windowless locked room, and find the source of what sounds like it is both possible and impossible.

VALUING OURSELVES AND VIEWING OTHERS

Some people put others up as a means of putting themselves down. Some people put others down as a means of putting themselves up. Can we learn to value the gifts and talents of others without putting others or ourselves down or up?

Each of us is like an orchestra. All the instruments are the sum of our life experiences. How they play together and the music created are unique to us. This music has never played before in the history of the universe. You are unique and wonderful. Value yourself. Learn about your talents and genius. Allow yourself the freedom to express your talents and genius. Never put others up as a means to put yourself down or put others down as a means of pulling yourself up. Why is this form of behavior so common? This is not a nice human dynamic; thus, people find it very difficult to talk about. Start with yourself. After you become familiar with these dynamics, search for how the culture supports making objects out of others. It is always useful to have a wise and caring friend who is benign (will not hurt you, trustworthy). Talk over these issues with a most trusted friend. When you have gained some wisdom on this topic, engage groups of people to talk about these issues.

Extensions

Notice how common a thing this is. What are the effects of putting others up or putting others down? Observe your own reactions and those of others. Look up the difference between being reactive and being proactive. If one is basing one's self-security and stability on putting others up as a means of putting oneself down or one is putting others down as a means of pulling oneself up, then is one being basically reactive or proactive in life? If you are reactive to life, can you be stable, secure, and at peace with yourself? Why do so many people try to have power over and against others? Why do we hurt each other so much? Is it necessary? Are there alternatives? Why do people try to put themselves down? Hint: sometimes it has something to do with finding one's place in a larger social system, losing one's courage to redefine one's place, and feeling powerless to do anything about this position one has accepted about oneself. There are other reasons also. Explore the issues. Be observant. Take careful notes on what you see. What are the patterns?

VEGETABLE FRUIT

What is the difference between a vegetable and a fruit?

Extensions

Once you know the difference between a vegetable and a fruit, list the various items that are definitely fruits and vegetables. Then list items that could be considered either one. Are there any examples of fruits that do not contain seeds for future generations? If so, how do they reproduce? Which are the only fruits with the seeds on the outside? Now switch from plants to animals. What is the difference between a mule and a donkey? Do they both contain the seeds or eggs of future generations? How do they each reproduce?

VELCRO

How is Velcro made? Who invented it? Were they looking for something else when they stumbled on the means to create this material? Did someone plasticize one of the weird hairs that grow out of the eyebrows of some people? Ever wonder if all the Velcro strands are identical? Are there two different kinds of Velcro filaments that always get hooked on each other? What would happen if you secretly put Velcro on the top of the football helmets of both opposing teams? Could there be a world-class interesting football game coming up? Imagine some other funny and hopefully harmless things to do with Velcro.

Extensions

See if you can find some other examples of successful products that were discovered unexpectedly. So often groups of persons or individuals who are deeply committed to a project experience some anomaly (unexpected event) in their process or results. Quite often, these anomalies are treated as noise (irrelevant material). Therefore, they are ignored. Sometimes these anomalies are taken as a sign that the methodology is not rigorous enough (variables are not being controlled). Anything that leads up to that anomaly is eliminated. Relieved of the burden of that impurity in methodology, the research group moves on. It takes a special kind of sensitivity and alertness to recognize aberrant (unusual) patterns that might mean something of importance but which are also totally unexpected. (*See* "Remembering, Anticipating, or Just Being Creative?") Taking notice of what is problematical, totally unexpected, or aberrant takes a special leap of human comprehension.

In your life, have there been any examples of unexpected things arising and you recognized them while others ignored them? Might this have happened when you were working with groups of people brainstorming on some project? Many ideas are put forth. A few of them become the center of attention. Maybe you were the one who noticed that one of the discarded or ignored ideas from the early part of the discussion might provide the way to solve a problem that the group is stuck on later in the process. This is noticing the irrelevant or ignored anomalies. Develop this art and sensitivity in your life. Those persons who sense and see the presence of some connecting idea, feeling, sentiment, intuition, construct, process, or image are the ones who can bring two or more diverse and seemingly disconnected or contradictory realms together into a larger integrated whole. Look for the in-between places that may contain the connecting stroke of genius. Where others see a dead end, you (or a group) may experience a dimension that fulfills a great need. This could be making connections that result in peace, the hungry being fed, ecological sustainability, nonviolence, or greater efficiencies and effectiveness in some process. Remain open. Cultivate the mind-set that allows for:

- open possibilities
- multiple frameworks of understanding that do not all fit together perfectly
- anomalies
- challenging questions

- rearrangement of fundamental biases
- awareness of our biases
- a willingness to grow beyond many of our biases
- a capacity to experience oneself at the most fundamental level as being on a journey

WAGON TRAINS

People went west on wagon trains in the United States. Were such vehicles used elsewhere for mass migrations of people? Where? Who? When? Did Americans invent this mode of transportation?

Extensions

Where do we find the earliest example of a wheel? What else are wheels used for other than for getting places and hauling things?

WAITING IN LINES

Have you ever noticed that some people act differently when they are in a long line? When we have to wait a long time, some people begin to react to the circumstances. What are some things you've observed?

Extensions

Do circumstances force us to act differently, or do we have certain underlying tendencies that emerge under certain circumstances? Are we different people with different characteristics, given a change in the social climate? Notice these patterns in your own life. How do you act differently in various kinds of circumstances?

Have you ever noticed that it is so much easier to see patterns that upset you in other people? Sometimes we tend to ignore, excuse, or rationalize (explain away) our own patterns! Why?

WARNINGS IGNORED

There are certain behaviors that will, for most people, result in unhappy endings: smoking, eating too much of certain kinds of fats, little or no exercise, exposure to nuclear radiation, or drinking saltwater if you are thirsty and afloat in a emergency raft after your boat has sunk. These are all extreme examples. What are some examples of less severe behaviors that aren't good for any of us? Have you ever caught yourself indulging in some behavior that you know is not good for you or for others? Under what conditions do you engage in such behavior? How do you rationalize (explain) it to yourself? How do you make excuses for yourself? What have you noticed about persons you've observed who engage in unsafe and dangerous behaviors? Are there any patterns that you've noticed? In terms of basic life wisdom and common sense, who are the people you listen to very carefully and who are the people you ignore?

Extensions

Under what conditions do you engage in behaviors that require sacrifice, delayed gratification, work, and perhaps no direct benefit to you personally? There are many examples of forms of behaviors that result in people changing their lives and living in regard to the needs of wider circles of people who are not necessarily related directly to their own family, clan, community, race, or nation. What are some examples of such behaviors? What are your values that encourage such behaviors? Actually, thoughts are just as real as actions. What are examples of judgments, beliefs, ideas, and ideals that require sacrifice, delayed gratification, work, and perhaps no direct benefit to you personally? This is the realm of mental or psychological effort that is related to growth, learning, altruism, justice, peace, and compassion.

WATER FROM UNEXPECTED PLACES

We've all been taught that rain happens as a result of an evaporation process in which ocean, lake, or river water evaporates, rises, and eventually becomes clouds that subsequently release their moisture in the form of raindrops that fall back to the Earth. Think of another source for rain. Remember to change the picture of everything you have been taught. Alter some elements of this picture totally and radically. Stop reading here and proceed only after you've formed some fresh, radically new ideas.

Rain can also rain down on us from outer space! What could be the possible source for such rain? Hint: the source is from the early days of the creation of the universe. Stop reading here and proceed only after you've formed some fresh, radically new ideas.

Comets are composed of water, ice, and dust left from the mysterious formation of the universe. As they hit the Earth's atmosphere, they melt (vaporize) and then precipitate (form) as raindrops. Usually, this water frozen in a comet would simply vaporize and not condense into raindrops. This happens from six hundred miles to fifteen thousand miles above the Earth's surface. If there were vapor from this source fifteen thousand miles up, would it drop to Earth? Might it eventually drop to Earth in any form?

Let's assume for a minute that vapors from melting comets would eventually drop low enough to condense in the form of raindrops. What is the height of the highest clouds? Compare the two distances of the origin of the cosmic raindrops with the clouds. Next, compare the variance (difference) of heights of the clouds. What is the range of heights (difference between minimum level and maximum level of clouds)? Next, compare the range of heights for the formation of raindrops from comets (14,400 miles). Draw a picture showing the Earth's surface with the variance of distances for clouds and the distances in which raindrops begin to form from comets. Make some assumptions about the formation of these special raindrops. State your assumptions. Can you use the same scale for both the clouds and the point of origin of the vapor from the comets?

Developing scales for any drawing is an interesting task. If two different phenomena of greatly different scales are to be included in a rendering (drawing) of some system, you have some challenges in creating the rendering of the system. Imagine drawing a graph or picture of the maximum possible distance covered in one certain time range by light, a microbe, a rocket, a hawk, the world's fastest jet, a comet, a snail, the speed of sound, an ant, a turtle, and a hungry child moving toward her favorite dessert. What would be several different ways of drawing this picture, being mindful of the need to compare the different elements of the picture with a comparable scale? First, rank-order them (from slowest to fastest). There are many possibilities for you. What are other pictures that you can draw illustrating the use of scales to compare different elements of the same system?

Back to comets hitting the Earth. These babies give off a lot of rain. Dr. Louis A. Frank, a physicist at the University of Iowa, estimates that over a ten thousand–to twenty thousand–year period, these dirty iceballs from space (comets) add approximately one inch of water to the Earth's surface. This may or may not strike you as being very significant. Look up how water volume is measured. Hint: find a unit of measurement called an acre-foot or cubic mile. Once you learn about how to measure large volumes of water, try to draw a picture illustrating this amount of water. Use scales and compare it to other known things that are very clear and obvious to you. For instance, compare the size of a mouse to the toenail of an elephant. Compare the tip of an average-sized nail, the tip of a needle, the tip of a hypodermic needle, the tip of the tool used in laser surgery, to the tip of an iceberg. Try comparing the size of a whale eye to that of both an elephant's eye and that of a large dinosaur of your choosing.

If you only have an 8.5-inch by 11-inch sheet of paper, you need to scale the items to fit your sheet. Think of several ways this could be done. How could you in the same sheet illustrate the circumference of these eyeballs and the circumference or diameter of a baseball, a beach ball, a golf ball, the Earth, and the sun? Is this impossible? Could you use images with different scales? How about showing a segment (piece) of the circle representing the object? The piece of the circle representing the sun (an arc) would look like a straight line (representing a very small segment of a curve). You could write in what proportion or percentage of the total curve this segment represents. The arc representing the eyeball of awhale would be much more curved of the page upon which you are drawing. Could you include the curve of the surface of nucleus in this same rendering? Could you include the curve of the limits of space-time in the same rendering? Is there a way to estimate the circumference of the limits of space-time if we know the approximate age of the universe?

Back to the comets and the dirty iceballs from outer space. When you hear about something accumulating over the period of ten thousand to twenty thousand years, change the scale of the picture. Now think in terms of geologic time (millions and billions of years). Guess what? On this scale, we learn that if the comets (big huge dirty iceballs) were pelting (hitting) the Earth at the same rate of five to thirty per minute, or up to about forty-three thousand a day, then over the course of geologic time, these comets may have added miles of water depth to the Earth's water supply! Where's all the water?

Extensions

The dirt in these iceballs from outer space also contains organic materials that may have contributed to the formation of life on our planet. Look up the definition of organic materials. Where could they have come from? How were comets formed? How could they have contributed to the formation of biological life on our planet?

WATER FLOWING UP OVER A WATERFALL?

Is it possible for water to regularly flow (out in nature) backwards, up, and over a waterfall? Hint: yes, in a particular bay on an ocean, and it is due to the tides. Find the bay! Hint: tides are especially pronounced (great) given certain kinds of land formations. Find out more about how land formations affect the local influence of tides. Then find a place with a waterfall right at the place where the tidal rise is great.

Extensions

What causes tides? Are all bodies of water affected by tides? Is there such a thing as a tidal wave that sweeps around the world regularly? Is this different than a wave caused by an earthquake (which used to be called a tidal wave)? How do the tides move around the world? Could the leading edge of the tides moving across the oceans be something like a wave? Since our bodies are mostly water, could we experience biological analogs (equivalents) of rising and falling tides within our own bodies? Could this have anything to do with why your bladder sometimes feels full and sometimes empty? Maybe Heisenberg's Uncertainty Principle would be a more likely explanation. Next time you have to go to the bathroom, quickly check to see what phase the moon is in at that moment. Maybe you've just been moonstruck.

WATERS OF LAKE SUPERIOR

Have you ever wondered how much water is actually contained in some huge body such as an ocean or a lake you can't see across? It is useful to play with images in your mind. In this case, you'll have to visualize some very big numbers. In ancient times, an unimaginably huge number would have been a thousand. This is where we get the word *myriad*, as in the sentence "There are a myriad of opportunities before you." (Compare the words *host*, *plethora*, *legion*, and *panoply*.) When I was a child, the unimaginably huge number was a million. In the late 1950s, there was a program called *The Millionaire*. If I remember right, every show began with an older man handing a younger man a check for a million dollars and the instructions as to who was supposed to receive the money. All you ever saw of the older man was an outstretched hand. The source of the unimaginably huge sum of money was a mystery. Then the younger man would go and deliver the check to totally unsuspecting individuals.

Today, what is an unimaginably huge number? We talk in terms of billions and trillions of miles when we discuss outer space. Nobody in her or his right mind can directly fathom or understand a trillion. To fathom something is to search the deep stuff of life. Look up *fathom* in an unabridged dictionary that gives the history of words. We look into the deep stuff of life. We need to go under the surface of what is given. We bring back treasures. One form of treasure is to know how to cultivate the use of images in trying to solve complex issues. If you start to understand the magnitude (size) of a trillion, will you be in your right mind any longer? You know that you have mental expansion issues going on in your life when you begin to comprehend a quadrillion. By the time you reach a quintillion, you have crossed over the edge into the realm of genius.

The largest freshwater lake in the world in terms of surface area is Lake Superior. If you go to an encyclopedia and look up lakes or Lake Superior, databases (information sources) will give you the figure of how much water is contained in Lake Superior. You may choose to figure out this volume issue by yourself. This is defined in terms of cubic miles or acre-feet. If the volume in your database is not measured in cubic miles, learn how to convert the measurement that is given into cubic miles. If you don't know how volume of anything is measured, look up *volume* and find out.

Now that you have the number of cubic miles of water in Lake Superior, we are left with another challenge. How do we envision a cubic mile of water? Go find a hill, intersection, or place with a broad view like a field. Develop some kind of measuring method (like twelve blocks equals a mile, or measure a mile length by riding in a car and watch the odometer very closely). Don't be the one driving while you are observing the odometer. You could always take the easy way and lay out marbles in a straight line. Then find out how many are in a mile. Borrow some from somebody and lay out one mile's worth of marbles.

Everybody will think something of you, but so what? You might use a little arithmetic and calculate how many marbles are in one inch and then do a little multiplication. This wouldn't be as fun as laying out one mile's worth of marbles. This way, you could get into a world book of records and into the doghouse with people who want their marbles back.

Once you have been able to gauge a mile of length from one vantage point, now—in your mind's eye—imagine what a mile of width would look like using the mile of length as your guide. Continue with the marbles and you'll become a marvel quickly, especially if you try to represent the length, width, and height of one cubic mile with marbles. There has to be some glue strong enough that would allow you to pile up one mile's worth of marbles. (*See* "Glue Limits.") Another and maybe more practical way to visualize one cubic mile is to stand near something very tall. Remember that a mile is over 5,280 feet. So if you are standing near a huge microwave transmission tower, find out or make some estimates as to how tall it is. You could use a form of mathematics called trigonometry to figure out the height of the tower. Have someone who knows trigonometry teach you how to figure this out. Now stand back and see what a cubic mile is. It is very helpful to be able to see or visualize your problem.

We are left with a further challenge. We are not able to visualize what thousands of these cubic miles would look like. When you drive between two distant places, try to get a feeling for the distance. If it is a thousand-mile trip, you could imagine a thousand of these cubic miles laid out end to end.

Another way of visualizing something is to put the challenge of visualizing many cubic miles in terms of something you can easily see or hold. Try to imagine a unit of measuring space that you can visualize easily and hold in your hand. Hold a golf ball in your hand. It is round and not cubic, but it is approximately one cubic inch in diameter. Therefore, if we know how many cubic miles of water are in Lake Superior, there is a relatively easy way to figure out how many cubic inches of water are in Lake Superior. Find out how many cubic inches are in one cubic mile and do some multiplying.

You would then be able to hold in the palm of your hand a golf ball and gaze out across the water of Lake Superior and know the meaning of a very large number (it is something much larger than a million, billion, or trillion). Can you guess in advance the approximate number of golf balls that would fit into Lake Superior (assuming they would replace or displace all the water)? Imagine standing on the coastline of the Pacific Ocean and asking the same kind of question while you are holding the proverbial (famous) golf ball in your hand. Sidelight: of any golf ball ever hit with a golf club, which one would be the most difficult to fetch (get)? Hint: the answer is somewhere in this book.

Once you've figured out how many golf balls would fit into Lake Superior, do the same analysis for the Pacific Ocean, the Atlantic Ocean, the Indian Ocean, and for the volume of water you would get if you melted the entire amount of snow and ice at Antarctica. In advance of finding the answers, make estimates as to how these various quantities would compare. Then do your analysis. Can you believe how large these numbers are? Try to find a database comparing the amount of freshwater to the amount of saltwater on the Earth's surface. In advance of your research, estimate what you think the comparison will be. Try to do this same estimation in terms of the number of atoms in any of these bodies of water. (*See* "Atoms—How Many Are in the Lake?")

Is there a greater volume of water in Lake Superior in the dead of winter or in the height of summer? This question relates to volume of materials in their solid versus liquid states. Lake Superior is never frozen solid, but (rarely) it does completely or almost completely freeze over.

If you assume that one cubic inch is approximately the size of one golf ball, go and try to borrow the number of golf balls that equals the number of cubic inches of water in Lake Superior. Now stack them up very neatly. How high would this pile go if it were to be a mile across and a mile long at the base? Would superglue hold them together? If you were to take the golf balls that are on temporary loan and create a perfect square of one thousand balls wide and long, and if you were to place one ball in every depression between four balls of the lower layer, you would create a second layer. It would be narrower than the first layer. What geometric form are you building? How many layers would it take to get to the top where there is only one ball at the pinnacle? How high would the structure be? There are formulas that would help you solve this problem.

Extensions

Take the same method and use it to estimate the number of grains of sand on a beach. Hint: take a very small area and approximate the number of grains of sand in that volume. Then measure the beach. Do this by measuring the average length of your step. How do you get an average figure? Look it up or ask somebody. Get the approximate length and width of the area being measured. Make certain assumptions about the depth of the sand. Now use the same method you used for Lake Superior and find out how many grains of sand there are on the beach. I'm sure any lifeguard would be quite interested in what you are doing when you try to determine the depth of the sand.

Other options: How many leaves are there on one tree? Think about this while you are raking them up in the fall or walking through a park in the fall. Now try to imagine how many trees there are in the world. Multiply the number of trees that drop their leaves by the number of leaves on average per tree. This gives you an estimate as to the number of leaves that fall to the Earth every year. Try to figure out the number of leaves or trees that need to be planted in order to affect the course of global warming.

Hint: what do trees absorb from the atmosphere and what do they put back into the atmosphere? What is a possible relationship between global warming and too few trees on the planet? You must make certain assumptions, of course. Are there too few trees or is their too much pollution? Could we benefit by having more trees on the surface of the Earth? Try it! P.S. Do trees pollute the air? Given the amount of air pollution from our current world population of humans of about five billion, what will the pollution be like when we are a world filled with nine billion people? This is the latest estimate of our population growth in a few years. How many trees will we need then? What is happening to our forests all over the world?

WATER TO DRINK

How many people in the world drink unsafe water? How far do some people have to go for water every day? What is in the water that people are drinking that is unsafe?

Extensions

What can be done to make healthful water available to more people (or all people)? How healthful is the water supply in the United States? Is the situation getting worse? What is happening to our worldwide water supply?

WEATHER REPORTS

One night I was sitting in my hotel room proofreading a document. I took a break and turned on the TV. The evening news program promised that it would be talking about new discoveries in what is causing the apparent changes in our climate. I turned the sound off and went back to work. Forty-five minutes later, the promised news analysis was broadcast. I turned on the sound. All the other news stories were ten to twelve minutes long. This one lasted three minutes, and all it said was that there are upper air disturbances causing some changes in weather patterns. The same statement was repeated about five times, and then the report ended without clarification (making clear or adding information) of the issue. Observe and analyze the quality of reporting in your local newspaper, any national newspaper, TV reporting, or radio news programs. In what ways are the reporters setting a wider context for the issues being presented? In what ways are the tools of cultural, historical, and scientific analysis being brought to bear on the topic? If the point of view of the report does not happen to match your point of view on some topic, was the reporting insightful and well presented in such a manner that it made you think?

Extensions

Have you ever had the experience of watching a weather report and you were left to wonder where the killer blizzard went two days later after it left your area? Have you ever wanted to know what is causing the bigger hurricanes, the floods, the droughts, and the inundations of rain in other areas?

We rarely get any insight into the larger or more encompassing patterns related to climate.

Look up El Niño. What might these phenomena have to do with weather patterns where you live? There is a related phenomenon named La Niña. Look it up also. When you find information on these phenomena, you'll probably find other information on the root causes of climate and weather changes.

WEIGHT OF OUR VALUES

We tend to accumulate things that we value. Look at what you and your family have lying around your house, garage, and yard. What does it all weigh?

Extensions

How much do the accumulated items of people in poorer countries weigh? What is necessary for our well-being and survival? How much could you get along without? To what degree is your happiness dependent upon having any of these items? Don't forget to calculate the weight of your home (house, apartment, duplex).

WH—HOW TO SAY IT

Listen carefully to someone who is saying such words as *when*, *where*, *why*, *whisper*, *wham*, *whip*, and *whistle*. Do they sound a little different from *walk*, *weep*, *wing*, and *wind*? If they do sound different, why is this so?

Extensions

Find words with the letter combinations *sch* in them. How is it pronounced? Find other interesting letter combinations that affect our pronunciation of words.

WHERE ON EARTH?

Where is the glabella and philtrum? Get out a real good atlas. Then again, maybe you want to look elsewhere. Remember to keep in mind that the way a question is asked predisposes us to certain limited answers. "Where on Earth" could be interpreted to mean where on my body are the glabella and philtrum. Hint: this is a piece of old cultural lore—the philtrum is the mark of an angel left at the moment of birth. This should really help you.

Extensions

Once you have located these two items, locate the septum and the fourth digit. How many fourth digits are there on average (for human beings)? Hint:

look out for crooked and deviated septums. Next, locate the xiphoid process. Also, try locating your hyoid bone. Have some fun with names. Enjoy the sounds. Look up some of the cultural lore related to some of these odd-sounding names.

WHOSE VOICE IS HEARD?

There are many reasons some persons become famous. Once they are famous, we listen to them. They become important to us. They become the markers from which we take our bearings (sense of direction) for demanding and complex issues. Other persons have great things to contribute to society, but they are never heard. Who are the persons we tend to listen to? Why do we ignore others who have great ideas or who are themselves great examples of how to live?

Extensions

Often, do famous people touch the deeper beliefs and sentiments (feelings) of wide circles of people? Are they famous because they touch us deeply, or do they touch us deeply because they are famous and thus we allow them to touch us deeply?

WHY "?" AND ( )?

Why do we place the end-of-the-sentence punctuation mark for quotations inside the quotation marks? He said, "This stuff isn't chocolate. It tastes like mud!"

Why do we then place the end of the sentence punctuation marks outside of the parentheses? He said he was home by midnight (we all knew better). What are the exceptions to this grammatical rule about placing the sentence punctuation mark outside the parenthesis? In several places in this book, the final punctuation for the sentence is included inside the parentheses. Why?

Extensions

Is there only one set of rules, or are there variations of the rules used by different writers? Is there one definitive (authoritative or final) book on grammar? If not, is grammar in part a matter of personal style and choice?

WOMEN AND MEN

Kids rule, parents drool. Somewhere this phrase arose. It's a humorous utterance with a serious background. When people feel controlled by others, they generally don't like it. Now a question: Do you think one sex prevails in power? Is it men or women? Does one gender "rule"? Give some examples. Support your case. This sounds like a question appropriate only for youth, but in fact many adults carry around with them everyday root judgments that are about as simplistic as believing that one gender really is more powerful, intelligent, motivated, capable, or gifted. Once we give credence (credit or belief) to something deep and primary, then our human tendency is to start gathering evidence to justify this crystallizing sentiment. It is amazing the difference these crystallizing sentiments can make in what we see in our world. Try to practice the art of becoming aware of the prime crystallizing sentiments that affect what you see in the world. Once you are able to be aware that you even have such influences operating in your life, your self-awareness will dramatically expand in ways that you can't imagine or predict. What are the ways you've experienced power being used between men and women?

Extensions

Is it necessary that one gender try to think of itself as being the most powerful in some area of our shared lives? Are there other ways of being more creative, loving, and just? What are some gifts that would arise if we treated each other as equals? What are we missing in life right now because of our ways of treating other persons of the opposite gender unequally, without love, or unjustly? What is it going to take to change these things? Does equality in terms of social, cultural, economic, and political power mean that we all have to be the same?

X FOR A KISS

Have you ever seen a letter marked with X's on it as a symbol for a kiss? Where did this custom come from? Before you read on, challenge yourself a little to find an answer.

Somewhere I ran across the curious historical gem: X's are from the medieval legal custom of marking the sign of St. Andrew. This was a cross used as a sign of integrity and honesty (commitment to carry through with an agreement). This sign was placed after the signature on binding contracts. The sign assured that the agreement was binding. It became the custom to also kiss the document as another sign of integrity and honesty. The cross can look like an X. The custom of signing the symbol of St. Andrew's cross was forgotten, and the association of the X with a kiss survived.

Extensions

Find other common symbols that we use and discover their sources.

ZIP CODES

ZIP codes are used to make delivering the United States mail more efficient. ZIP is an acronym (a word in which every letter is a first letter of other words). What does the acronym stand for?

At first, ZIP codes were five numbers. Then the U.S. Postal Service developed a system with a four-digit extension beyond the basic five numbers. This is designed so that a letter can be delivered to an exact spot.

Look up your ZIP code and its extension. How precise is this nine-digit sequence? If you had nothing on the envelope except the nine-number ZIP code, would it get to your house? Might the nine-number ZIP code identify a small area like your block? Research this and get the answer.

Try to locate the information as to where unique number combinations are located in the country. Try these for a start: 11111-1111 through 99999-9999. Try a number combination like 07041-7760. What is unique about this sequence? Try a code like 11221-9620. Try 04121-9440. Try 12071-9410 and 07041-9690. What do all these sequences hold in common? Where are they located on the map? Hint: try your birthday as a code and then add a zero at the end. Try applying other code sequences to ZIP code format. Then find where they are on a map. Make a game out of it, and challenge a group to find some of the solutions. Try out any kind of sequence you can think of (prime numbers, telephone numbers, or assign numbers to the letters of your name).

Extensions

You could construct secret codes using place names and mailing addresses to stand for sequences of numbers. You might invent a game out of these activities that might catch on and make you rich. Who knows? How does the system of letters and numbers work for the postal system in Canada?

About the Author

Curtiss DeMars-Johnson has devoted his life to encouraging others to take imaginative and intellectual leaps beyond the routines preoccupying our lives and to venture the challenge of discovering vastly richer ways of using our gifts to face our individual and shared challenges. He is a counselor, teacher, and a group facilitator. He has worked in the area of organizational development, group process, individual and group learning, goal setting, conflict management, personal growth, cultural change, non-violent and creative responses to social issues, and creativity as a means of inspiring the discovery and use of latent resources for positive change. He has worked with groups composed of persons with diverse cultural, racial, ethnic, gender, age, career, religious, and political backgrounds. He has been a public school teacher, parish minister, and is now dedicated to writing, teaching, group facilitation, and organizational development.

www.ingramcontent.com/pod-product-compliance
Ingram Content Group UK Ltd.
Pitfield, Milton Keynes, MK11 3LW, UK
UKHW022314150926
475604UK00003B/141